SINGLE AND MULTIPLE STIMULUS STATIC PERIMETRY IN GLAUCOMA; THE TWO PHASES OF PERIMETRY

ACADEMISCH PROEFSCHRIFT

TER VERKRIJGING VAN DE GRAAD VAN

DOCTOR IN DE GENEESKUNDE,

AAN DE UNIVERSITEIT VAN AMSTERDAM

OP GEZAG VAN DE RECTOR MAGNIFICUS DR. A. DE FROE,

HOOGLERAAR IN DE FACULTEIT DER GENEESKUNDE

IN HET OPENBAAR TE VERDEDIGEN IN DE AULA VAN DE UNIVERSITEIT

(TIJDELIJK IN DE LUTHERSE KERK, INGANG SINGEL 411, HOEK SPUI)

OP DONDERDAG 4 OKTOBER 1973, DES NAMIDDAGS TE 5 UUR

door

ERIK LOUIS GREVE

geboren te Amsterdam

DR. W. JUNK B.V. – PUBLISHERS – THE HAGUE

1973

Promotor: PROF. DR. R. A. CRONE

Co-referent: PROF. DR. G. VERRIEST

© Dr. W. Junk B.V. – The Hague – 1973
ISBN-13: 978-90-6193-002-0   e-ISBN-13: 978-94-011-7765-8
DOI: 10.1007/978-94-011-7765-8

'The limits of our
visual field are not
the limits of the world'

ACKNOWLEDGEMENTS

My deepest gratitude goes to my promotor Professor CRONE for his stimulating advice and constructive criticism during the years of research and compilation of the manuscript.

The perimetric department of our Eye Clinic would not exist without his support.

I gratefully acknowledge the help and advice of Professor VERRIEST. His knowledge added much to my understanding of the importance of visual psychophysics in visual field examination. Our cooperation in a Dutch manual for perimetrists provided a great deal of experience.

The first part of this study could be performed thanks to the assistance of my military superiors during the years I was working in the Military Hospital 'Dr. A. MATHYSSEN'. I am thankful for the opportunity given to me by the chief of the Military Hospital Colonel Dr. J. J. VAN BESOUW and by the chiefs of the Ophthalmological Department Lnt-Colonel Dr. C. H. G. BOTERMANS and Dr. J. VAN DER LEY. The personal encouragement and actual help I received from the head of the Department of Medical Scientific Affairs (Office of the Surgeon General RNAMC), Lnt-Colonel Dr. R. G. NYPELS has made it possible to complete my studies during my service in his department.

I would like to express my indebtedness to Professor HAGEDOORN who suggested and stimulated my first steps in the province of visual field examination. I realise the great importance of the support of Professor BLEEKER, Dr. DAKE and Dr. MESKER during the difficult period of introducing more elaborate methods of visual field examination in our Eye Clinic.

I am deeply appreciative to many of my colleagues in the Eye Clinic for their understanding and indispensable cooperation.

I have learned very much from the long discussions with Professor AULHORN and Professor FANKHAUSER. I am grateful for the hospitality of the Tübinger Eye Clinic where I had the chance to learn from the tremendous experience that Professor AULHORN and Professor HARMS have gathered.

I am indebted to Dr. SPEKREIJSE and Dr. VOS for their lessons in visual physiology, and to Dr. WIJNANS for his statistical advices.

Mrs. KATHLEEN BOET translated the manuscript into English. However she did much more than that. Her critical reading of the whole text made a valuable contribution to the clearness of the manuscript.

This study would not have been possible without the help of my collaborators in the Perimetry Department: in the beginning G. F. KINDS and later W. M. VERDUIN, Miss M. LEDEBOER and P. RISON.

Although written by me this study is to a large extent also theirs.

In the various stages of the compilation of this monograph Miss LIESBETH BURGMAN, Miss BETTY COENEN, Miss DORINE DE JONG, Miss ANNELIES KAISER, Miss CATO OTT and Miss LOEKE SCHREUDER helped in typing, reading and correcting. Their enthusiastic assistance has been a great support.

Mr. A. BLIJLEVE, medical draughtsman, prepared the illustrations and the cover design with great dedication. To him and to Mr. C. ZEILSTRA of the photography department I am much indebted.

In the first two years of my investigation I received financial support from the Organization for Health Research TNO (Project GO 691–77) for which I express my gratitude.

Dr. W. Junk b.v. – Publishers have assisted me in every possible way to realise the publication of this book.

One of the most unhappy experiences during my work on this study is the realization that it is one's family that suffers most. I am more than grateful for their patience and understanding.

I gratefully acknowledge the assistance given by numerous authors and publishers in consenting to the reproduction of illustrations.

ARMALY, H. F.

AULHORN, E.

BARGMANN, H.

BOYCOTT, B. B.

DOWLING, J. E.

ENOCH, J. M.

FRANCOIS, J.

FANKHAUSER, F.

GLOSTER, J.

GOUGNARD, L.

HARRINGTON, D. O.

HARMS, H.

MEYTHALER, H.

MOSES, R. A.

OPPEL, O.

PIRENNE, M. H.

SCHMIDT, TH.

SLOAN, L. L.

TRAQUAIR, H. M.

VERRIEST, G.

S. Karger (Basel)

Brit. Med. Journal (London)

Springer (Heidelberg)

Academic Press (London)

Amer. J. Ophthal. (Chicago)

C. V. Mosby (St. Louis)

Pergamon Press (Oxford)

George Thieme (Stuttgart)

Henry Kimpton (London)

American Medical Ass. (Chicago)

Proc. Roy. Soc. (London).

CONTENTS

SINGLE AND MULTIPLE STIMULUS STATIC PERIMETRY IN GLAUCOMA; THE TWO PHASES OF PERIMETRY

CHAPTER I

INTRODUCTION

In this study an attempt will be made to give a survey of the present-day methods available for visual field examination in glaucoma. The conclusions are primarily concerned with routine visual field examination, such as can be performed in a large eye clinic. Special methods of visual field examination, such as the examination of spatial summation and adaptoperimetry, will be considered where necessary in order to justify the choice of the routine method. Special attention will be paid to glaucomatous visual field defects. These defects form a large proportion of the cases for visual field examination which present themselves at our department.

The object of this study is to decide the contribution of the various methods of perimetric investigation in the practice of visual field examination. For this purpose the visual field examination in glaucoma is expressly divided into two phases: a detection phase and an assessment phase. The different functions of kinetic perimetry and static perimetry are emphasized.

In particular, the merits of multiple stimulus static perimetry are expounded. The theoretical background of this method is discussed and the usefulness of this method in practice is demonstrated by means of a study of 1372 visual fields of glaucoma patients.

The importance of the determination of the difference threshold is emphasized. On this basis it is possible to achieve an exact measurement of the intensity of defects.

On the grounds of our own experience and study of the literature a conclusion will be drawn concerning the optimum examination method. In order to reach this conclusion, a number of fundamental principles are first described.

1

In recent years interest in accurate quantitative visual field examination has increased.

Since the pioneering work of VON GRAEFE (1815) on campimetry and AUBERT & FÖRSTER (1857) on perimetry, visual field examination has undergone a tremendous evolution. As usual this evolution has not taken place smoothly. Years pass before new ideas are introduced and generally accepted. Then a period of acceptance is passed through before new and better ideas begin to be advanced. BJERRUM, RÖNNE and FERREE & RAND have made important contributions to the improvement and standardization of visual field examination in the period up to 1940. The well-known names of EVANS, TRAQUAIR, PETERS, WALKER and MALBRAN are also associated with this period. A survey of this older literature is given in DUBOIS-POULSEN's standard work (1952).

Visual field examination made an important leap forward shortly after the second World War. GOLDMANN introduced his perimeter in 1945, by means of which it became possible to apply the principles of quantitative kinetic 'Lichtsinnperimetrie' to routine visual field examination.

In 1939 SLOAN drew attention to the value of static perimetry. Through the work of HARMS & AULHORN (1940–1972) static perimetry has become well known. These authors' investigations have led to the construction and introduction of the Tübinger perimeter. In the meantime the Goldmann perimeter is used in all parts of the world. The distribution of the Tübinger perimeter is dependent on the interest shown in static perimetry, for which this instrument is specifically constructed. The distribution of the Tübinger perimeter is restricted mainly to large ophthalmological centres.

Although both perimeters have become well known, the principles on which they are based are often not recognized. These principles lie in the province of visual physiology. Visual field examination cannot possibly be performed well without knowledge of a number of fundamental principles of visual physiology. In numerous publications GOLDMANN, HARMS & AULHORN, FRANÇOIS & VERRIEST, FANKHAUSER, SCHMIDT, DUBOIS-POULSEN & MAGIS have tried to make the physiological basis of perimetry more widely known. Since DUBOIS-POULSEN's standard work 20 years ago no complete survey of this subject has been published. AULHORN & HARMS have recently published a survey of their own work.

Perimetry has occasionally been called the step-child of ophthalmology. It is hoped that this work will lead to a better understanding of the many good qualities and possibilities of this step-child. At the moment it appears that a period of acceptance of static perimetry as indispensable companion to the already accepted quantitative kinetic perimetry has arrived.

CHAPTER II

SOME BASIC FACTS FROM VISUAL PHYSIOLOGY

VISUAL FIELD EXAMINATION IS A THRESHOLD MEASUREMENT

The 'visual field' is that portion of space that is visible to the fixating eye. Visual field examination is the examination of the *function* of the visual system in this whole field and not only the determination of the limits of the field, as is often wrongly thought. A distinction is usually made between the function of the centre of the visual field and of the peripheral visual field outside it. Examination of visual function usually means the function of the central visual field by means of visual acuity or colour vision, for instance. It is true that central vision has a dominating function in the visual system, yet it is astonishing that the clinical examination of function is usually limited to this very small part (1/15,000) of the visual system. When assessing the function of the visual system examination of the visual acuity and the visual field must always go together. It is not possible to examine all the $\pm$ 15,000 square degrees of the visual field. In visual field examination therefore a random sample is taken, which gives as much insight as possible into the function of the visual system. This means that a number of positions in the visual field are selected and their function is recorded.

Thus, in practice visual field examination is the examination of the function of a number of selected places in the visual system. Recording the function in the visual field has not only intrinsic value but can also be of diagnostic importance.

Visual field examination is one of the psychophysical methods of examination. A physically defined stimulus leads to a psychic sensation, which in turn gives rise to a reaction in the form of pressing a switch or giving a verbal answer.

4

The sensation produced by a given stimulus is used to determine the integrity of the visual system. A 'stimulus-response' equation ($R = f(S)$) indicates how a measurable aspect of the response R varies as a function of the stimulus S. 'The measure of the response is graded with the measure of the stimulus'[1]. In visual field examination the minimum light stimulation is measured which is needed to produce a response. When assessing the function of the visual system in this way, the threshold stimulation necessary for a response is used. Man is able to react with reasonable reproducibility to threshold stimuli.

The threshold stimulation can take place in absolute darkness (absolute threshold) or against a background of given luminance. In the latter case the minimum contrast (or threshold contrast) between stimulus and background is under consideration This is known as the increment threshold or luminance difference threshold[2]; the term difference threshold will be used in this study. The difference threshold is the smallest measurable difference in luminance between a stimulus and a field of comparison (the background).

The function of the visual system which is measured by means of visual field examination is the light sensitivity. For reasons which will be given later the differential light sensitivity is measured with white light. The difference threshold is the measure of the differential light sensitivity. The differential light sensitivity is the reciprocal of the difference threshold. Measuring the difference threshold is the essence of visual field examination. DUBOIS-POULSEN[3] has expressed this as follows: 'La mesure des seuils est donc le seul moyen que nous possédions de relier les quantités physiques exprimant le stimulus aux quantités physiologiques sensorielles'.

The differential light sensitivity is a fundamental function of the visual system.

Visual field examination consists of the determination of the differential light sensitivity of an adequate number of positions in the visual system by means of difference threshold measurements.[4]

METHODS OF MEASUREMENT.

Every threshold value is subject to variability. The two most important psycho-physical methods of determining the difference threshold are the '*method of constant stimuli*' and the '*method of limits*'.

---

[1] GRAHAM 1966.

[2] BLACKWELL 1972

[3] DUBOIS-POULSEN 1952.

[4] The absolute light sensitivity can also be determined by measuring the absolute threshold. This will be considered in connection with adaptoperimetry.

5

In the 'method of constant stimuli' a stimulus is presented a number of times at various luminance levels and the subject is asked to react the moment he sees the stimulus. For a given stimulus value a percentage of positive reactions is obtained as compared with the total number of times the stimulus is presented. This information is usually plotted as a 'frequency-of-seeing curve', in which the abscissa is the logarithm of the luminance and the ordinate the percentage of positive reactions (Fig. 1). The result is an S-shaped curve between 0% and 100% frequency of seeing.[5]

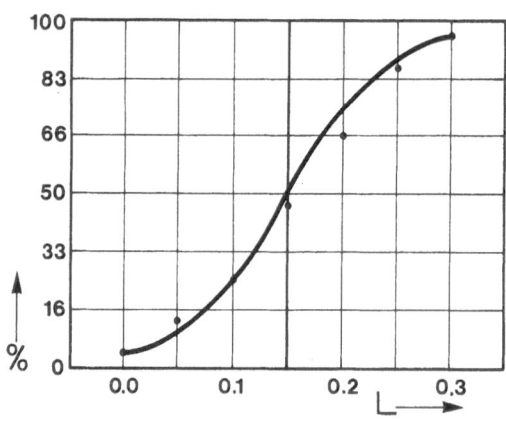

Fig. 1
Frequency-of-seeing curve
abscissa: arbitrary luminance steps of 0.05 log units
ordinate: frequency of seeing in percent

The threshold value could best be represented by this S-curve, but usually an arbitrary percentage is chosen as the threshold (e.g. 50%). The transition from no perception to perception is gradual. From an S-curve like this it appears that in a given stimulation area there is a certain probability (1%–99%) that the stimulus will be perceived.

In the 'method of limits' the luminance of the stimulus is increased until the subject perceives the stimulus (or the other way round: the luminance of the stimulus is decreased until the subject stops seeing it). From the above observations on 'frequency-of-seeing' curves it will be clear that the subject will not always perceive the stimulus at the same level of luminance, although the variability is limited.

From a number of observations the average value is taken as the threshold

---

[5] See also chapter VII.

value. In simplified form this method is used in perimetry. In practice the difference threshold is examined in two ways: kinetic and static. Both methods are based on the principle that an infraliminal stimulus is presented and that the stimulation is then increased, either continuously or in steps, until the threshold level is reached.[6]

FACTORS WHICH DETERMINE THE DIFFERENCE THRESHOLD

Before considering the methods of investigation, the factors which determine the level of the difference threshold will be discussed. These include the receptor and neural mechanisms which are involved in light perception. As the object of this study is to give a survey of the practice of visual field examination, observations on the receptor and neural mechanisms will be limited to the facts necessary for the comprehension of visual field examination.

The factors which influence the level and variation of the difference threshold can be subdivided into the following 5 groups:
1. Physical characteristics of the stimulation;
2. Preretinal factors;
3. Receptor and neural factors;
4. Psychological factors;
5. General health.

In Table I an attempt has been made to show the relationship between these factors. The stimulation passes from left to right through the optic system of the eye and gives rise to an electrical impulse in the receptors, which is integrated by the neural system.

The stimulus and the background are usually easily measurable physical quantities. The preretinal factors, the optical system of the eye, determine the final stimulation at the retinal level. These factors will be discussed after the normal visual field has been described.[7]

The distribution of the receptors over the retina and their function are considered under the subheading receptor mechanisms. The transmission and integration of impulses generated by light stimulation of the receptors through the cells of the retina, geniculate body and the cortex will be considered under the subheading neural mechanisms. Psychological factors will be considered only in connection with the multiple-stimulus method. Finally, the subject's general

---

[6] The reverse order (i.e. supraliminal to liminal) has certain disadvantages which will be described later.

[7] Chapter IX.

7

TABLE I

Factors that determine the level of the difference threshold

Physical characteristics of stimulation	preretinal factors	stimulation at the retinal level	receptor and neural mechanisms	psychological factors	
position of the stimulus in the perimeter		position of the stimulus on the retina	anatomical differences in the visual system	understanding	> μμ >
luminance level before the examination	pupil size; transparancy of media; ametropia; accomodation	retinal illumination before the examination: preadaptation level		interest	> μμ >
background luminance		retinal illumination adaptation level	adaptation	cooperation	> μμ >
contrast		retinal contrast		fear	> μμ >
stimulus luminance		retinal illumination by the stimulus	spatial interaction	training	> μμ >
stimulus size		size and sharpness of the image		general health	> μμ >
stimulus sharpness					> μμ >
presentation time			temporal interaction / local adaptation		> μμ >
movement			sensitivity to movement of the visual system	reaction time	> μμ >
chromaticity of stimulus		retinal chromaticity	specific sensitivity for colour		> μμ >
fixation target			conditions of fixation		> μμ >

health is an important factor which should be mentioned but needs no further consideration here.

PHYSICAL CHARACTERISTICS OF THE STIMULATION

The physical characteristics of the stimulation are determined by the instrument with which the visual field examination is carried out. The characteristics will be considered here in general. In Chapters VI and VIII a number of instruments will be described, with consideration of these characteristics. When one measures threshold values in a patient, and wishes to compare these values with those of normal subjects or of the same patient at an earlier investigation, an accurate, standardized, reproducible method of measurement must be available. The physical characteristics of the stimulation must thus be known and measurable. Regular standardization of the physical characteristics provides a guarantee for the reproducibility of the stimulation and is a first essential in visual field examination (and in every other psychophysical investigation).

The number of positions in the visual field to be examined and the distribution of these positions are of vital importance. The apparatus in use must be able to present a stimulus at any given point. The number of positions and their distribution will be considered in Chapter V.

Determination of the position of the stimulus.

The position of the stimulus is recorded on the basis of the eccentricity (η), expressed as the angle (in degrees) which the stimulus makes with the fixation axis, and of the meridian in which the stimulus is presented[8].

The position of the object in space is a guide to the position of the object on the retina. One millimeter on the retina represents approximately 4 degrees in the visual field. These values vary to some extent, dependent upon the eccentricity, the optics of the eye and the refraction. A stimulus which, in a given meridian, makes a given angle with the fixation axis, will usually reach approximately the same position on the retina in different subjects. The variation in position between individuals may be one of the reasons for the variation in the level of the threshold.

In visual field examination the position of the stimulus in space means the position of the stimulus on the perimeter background. In the usual projection-

---

[8] To record the results of a visual field examination the positions examined must be registered on paper. One comes here onto the grounds of cartography with its own specific problems.

perimeters (and -campimeters) the determination of the position depends on a projection system and a system which registers the position.

The registration of the positions is to a large extent dependent on the accuracy of the perimetric chart (and in particular on the size of the chart), and on the transmission from the chart to the projector. If the registration of the position is less accurate, and especially less reproducible, the results, particularly when small visual field defects are concerned, will be affected.

Level of luminance before examination.

This is a physical factor which is usually not precisely known. This unknown factor is not important if the patient is allowed enough time to adapt to the background luminance.

Background luminance.

The background luminance must fulfil certain requirements regarding level, uniformity, constancy and measurability. The level of the background luminance determines (together with the preretinal factors) the adaptation level of the eye being examined[9]. Internationally, luminance is expressed in candles per square metre (cd/m^2). In ophthalmology the apostilb (asb) is often used. The luminance values of the Tübinger and Goldmann perimeters are expressed in apostilb. One apostilb is π cd/m^2.

Uniformity is necessary because all positions in the visual field should be examined under similar conditions. Uniformity is easy to obtain in hemispherical perimeters by illuminating the inside of the hemisphere with one light source. Reflection occurs according to the principle of Ulbricht's sphere, so that the whole hemisphere has practically the same illumination except for the immediate environment of the source of light.

Constancy of the background luminance is necessary because the degree of stimulation is dependent upon the contrast between stimulus and background and because the adaptation level should remain constant within certain limits[10].

---

[9] The choice of adaptation level will be considered later; chapter IV.

[10] The constancy of the background luminance is dependent upon fluctuations in the voltage. The effect of this fluctuation can be eliminated by the inclusion of a current stabilizer. This is provided in the Tübinger perimeter and the Goldmann perimeter for static perimetry. The majority of lamps used in perimeters give less light as time goes by. The resulting decrease in luminance is compensated by increasing the current by means of an adjustable resistance (Goldmann perimeter, Tübinger perimeter). If the decrease in luminance is due to localized blackening of the lamp this must be turned or replaced.

It is impossible to obtain uniformity and constancy of background in arc-shaped perimeters.

The luminance can be measured with a luxmeter or a luminancemeter. The Goldmann and Tübinger perimeters are equipped with such a standardizing apparatus.

Luminance of stimulus.

For the luminance of the stimulus the requirements of constancy, measurability and uniformity are just as important. The luminance of the stimulus should be able to be altered in steps. In practice this is achieved by means of neutral density filters. It is important that these filters do not essentially alter the spectral composition of the lamp-light and that the steps of luminance are correct, i.e. that they are all of the same size. Also the density of the filters should not alter in the course of time. The size of the steps is determined by the variation of the differential sensitivity, and by the significance of the intensity of relative defects[11].

The usual size of the steps is one tenth (0.1) logarithmic unit. An increase of luminance of 0.1 log unit corresponds approximately to an increase from 100% to 125%[12].

The luminance of the stimulus and the luminance of the background determine the contrast. In visual field examination contrast is expressed as:

$$\frac{\text{L stimulus} - \text{L background}}{\text{L background}}$$

---

[11] These factors affecting the choice of the size of the steps will be discussed in Chapter VII.

[12] In the following table some logarithmic steps of luminance with the corresponding increase or decrease in luminance are given in percentages.

Increase in luminance	Percentage	Decrease	Percentage
0.1 lu	125%	0.1 lu	80%
0.2 lu	160%	0.2 lu	63%
0.3 lu	200%	0.3 lu	50%
0.4 lu	250%	0.4 lu	40%
0.5 lu	315%	0.5 lu	31%
0.6 lu	400%	0.6 lu	25%
0.7 lu	500%	0.7 lu	20%
0.8 lu	630%	0.8 lu	16%
0.9 lu	800%	0.9 lu	12%
1.0 lu	1000%	1.0 lu	10%

The smallest perceptible difference of luminance, L stimulus – L background, is expressed as ΔL. ΔL represents the difference threshold luminance. The differential light sensitivity can be expressed as $\dfrac{L}{\Delta L}$.

Size of stimulus.

The size of the stimulus is expressed as the angle in degrees which the stimulus subtends at the eye. The assumption is made that the stimulus is round. When this is not the case (as in the Goldmann perimeter) the area is given or the equivalent angular size[13]. If the diameter of the stimulus and the distance between the stimulus and the eye are known, the angular size in degrees (α) can be calculated according to the formula:

$$\alpha = \frac{\text{diameter of stimulus}}{\text{distance}} \times \frac{180}{\pi}$$

The sizes of the stimuli must also be kept constant. The size of the stimulus used is decided by the quality of the optic system of the eye, the resolving power of the retina and the size of the defects in the visual field[14].

The size of the stimulus is dependent upon the distance between the eye and the background upon which the stimulus is projected. Therefore this distance must remain constant. The shorter this distance is, the greater will be the effect of backward and forward movements of the head on the size of the stimulus. With the usual distance of 30 cm the subject's head must be fastened in order to prevent these movements.

Sharpness of stimulus

The sharpness of the stimulus is a question of the distribution of the luminance over the surface area, and especially the edges of the stimulus. Sharp definition means that there is a steep luminance gradient at the boundary between stimulus and background. If the edge of the stimulus is not sharply defined the stimulation is reduced, with the result that the difference threshold is altered.[15] The stimulus must always be sharply defined against the background.

Presentation time.

The presentation time is important in static visual field examination. A presenta-

---

[13] see e.g. ENOCH et al. 1970.
[14] see Chapter IV.
[15] see Chapter IX.

tion time of short duration is not so easy to measure as the luminance and size of an object. This problem is usually avoided by choosing a presentation time which is so long (0.5 s or more) that variations in the time do not affect the size of the stimulus. If short presentation times are used, electromagnetic shutters or flash-lamps must be considered. For electromagnetic shutters reliable presentation times are generally not much shorter than 0.005 seconds.

The reproducibility of the presentation time is the most important point with electromagnetic shutters.[16]

A slight change in the presentation time which may occur in the course of years only affects the recorded level of light sensitivity in the whole visual field and does not affect the relative intensity of the defects.

An advantage of electromagnetic shutters is that the luminance of the light source can be standardized in the normal way (with the shutter open).

The possibilities of Xenon flash-lamps are considered in connection with the Visual Field Analyser.[17] Neither the presentation time nor the luminance of a Xenon flash-lamp can be measured in the ordinary way.

Movement.

The speed, acceleration and direction of movement in kinetic visual field examination are easy to measure. The difficulty lies in the fact that the movement is guided by hand. This makes it very difficult to keep the movement factors constant. As will be described elsewhere the visual system is specifically sensitive to movement.[18]

Differences in speed, acceleration or direction result in an altered difference threshold. The biggest problems of movement standardization arise during the examination of visual field defects. Defects are usually examined in all possible directions and in practice it is impossible to reproduce all these directions (and speeds) accurately by hand.

For experimental purposes automatic transporters have been constructed, but these are not much used in practice.[19] One is confronted here with the prob-

---

[16] We have been using a Compur shutter for 3 years, and it has never been defective. The variation in the presentation time of various presentations is even after 3 years very slight.

[17] see Chapter VIII.

[18] see this Chapter II: page 42.

[19] DUBOIS-POULSEN 1959.

lem of the imperfect standardization of movement, which introduces a factor of inaccuracy into kinetic field examination.[20]

Chromaticity of the stimulus.

Visual field examination with coloured objects will not be discussed here. As the sensitivity of the visual system differs for different wavelengths, the colour and the spectral composition of the stimuli should remain constant. This must be taken into consideration when the luminance of white light is altered; variable resistances are not suitable for altering the luminance. If filters are used they should leave the colour and spectral composition of the light source unchanged.

Fixation target.

The fixation determines the position of the stimulus in the visual field. For photopic visual field examination the fixation target must fulfil the following criteria:

1. the fixation target must be bright enough to be seen clearly and easily, but not so bright that it has a dazzling effect or influences the state of adaptation of the central retina;
2. the fixation target must be as small as possible, so that it only occupies a small space. It should be small to avoid shifting of fixation within the target, but big enough to be clearly seen. It must be sharply differentiated from the background.

Small details of the fixation target must be easily visible in order to encourage accommodation. In the Tübinger perimeter the fixation target is the only object which stimulates accommodation. In the Goldmann perimeter the fixation target is surrounded by a dark ring of 2° diameter, which also encourages accommodation. It is very difficult to accommodate well onto the level of a structureless homogeneous background without an adequate fixation target. For mesopic and photopic visual field examination a red fixation target is required because the eye in these circumstances only retains its greatest sensitivity at the centre for red light. Furthermore a red colour is convenient to differentiate the fixation object from the stimulus.

When the difference threshold at the fovea is to be determined, four small points, forming the corners of a square, can be used. The eye is capable of fixating onto the centre of this square.

---

[20] see also Chapter III. SCHMIDT and SCHMIDT-BERGHOFER (1961) demonstrated an instrument with which the pantograph of the Goldmann perimeter can be kept moving at a constant speed. The direction of examination is determined by the investigator.

Summarizing, standardization of the physical characteristics of the stimulus requires the following conditions:
1. It must be possible to present the required number of stimuli at any desired position;
2. cartographic accuracy;
3. uniformity, constancy and measurability of all luminance values;
4. constant and even steps of stimulus luminance; steps of 0.1 log unit should be possible;
5. sharp definition of the stimulus;
6. constancy of presentation time;
7. standardized movement (as far as possible);
8. constant colour and spectral composition of white stimuli;
9. adequate fixation target.

RECEPTOR AND NEURAL MECHANISMS.

Anatomical considerations.

The topography of the light sensitivity of the visual system is determined by the presence of two sorts of receptors, by the heterogeneous structure of the retina, by the possibility of interaction at different levels of the visual system and by the adaptation of this interaction to different states of stimulation.

In the pars optica retinae 3 sorts of cells can be distinguished:[21] receptors, conducting cells and associative cells.

The distribution of the receptors, the rods and cones, over the retina is shown in Fig. 2[22]. The greatest density of the cones is in the centre of the retina and decreases rapidly towards the periphery.[23]

The greatest density of the rods is at 18° and they are absent at the fovea centralis. The density of the cones at the fovea is about the same as the density of the rods at 18° eccentricity.

The conducting cells are the bipolar cells and the ganglion cells. Direct transmission takes place from the receptors to the bipolar cells and from there to the ganglion cells.[24] Fig. 2 also shows the density of the ganglion cells in the hori-

---

[21] POLYAK 1941.

[22] after ØSTERBERG 1935.

[23] MARKS & LIEBMANN 1965. The shape and size of the cones is very variable throughout the retina, but it is improbable that variations in absorption are associated with this.

[24] Many different sorts of bipolar cells and ganglion cells have been described; a detailed description is outside the scope of this work.

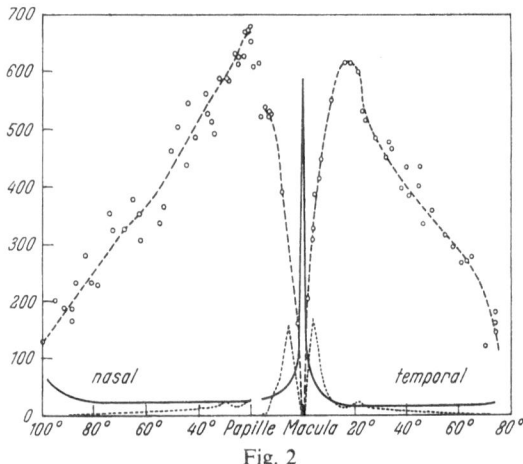

Fig. 2

Distribution of rods, cones and ganglion cells along the horizontal meridian of the retina
abscissa : eccentricity
ordinate: number of cells per 400 μ^2
——————— cones
- - - - rods
--------- ganglion cells

zontal meridian.[25] There are no ganglion cells in a central area of 420–460μ.

In order to understand the topography of the light sensitivity the following facts are of importance (see also Fig. 3).

In the fovea the number of cones, bipolar cells and ganglion cells is the same. In the rod-free fovea this is the only conducting system. An impulse coming from one cone can via this individual conducting system be carried to the lateral geniculate body, although even at the fovea the passage of the impulse probably does not follow this one-to-one relationship. Outside the fovea several cones are connected with the bipolar cells, so that convergence of signals takes place. The rods also form a group from which signals converge on a common bipolar cell.

Outside the fovea there are mixed groups of cones and rods from which impulses can be conducted to a common bipolar cell. If the number of ganglion cells is divided by the total number of cones and rods, it appears that there are on the average 4–6 cones and 100 rods per ganglion cell nerve fibre.

The various dendrites of the bipolar and ganglion cells have a very variable branching pattern (see Fig. 3). The dendritic fields in the central retina cover a smaller area than in the peripheral retina. The dendritic fields of various cells overlap each other.

The associative cells are the horizontal cells and the amacrine cells. The

---

[25] OPPEL 1967.

16

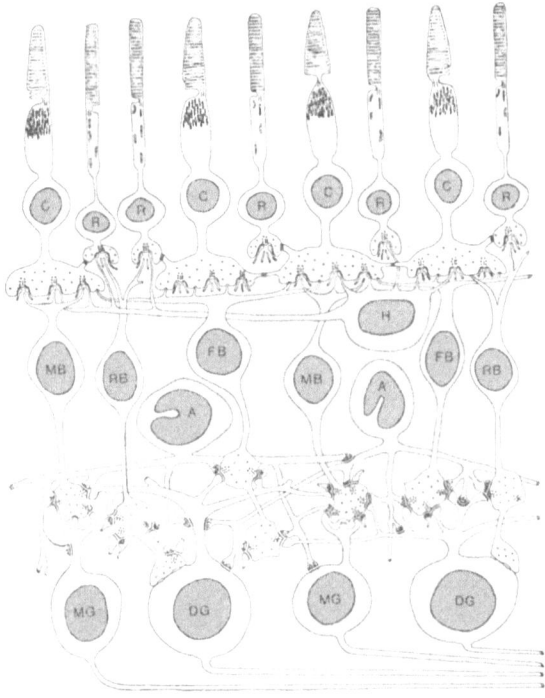

Fig. 3

Schematic representation of connections between receptor cells (R and C), horizontal cells (H), bipolar cells (MB, FB, RB), amacrine cells (A) and ganglion cells (MB, DG).

horizontal cells make contact with both rods and cones. The amacrine cells make contact with bipolar cells and ganglion cells. The dendritic fields of these cells, unlike the bipolar and ganglion cells, have the same size in the central and the peripheral retina.

From these facts two striking points emerge: 1) the convergence from receptors onto conducting cells becomes greater on moving from the centre to the periphery of the retina; 2) numerous anatomical possibilities for lateral contacts are exhibited. These points, together with the distribution of the receptors over the retina, form the anatomical basis for the topography of the light sensitivity and the interaction on which this is based. The maximum extent of a dendritic field is 1 mm. This corresponds to $\pm$ 4° in the visual field. On the basis of these facts spatial interaction should be limited to an area with a maximum diameter of 4°, unless there are synaptic contacts between the various dendritic fields.[26]

---

[26] DOWLING & BOYCOTT (1967) think that some amacrine cells make contact with each other.

Definition and mechanisms.

The differentiation between the rod and cone systems is functional as well as morphological. One of the most remarkable properties of the visual system is that it can alter its light sensitivity over a large range of levels of retinal illumination: *adaptation.* Adaptation is the ability of the visual system to alter its light sensitivity as a function of the illumination level of the moment, the previous illumination level and the time between the two.

When discussing the adaptation, four points will be considered:[27]

1. accessory mechanisms;
2. temporal adaptation;
3. steady state adaptation;
4. the relationship between 2 and 3: the concept of equivalent background.

The adaptive ability is based upon changes in the diameter of the pupil, the duplicity of the receptors, changes in the concentration of photochemical substance in the receptors, and neural interaction. The retinal illumination can be reduced by narrowing the pupil. The effect of narrowing the pupil, however, is at most one log unit, whereas it appears that the adaptive ability covers a range of luminance of more than 10 log units. Even when the diameter of the pupil is artificially kept constant adaptation occurs.

As is well known, three ranges of adaptation are distinguished: in the photopic range (high retinal illumination) the cone system is active; in the scotopic range (low retinal illumination) the rod system is active. In the interjacent mesopic range both receptor systems are active, i.e. the light threshold is for both receptor systems about the same. The difference in the light sensitivity is regarded as one of the most striking differences between the rod system and the cone system. The absolute threshold for the rod system is lower than for the cone system, i.e. the absolute light sensitivity of the rod system is greater. When the conditions are favourable for the cone system – optimal wavelength, small stimulus, short presentation time – the human fovea is only slightly less sensitive than the periphery at 15° eccentricity, where the sensitivity of the rods is maximum. If however light of 527 nm, a large stimulus, and a longer presentation time are used, the light sensitivity of the rod system is 10^4 times as great as that of the cone system. Thus the great advantage of scotopic vision appears to lie in greater spatial and temporal summation, which results from properties

---

[27] BARLOW 1972.

of the neural connections between receptor and ganglion cells.[28] At a high level of retinal illumination the light sensitivity of the visual system is determined by the cone system. By switching from rod system to cone system the visual system can adapt itself to either low or high levels of retinal illumination. Changes in dynamics within the two systems make further extension of the adaptation possible. The cone system exhibits slight spatial interaction; the rod system exhibits great spatial interaction. Adaptation within the cone system takes place more quickly than in the rod system.

In addition to the rapid neural adaptation there is also the slow photochemical adaptation. The logarithm of the light sensitivity of the rod system during dark adaptation is proportional to the rhodopsin concentration.[29]

Temporal adaptation; adaptometry.

When investigating the temporal adaptive capacity the change in light sensitivity is registered as function of the time which has elapsed since the last change in adaptation level. Adaptation to a higher retinal illumination takes place rapidly; more time is needed to adapt to a lower retinal illumination.

Adaptation to lower illumination levels is usually expressed in the classical dark adaptation curve (Fig. 4); in this curve the logarithm of the light threshold

---

[28] BARLOW 1972.

[29] The connection between the photochemical and neural effects which determine the light sensitivity at various levels of adaptation was postulated by RUSHTON (1965) as follows: 'In dark adaptation, log threshold for rods is proportional to the amount of rhodopsin bleached. It also depends upon the size of the test flash and upon bleaching of the neighbouring rods. Each rhodopsin molecule while in a bleached state sends a continued signal of "dark light" to the summation pool. This total background of dark light adds simply to the bright background field (if any) and the dark adapted threshold in the increment threshold against this background'. Originally it was thought that there was a linear relationship between the rhodopsin concentration and the light sensitivity. It has however been shown that 7 minutes after intense bleaching 50% of the rhodopsin has already been regenerated, while the threshold is still many hundred times as high as the absolute threshold (RUSHTON, CAMPBELL, HAGINS & BRINDLEY, 1955). It also appeared that a pre-adaptation which hardly caused any bleaching of rhodopsin still gave rise to a marked elevation of the threshold (RUSHTON & COHEN 1954). The fact that differences in height and duration of the pre-adaptive luminance lead to differences in the shape of the dark adaptation curve, and the differences in the curve when different sizes of stimulus are used, suggest a reorganization of the neural interaction during dark adaptation. In electrophysiological experiments it has been clearly proved that reorganization of the receptive fields occurs when the adaptation level changes (HART-LINE 1957).

19

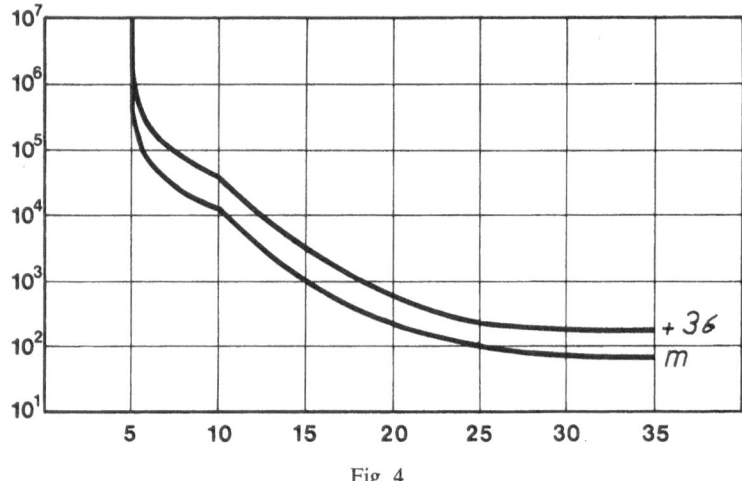

Fig. 4

Dark adaptation curve (Goldmann–Weekers apparatus)
abscissa: time after beginning of preadaptation
ordinate: luminance of stimulus in log units
Mean curve and 3 × standard deviation (upper curve)

s plotted against the duration of adaptation.[30] After pre-adaptation (i.e. after a period of very high retinal illumination) the course of the recovery of light sensitivity is investigated by determination at regular intervals of the light threshold either in complete darkness or against a given background. At a certain moment a stable adaptive condition, and thus constant light sensitivity, is achieved.

The time which elapses between the end of the pre-adaptive state and the stabilization of the adaptive condition is dependent upon the level of the pre-adaptive luminance and the duration of the pre-adaptation and upon the level of luminance which has to be adapted to. The higher the pre-adaptive level and the longer the pre-adaptive time, the longer it will be before the eye is adapted.[31] For white light and an object of a certain minimum size the dark adaptation curve has a biphasic shape.[32] From the curve it appears that at least 30 minutes are necessary for adaptation to complete darkness. The dip in the curve, point α, divides the photopic and the scotopic portions of the curve. The more or less abrupt transition from the photopic to the scotopic system is usually considered to be an argument in favour of the independent working of the two systems.

---

[30] originally difference threshold, later absolute threshold (see page 00).
[31] for further information see BARTLETT 1966.
[32] KOHLRAUSCH 1922.

According to this theory the threshold is determined by the system with the greatest light sensitivity[33]; the only point where the sensitivity of the cone system is the same as that of the rod system is point α.

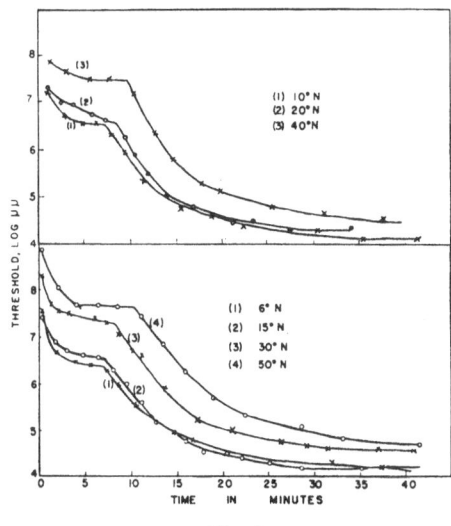

Fig. 5

Dark adaptation curves at several locations in the nasal visual field; preadaptation of 1100 mL.   abscissa: time after beginning of preadaptation
ordinate: luminance of stimulus in log units

The point alpha is not situated at the same point of time for every position (Fig. 5). In the periphery point alpha is reached several minutes later than in the central visual field. This signifies that the whole visual system does not change over from the photopic system to the scotopic system under the same adaptive conditions. In the whole 30° visual field, however, point alpha is reached more or less simultaneously.

Adaptation and the two receptor systems.

The light sensitivity of a given position is determined by the density of the receptors there, by the adaptation level, i.e. the dominating receptor system, and by the degree of spatial and temporal interaction within this system. As only cones are present at the fovea the light sensitivity at the centre of the visual field is determined by the cone system alone. The distinction between the functions of the rod and cone systems is based, among other things, on the colour

---

[33] STILES 1959.

vision [34], the *Stiles-Crawford* effect[35], experiments with rod-monochromats and patients with congenital night blindness. The visual acuity is low when only the rod system is active; when the cone system is functioning the visual acuity is high. The capacity of the rod system for spatial and temporal integration is greater than that of the cone system.

For practical visual field examination it is important to know 1) how sharp the transition is between the fields of activity of the two systems and 2) how much difference there is between the sensitivity of the rod and the cone systems at different levels of adaptation.

Strict differentiation of the function of the two receptor systems is probably not justified. The fact that the threshold for one receptor system in a given range of adaptation is lower than for the other receptor system does not mean that the light sensitivity is determined exclusively by the latter system.

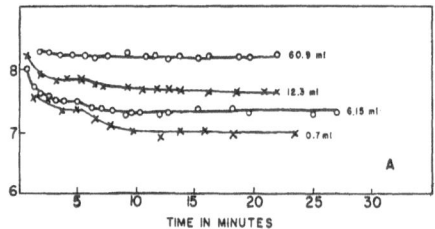

Fig. 6

Adaptation to four different levels of luminance (expressed in millilamberts) measured at 15° eccentricity in the nasal field.
abscissa: time after preadaptation in minutes
ordinate: luminance of stimulus in log $\mu\mu$L

The rod system is not saturated until the luminance is 120 –300 cd/m².[36]

When adapting to a given level of luminance instead of to complete darkness it is found that the dip in the dark adaptation curve does not disappear until a level of $\pm$ 200 cd/m² is reached (Fig. 6).[37] This could indicate that the rod system can still function at high adaptive levels. At mesopic adaptive levels

---

[34] The relative sensitivity of the rod system is maximum at 505 nm, and at 555 nm for the cone system. The rod system is not associated with colour response whereas the rod-free fovea has a highly developed colour-sense which must arise from the cones.
[35] Cones are sensitive to the direction in which the light strikes them, rods are not (STILES & CRAWFORD, 1933).
[36] AGUILAR & STILES, 1954; FUERTES, GUNKEL & RUSHTON 1961; MANDELBAUM & NELSON 1960.
[37] SLOAN 1947, 1950.

(0.01 – 0.1 cd/m²) the cone threshold and the rod threshold lie close together[38]. Even at high levels of adaptation the difference in sensitivity between the rod system and the cone system is only very slight. If one of the systems should fail this would only cause a slight change in the light sensitivity.[39]

From the fact that at the beginning of the scotopic period colour is still discerned, it appears that the cones are still functioning to some extent.[40]

With certain presentation times it appears that stimuli of 510 nm at photopic luminance levels are desaturated, a result of activity of the rod system.[41]

Electrophysiological experiments have shown that ganglion cell responses may be found coming simultaneously from rods and cones.[42] Under photopic conditions the rod activity is inhibited by the activity of the cone system when impulses from these two systems reach a ganglion cell within a certain interval.

The final sensation over a wide range of adaptation is probably produced by interaction between the two systems.[43] If the limits of the mesopic area were to be based on the simultaneous functioning of rods and cones, a very large area of adaptation would have to be called mesopic.[44] A sharp division between the function of the rod and the cone system at various adaptive levels does not appear to exist; there is a gradual transition from dominant cone to dominant rod function.

Steady state adaptation.

As distinct from the examination of temporal adaptation, in the examination of steady state adaptation the visual system is allowed to reach a condition of equilibrium. The light sensitivity is measured as a function of a given background luminance to which the eye is adapted.

The results of measurements of the steady state adaptation can be recorded as the classical curves in which the difference threshold of one position is plotted as function of the background luminance, or as perimetric sensitivity curves at various levels of background luminance (adaptoperimetry).

---

[38] DANNHEIM 1967.

[39] SLOAN 1950.

[40] MOTE & RIOPELLE 1953; VERRIEST 1960; BARTLETT 1966.

[41] VERRIEST 1960.

[42] GOURAS 1965, 1966, 1967, in monkeys.

[43] see recent discussion by WALTER 1971, which also covers GOURAS' work.

[44] see also WALD 1961; WALD concluded that there is a large transitional area between rod and cone function. His conclusions were based on the desaturation of colour in the photopic part of the dark adaptation curve, on the peripheral spectral sensitivity curve and on the occurrence of the Stiles-Crawford effect under certain scotopic conditions.

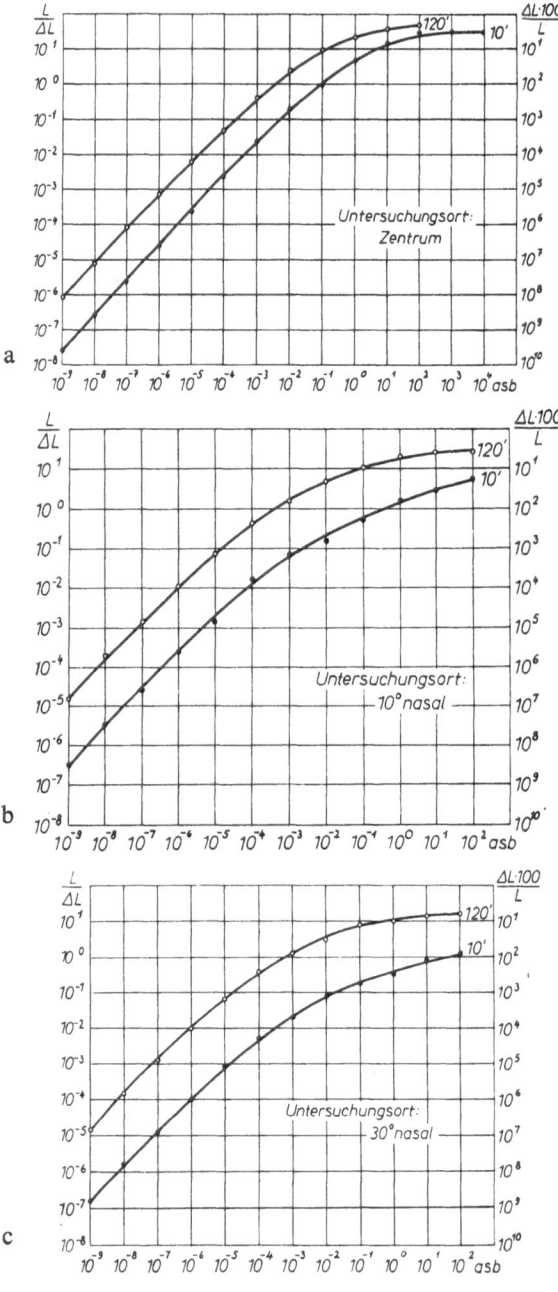

Fig. 7

The relation between log $\frac{L}{\Delta L}$ and log L, as measured for 3 different positions in the visual field (0°, 10°, and 30° nasal).

24

Adaptation and difference threshold.

When the light sensitivity $\dfrac{L}{\Delta L}$ is plotted against the background luminance a curve results as shown is Fig. 7[45]. In this curve we can distinguish a horizontal part, a part which makes an angle of 45° with the abscissa and a transitional part. The horizontal part shows that, with a background luminance of between 100 asb and 1000 asb (31.5 –315 cd/m²), the differential light sensitivity $\dfrac{(L)}{(\Delta L)}$ remains constant[46] (central visual field, 10′ stimulus). This is approximately the luminance at which the rod system is saturated. The foveal curves show that there is some decrease in light sensitivity between 100 asb and 10 asb. When the background luminance is reduced further the differential light sensitivity decreases with increasing rapidity. In the 45° part (L between 0 asb and $\pm\,10^{-2}$ asb; central visual field) the differential light sensitivity $\dfrac{(L)}{(\Delta L)}$ decreases with decreasing background luminance and the difference threshold (ΔL) remains constant. In the transitional area the difference threshold increases until the horizontal part is reached where the increase is proportional to the increase in background luminance. The exact shape and position of the transitional area is dependent upon the position being examined and the size of the stimulus. In the foveal curve, the background luminance at which the transitional part changes into the 45° part corresponds with the point alpha in the dark adaptation curve: the central difference threshold has reached its final value.

In the curves for the periphery the transition to the 45° part takes place much later. The difference threshold continues to decrease until the background luminance has been reduced to 10^{-12} asb ($10^{-12.5}$ cd/m²). This background luminance is called physiological darkness.[47] The difference threshold is then the same as the absolute threshold. This corresponds with the final threshold of the scotopic part of the dark adaptation curve.

Adaptation and topography of the light sensitivity; adaptoperimetry.

The topography of the light sensitivity in the horizontal meridian at different background luminances is shown in Fig. 8.[48] Here again three parts can be distinguished: photopic, scotopic and mesopic.

---

[45] AULHORN et al. 1966.

[46] Law of Weber-Fechner: $\dfrac{\Delta L}{L} = C.$

[47] AULHORN et al. 1966.

[48] see also HARMS 1949.

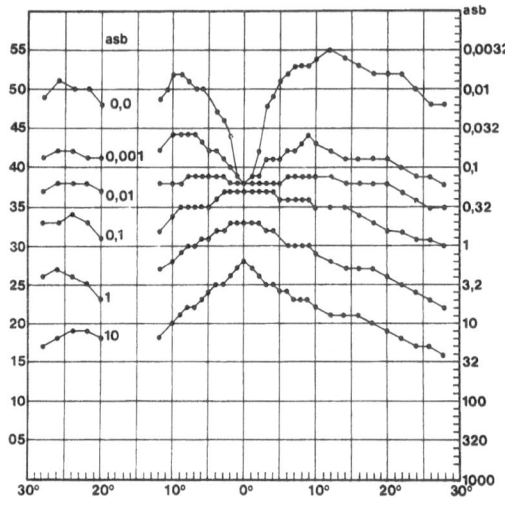

Fig. 8

Topography of light sensitivity in the horizontal meridian of the 30° (radius) visual field at different background luminances (levels of adaptation); the background luminance in asb is indicated for each curve
abscissa: eccentricity
ordinate: luminance of stimulus in asb.

Photopic level.

At the photopic level the light sensitivity decreases from the centre to the periphery. This decrease is more or less linear over a large area, if the threshold luminance increases logarithmically.[49]

The topography of the photopic light sensitivity is often visualized three-dimensionally as an 'island of vision in the sea of darkness' (Fig. 9).[50]

The photopic curves of sensitivity in Fig. 8 are meridional vertical sections through the 'island of vision'. Such curves represent the change in light sensitivity as the eccentricity increases. The term 'sensitivity curve' will be used for these curves. The topography of photopic light sensitivity is characterized by maximum sensitivity in the central visual field.

The topography of the light sensitivity can also be recorded as isopters, analogous to contour lines in cartography: lines joining points of equal light sensitivity. A horizontal section through the 'island of vision' produces an

[49] $S = A.e.^{-m}$: MAGIS 1956.
[50] Traquair's Clinical Perimetry, 1937.

26

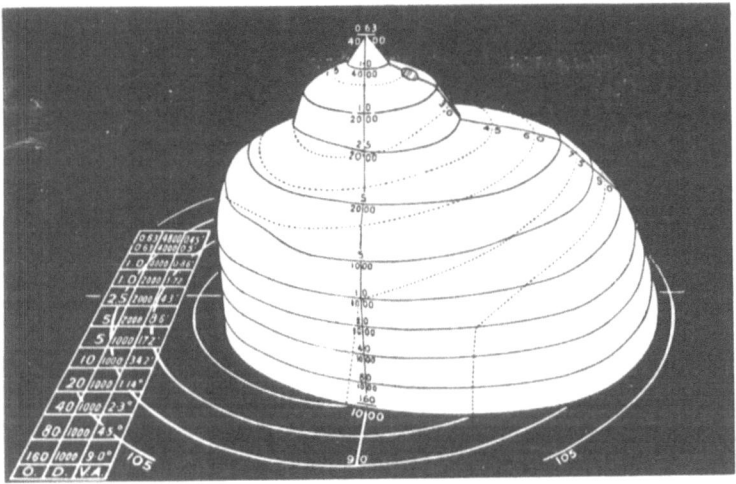

Fig. 9
The island of vision in the sea of darkness.

isopter. These are the two customary ways of recording the topography of the light sensitivity which are used in perimetry.[51]

It would of course be possible to give each position examined a mark, indicating the function of the position, analogous to visual acuity determination. The result is then a chart with a number of figures spread out over the visual field.[52]

Scotopic level.

At the scotopic level the shape of the sensitivity curve is different. The change with respect to the photopic curve is most marked in the central and intermediate visual field.[53] In the periphery outside the 30° parallel the shape of the sensitivity curve remains the same at all levels of adaptation.[54]

Maximum sensitivity at the scotopic level has shifted from the centre to the 20° parallel. There is a relative scotoma in the centre. The shape of this scotopic

[51] see also Chapter III.

[52] This method is employed in one of the instruments used by us for multiple stimulus presentation, the Visual Field Analyser.

[53] The visual field is divided into a central area within the 10° parallel, an intermediate area or Bjerrum area between the 10° and the 30° parallel, and a peripheral area outside the 30° parallel.

[54] SLOAN 1939, JONKERS 1954.

27

sensitivity curve is comparable to the shape of the curve in Fig. 2[55], which represents the density of the rods in the horizontal meridian.

Mesopic level.

Between the typical photopic sensitivity curve and the typical scotopic sensitivity curve lies a series of transitional forms. In Fig. 8 these can be found in the area between 100 asb and 0 asb ($\approx 10^{-12}$) asb. The curves with background luminance of 1 asb still have a central sensitivity peak, but this is not so obvious as at 100 asb. The curve with background luminance of 0.001 asb shows a relative central scotoma but this is not so pronounced as at 0 asb. This whole transitional area could be called mesopic, but in order to fix definite limits for visual field examination at mesopic adaptation levels, we follow BAIR's definition[56] of the mesopic sensitivity curve as the curve in which the sensitivity is uniform throughout the whole area within the 20° parallel, i.e. where the curve is horizontal in the 20° area. This area is isoliminal.

In the curves in Fig. 8 this point is reached at a background luminance of 0.01 asb. When the background luminance is decreased further the foveal threshold does not become lower. This condition of adaptation is comparable to the point alpha in the dark adaptation curve.[57]

The level of adaptation at which the 20° area is isoliminal varies with the size and spectral composition of the stimulus (see Fig.10).

Equivalent background; the relationship between adaptometry and adoptoperimetry.

Both changing and constant levels of adaptation have been discussed above. In the usual (temporal) examination of dark adaptation, adaptometry, after pre-adaptation the change in threshold of a given position is measured as function of the time. In adaptoperimetry[58] (steady state) the light sensitivity of various positions, usually along one meridian, are examined at photopic, mesopic and scotopic background luminances. In adaptometry the adaptive state, and thus the threshold, alters continually, whereas in adaptoperimetry the adaptive

---

[55] see page 16.

[56] BAIR 1940.

[57] On the understanding that the background luminance concerned is added to the equivalent background of the point alpha.

[58] Adaptoperimetry was described by HARMS in 1949.

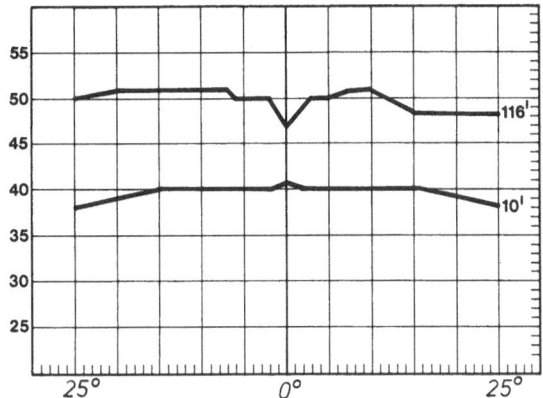

Fig. 10

Sensitivity curves measured at a mesopic level of adaptation (0.01 asb) with 2 different
stimulus sizes.

abscissa: eccentricity
ordinate: filter position of Tübinger perimeter

state is constant during the examination at a given background luminance.
There is a relationship between the two methods: the thresholds which are
measured during adaptometry are the same as the thresholds against a hypo-
thetical 'equivalent background'.

The principle of 'equivalent background' is known from the psychophysical
literature.[59] The equivalent background is the background that elevates the
difference threshold to the value of the threshold with zero background at a
certain time during dark adaptation. The thresholds measured in adaptometry
are presumably the difference thresholds against an equivalent background of
a positive after-image, produced by the pre-adaptation.[60] In the explanation of
the relationship between adaptometry and adaptoperimetry the influence of the
time factor has not been mentioned. In adaptoperimetry the subject has plenty
of time to adapt to the constant background luminance. In adaptometry the
state of adaptation depends on the speed of adaptation. The two conditions –
real background and equivalent background– are not in all respects comparable.[61]
The idea of equivalent background, however, is useful for indicating the relationship between adaptometry and adaptoperimetry.

---

[59] CRAWFORD 1947; RUSHTON 1963, 1964, BARLOW 1972.

[60] This has been shown by BARLOW & SPARROCK (1964) in a particularly attractive
experiment.

[61] BARLOW 1972.

An interesting consequence of the principle of equivalent background is that the time-consuming dark adaptation examination (duration 45 minutes) of only one or two positions can be replaced by adaptoperimetry at various levels of adaptation. The latter method provides information about a larger number of positions: in the same examination time a better impression is obtained of the adaptive function of various parts of the visual system. Cases in which the sole anomaly is delayed adaptation without alteration in the threshold are the only ones which are not detected by adaptoperimetry[62].

Conclusion:

1. Isolated activity of the cone system or the rod system is only certain when the retinal illumination is either very high or very low.
2. In the intermediate area of retinal illumination it is probable that combined action of the two receptor systems is responsible for the light sensitivity.
3. At the low photopic and mesopic constant adaptation level there is little difference in sensitivity between the cone and the rod system, as is shown by the dark adaptation curve.
4. It is not possible to define the mesopic level sharply. In visual field examination we define the mesopic level as the adaptive condition in which the light sensitivity in the area within the 20° parallel is uniform.
5. The differential light sensitivity reaches a maximum at the photopic level. Above ± 315 asb ($100 \, \text{cd/m}^2$) no further change in the differential sensitivity occurs when the background luminance is increased. The differential sensitivity decreases as the background luminance decreases.
6. Under different adaptive conditions both the light sensitivity and the topography of the light sensitivity within the 20° parallel change.
7. In adaptometry there is an 'equivalent background' corresponding to each point of time after the end of the pre-adaptation. In this way adaptometry is directly comparable to adaptoperimetry.
8. For visual field examination it is important to know that an adaptation time of 5–10 minutes is needed for photopic adaptive levels, and that at least 30 minutes is needed for scotopic adaptive levels.

On these conclusions, together with a discussion of the literature on visua-field examination, the choice of adaptation level for routine visual field examinal tion will be based.[63]

---

[62] We do not know if such cases have been found in practice.
[63] Chapter IV.

Spatial interaction.

Psychophysical findings.

It has been known for a long time that there is a reciprocal relationship between the threshold luminance and the size of the stimulus. Within certain limits there is summation of the effects of the light stimuli falling on different parts of the retina, so that the total effect is the sum of the separate effects. This interaction is chiefly made possible by the extensive lateral connections between the retinal conducting and associative cells, and perhaps also by integration at higher levels.

Laws of summation.

The relationship between threshold luminance and size of stimulus is usually expressed in the perimetric literature by the formula $\Delta L \times S^K = C$, where S is the size and ΔL the threshold luminance of the stimulus. In this formula K is the coefficient of summation. [64]

If spatial summation is complete this signifies that the threshold light flux for the sizes of stimulus used is constant. In this case the coefficient of summation K equals 1. The formula then assumes the form of the well-known Ricco's law[65]: $L \times S = C$. The limited validity of Ricco's law has led to the formulation of several other laws, the best known of which are Piper's law[66] and Pieron's (or Elsberg-Spotnitz') law[67]:

Piper: $L \times \sqrt[2]{S} = C$, where $K = 0.5$

Pieron: $L \times \sqrt[3]{S} = C$, where $K = 0.3$

In the case of the last two laws partial spatial summation is indicated. The significance of Piper's and Pieron's laws is limited because actually all stages of partial summation can occur if the right conditions are chosen.

Summation and inhibition.

The term 'spatial summation' is misleading as it gives the impression that when light stimuli interact the only effect is a greater or lesser degree of summation. As will appear later this is not the case and a sensation of light at threshold level must be seen as the result of the interaction of summation and inhibition.

---

[64] A disadvantage of this formula is that the size of K depends on the size of S.

[65] RICCO 1877.

[66] PIPER 1903.

[67] PIERON 1929, French literature, ELSBERG-SPOTNITZ 1937 Anglo-Saxon literature.

Partial summation thus indicates that inhibitive interaction mechanisms are also at work. Only in the case of complete summation (K = 1) inhibitive interaction is not involved[68]. The literature on visual psychophysics deals extensively with spatial summation.[69]

The majority of psychophysical experiments on spatial summation are performed by one of the following two methods:

1. The light sensitivity (thus the threshold luminance) of a given position is examined with various sizes of stimulus. A graph can be drawn of the threshold luminance against the stimulus size: we call this a summation curve (Fig. 11).[70]

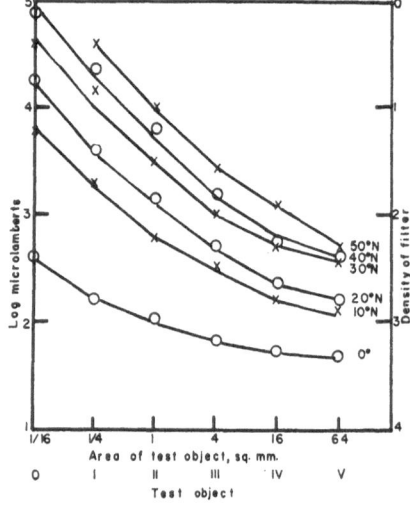

Fig. 11. Spatial summation curves of a normal subject for the fovea and for various locations in the nasal visual field.

abscissa: luminance in log units, ordinate: area of test object (Goldmann perimeter)

2. Using, as a rule, the method of constant stimuli, an examination is made of the effect of the presence of a stimulus on the perception of a second stimulus in the vicinity as function of the distance between them. Summative interaction is revealed by increased frequency of seeing of the stimulus as compared with the results with one stimulus alone.

---

[68] see SPEKREIJSE, WAGNER & WOLBARSCHT 1972.

[69] GRAHAM & MARGARIA, 1935; GRAHAM & MOTE, 1939; GRAHAM & BARTLET 1939; WEINSTEIN & ARNULF 1946; BLACKWELL 1946; BROWN 1947; BOYNTON 1951; BOUMAN & VAN DEN BRINK 1952; BRINDLEY 1954; VAN DEN BRINK & BOUMAN 1954; VAN DEN BRINK 1957; 1965; BARLOW 1958; WEALE 1958; HALLET et al., 1962; THOMAS 1963; 1965; GLEZER 1965; HALLET 1965; VAN DEN BRINK & REYNTJES 1966; KISHTO & SAUNDERS 1970.

[70] SLOAN 1961.

The first method is applied in perimetry.[71] We know of no perimetric literature on the second method.[72] From the psychophysical literature it appears that at the scotopic level spatial summation occurs over a retinal area varying from 4' at the fovea to 2° in the periphery (35°)[73]. The conditions under which the various authors obtained their divergent results are difficult to compare.

Most of the psychophysical experiments have no direct connection with perimetric studies, either because they are concerned with the absolute threshold instead of the difference threshold, or because only one position is examined (in many cases the fovea). We shall therefore only mention the general conclusions drawn:

1. Spatial summation is greater at the periphery of the visual field than in the centre. For the absolute threshold the area of total summation hardly increases from $\pm$ 3° eccentricity to the periphery. Only at the fovea the area of total summation is definitely smaller.[74]
2. Spatial summation decreases as the eye becomes more adapted to light; summation is poorer under photopic than under scotopic conditions.
3. Spatial summation varies with the colour of the stimulus.[75]
4. Spatial summation is greater when the presentation time is short than when it is long.[76]

WESTHEIMER[77] examined spatial summation by a method in which supraliminal luminances could be used, a fact which has proved important for the demonstration of inhibition. This method differs from the methods described above and will be mentioned again when the work of ENOCH et al.[78] is considered, who adapted WESTHEIMER's method for perimetry.

Electrophysiological findings.

In psychophysical experiments the sensitivity is usually measured by the luminance of either the difference threshold or the absolute threshold. These threshold luminances are lower than the luminances generally used for electrophysio-

---

[71] see Chapter IV.

[72] GOLDMANN (1946) investigated the distance between two stimuli at which they can still be seen separately.

[73] see HALLET 1963; GLEZER 1965; etc.

[74] GLEZER 1965.

[75] BRINDLEY 1954; KISHTO & SAUNDERS, 1970.

[76] BARLOW 1958.

[77] WESTHEIMER 1965, 1966, 1967, 1968.

[78] ENOCH et al. 1970.

logical examination[79]. When comparing the results of these two methods of examination this must be take into account.[80]

In psychophysical experiments an overall response is measured and no differentiation is made between spatial summation at the retinal level, in the lateral geniculate body or in the cortex; the summative capacity of the whole visual system is measured.

Receptive field.

HARTLINE[81] introduced the concept of the receptive field into neurophysiology and pointed out some fundamental properties of receptive fields, including the possibility of spatial summation. Most is known about the receptive fields of the retina. A retinal receptive field is that portion of the retina which, when stimulated by light, produces a response in one nerve cell. A receptive field represents the total area of the visual field in which neural interaction can take place. The receptive field may be that of a ganglion cell, of a cell in the lateral geniculate body or of a cortical cell. By tapping the responses from individual cells or nerve fibres in animals it has been possible to determine the properties of receptive fields at different levels. Responses from bipolar and amacrine cells[82] have up to now proved difficult to obtain, so that most of the information about retinal receptive fields has been obtained from tapping horizontal cells[83], ganglion cells or optic nerve fibres.

In his classic description of the retinal receptive fields KUFFLER[84] has shown that, dependent on the position of stimulation in the receptive field, an 'on-response' (excitation) or an 'off-response' (inhibition) can follow light stimulation. Two types of receptive fields were distinguished. The first type has a round 'on' centre surrounded by a concentric zone which gives an 'off' response. The second type is the other way round: an 'off' centre and an 'on' periphery.

In the retina and the lateral geniculate body the receptive fields are usually round. The periphery of the receptive fields in the lateral geniculate body has an increased capacity for inhibiting the impulses in the centre of the receptive field. This means that the geniculate body cells are even more specialized than the ganglion cells in their reaction to spatial differences in illumination: con-

---

[79] see WHITTLE & CHALLANDS 1969.

[80] see page 35.

[81] HARTLINE 1938; 1940a en 1940b.

[82] With the exception of WERBLIN & DOWLING 1969; KANEKO 1970.

[83] NORTON et al. 1968.

[84] KUFFLER 1952.

trast. Their function is to accentuate the difference – which is already present in the retinal ganglion cells – between the responses to a small stimulus and to diffuse illumination (background).

The receptive fields in the cortex have a more complex form (e.g. rectangular).[85] The visual cortex has a great variety of functions. The impulses from the lateral geniculate body are regrouped in such a way that lines and contours form the most important stimulation. Orientation, the exact position on the retina and movement are also important factors[86]. In many cortical cells the simple objects used in perimetry produce no demonstrable electrophysiological reaction. Only a few cortical cells can be stimulated by changes in luminance, whereas changes in contrast form a stimulus for nearly all the cells.[87] The cortex is the most important level at which binocular impulses converge. The existence of binocular summation has been demonstrated.[88]

Summation area and receptive field.

It is clear that the receptive field resembles in many respects the areas in which interaction can be demonstrated in psychophysical experiments. Within certain limits, receptive fields exhibit constancy of light energy, i.e. interchangeability of luminance and size of stimulus. It appears that Ricco's law also applies to supraliminal luminances. Both the psychophysical interaction area and the receptive field increase in size at all levels from the centre to the periphery of the visual system; both increase in size during dark adaptation. During adaptation the peripheral inhibition disappears and leaves the receptive field with summative responses only [89].

One of the arguments against the equivalence of receptive field and psychophysical interaction area was the fact that the peripheral inhibition is difficult to demonstrate in psychophysical experiments. Recently this has been achieved[90].

As was already mentioned, electrophysiological experiments are carried out with supraliminal luminances. It appears that peripheral inhibition can only be demonstrated with supraliminal luminances.

---

[85] HUBEL & WIESEL 1963;

[86] The specific sensitivity for movement will be considered later; page 42.

[87] Possibly the great difference in amplitude of the visual evoked response in man for changes in luminance and in contrast is based on the same phenomenon (Spekreijse, personal communication).

[88] BATTERSBY & WAGMANN 1962; BLAKEMORE 1969 (cat.); SPEKREIJSE et al. 1972 (man).

[89] BARLOW et al. 1957.

[90] GLEZER 1965; WESTHEIMER 1965.

In psychophysical experiments performed at threshold level, inhibition at the periphery of the interaction area cannot be demonstrated.

The properties of the psychophysical interaction areas as described above, resemble most closely the properties of the receptive fields of retinal ganglion cells and cells of the lateral geniculate body. The complicated relationship between the neuro-anatomical structure of the visual system, the psychophysical interaction areas, and the receptive fields found with the help of electrophysiological methods, has become clearer in the last twenty years. Data obtained from anatomical, psychophysical and electrophysiological experiments enable us to form an idea of the mechanisms involved in bringing about light sensitivity[91]. The receptive fields, and also the areas in which interaction between light stimuli takes place, are most extensive at the scotopic level. At the scotopic level the visual system has a relatively coarse structure with large receptive fields, which, by summation, create the ability to see weak light stimuli. As the quantity of light falling on the receptive field becomes larger, the area in which summation can take place becomes smaller.

When stimuli are used which lie above the threshold of the cone system it appears that the electric recordings from receptors and bipolar cells (ERG) have both photopic and scotopic components but that the recordings from the ganglion cells have only photopic components.[92] The faster cone signal appears to render the ganglion cell refractory for a short time, thereby preventing the slower rod signal from exciting it. Thus the findings of electrophysiological experiments indicate interaction of the two receptor systems.[93] The light sensitivity is determined by the size of the receptive field. When the receptive field is larger, more light stimuli will be transmitted to one ganglion cell and the chance will be greater that the threshold is passed. The reorganization of the receptive fields is the basis for the change in light sensitivity when the adaptation level changes.

From a consideration of the structure of many of the receptive fields, consisting of an 'on' centre and an 'off' periphery, it follows that summation of the light energy of small stimuli occurs, because these stimuli fall within the area of total summation. The threshold then has a minimum value. As the stimuli become larger they fall partly on the peripheral parts of the receptive field which give rise to inhibition. The difference threshold must then have a higher value than that corresponding to the surface enlargement in comparison with the

---

[91] see e.g. DOWLING & BOYCOTT, 1967.

[92] GOURAS & LINK, 1966.

[93] see page 23.

smaller stimulus. Time is needed for development of the peripheral inhibition, so that the central receptive fields appear smaller when the presentation time is longer.

Temporal interaction.

Psychophysical findings

The relationship between luminance and presentation time of a stimulus is usually expressed in terms of a greater or lesser degree of temporal summation. As is the case with spatial summation this term does not express correctly the mechanisms involved in temporal interaction. The interaction can be either summative or inhibitive. Temporal interaction is based on chemical, neuro-retinal and central factors.[94]

A range of psychophysical experiments on temporal interaction have been performed in the course of the years. Most of the literature on this subject up to 1970 has been summarized in the recent 'Bibliography of work on flashing lights'.[95]

SWAN[96] was the first to discover the reciprocal relationship between luminance and presentation time, which holds for short presentations, although the name of BLOCH[97] is usually connected with this discovery. Temporal interaction can be expressed in a similar formula to that for spatial interaction:
$\Delta L \times t^K = C$. When K, the summation coefficient, equals 1, the product of luminance and presentation time is constant, indicating a constant sensation. This constancy is known as Bloch's law and applies to a certain length of time: the critical time (t_c), also called Bloch's time ($\Delta L \times t = C$ for $t \leqslant t_c$).

When the presentation times are shorter than the critical time, the threshold is determined by the luminous flux of the stimulus only. Flashes which have the same luminous flux produce the same effect. A given amount of light energy, within the critical time, always gives the same effect regardless of its distribution over the presentation time.[98] Bloch's law holds even for flashes of very short duration and thus of very high luminance.[99]

---

[94] see e.g. BATTERSBY & SCHUCKMAN 1970.

[95] HARGROVES & HARGROVES 1971.

[96] SWAN 1849.

[97] BLOCH 1885.

[98] DAVY 1952; LONG 1951.

[99] BRINDLEY 1952; this means that saturation occurs after integration.

Data from the literature.

The results of psychophysical experiments are usually expressed logarithmically as 10 log luminance against 10 log presentation time or as the 10 logarithm of the product of luminance and presentation time against 10 log presentation

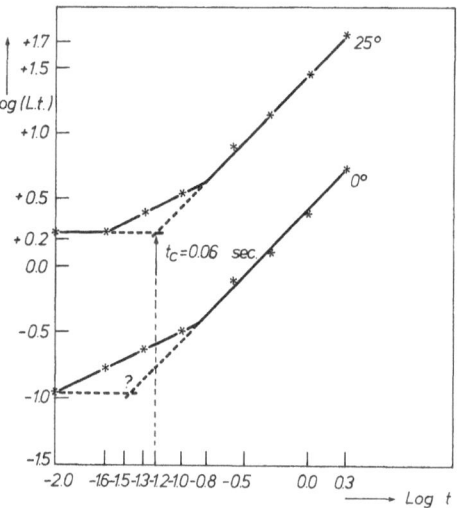

Fig. 12
Temporal summation curves of a normal subject at the fovea and 25° eccentricity.
abscissa: log.L.t.
ordinate: log.t.

time (see Fig. 12). In the latter case the relationship between luminance and presentation time is expressed for a short time as a straight line parallel to the abscissa. This straight line represents the constancy of the product $\Delta L \times t$, i.e. total temporal summation. When the critical time is exceeded the relationship is expressed as a line which makes an angle of 45° with the abscissa (slope = 1); this indicates that temporal summation no longer occurs and that the effect of the stimulus in this area is dependent on the luminance alone ($\Delta L = C$). Between these two situations – total summation and absence of summation – a transitional zone of partial summation can be found ($0 < K < 1$).

When the presentation time is long, far above the critical time, the perception of a stimulus is limited by local adaptation.[100] Experiments on temporal summation, like those on spatial summation, can be subdivided into two groups. In the first group of experiments the threshold luminance is measured for various

---

[100] see page 41.

presentation times; in the second group the frequency-of-seeing of two light flashes is measured as function of the interval between the flashes.

By means of these two groups of experiments it has been shown that, at certain intervals, inhibition can occur between two successive stimuli.[101] The general conclusions which may be drawn from the psychophysical literature[102] are as follows:

1. Temporal summation is greater at the periphery of the visual field than in the centre. The differences, however, are much smaller than in the case of spatial summation.[103]

2. Temporal summation becomes greater as the eye becomes more adapted to darkness. The critical time is inversely proportional to the background luminance;[104] at the centre the t_c under photopic conditions is 0.02–0.03 s and under scotopic conditions 0.2 s[105].

3. Although no agreement has been reached in the literature it is generally assumed that temporal summation becomes greater as the size of the stimulus becomes smaller. With large stimuli the t_c is shorter and the transition from total temporal summation to absence of summation is more gradual.

   At the fovea the t_c for a 1.5 min stimulus is $\pm$ 0.1 s, for a 10 min stimulus $\pm$ 0.05 s and for a 1° stimulus 0.03–0.04 s.[106]

4. With small stimuli the temporal summation is not affected by different wavelengths of the stimulus. With large (45 min) foveal stimuli the wavelength does have an effect: temporal summation is better for blue than for red stimuli[107].

5. Interocular temporal summation, indicating a central mechanism, has been demonstrated by means of supraliminal and subliminal stimuli[108].

   The results of psychophysical experiments have been confirmed by electro-

---

[101] BLACKWELL 1963, IKEDA 1965.

[102] a.o. BLONDELL & REY, 1911; GRAHAM & MARGARIA 1935; KAR 1936; GRAHAM & KEMP 1938; KELLER 1941; BOUMAN & VAN DEN BRINK 1952; VAN DEN BRINK & BOUMAN 1954; BIERSDORF 1955; BARLOW 1957, 1958; CLARK 1958; BAUMGARDT 1959; BAUMGARDT & HILLMANN 1961; SPERLING & JOLLIFFE 1965; ROUFS 1966; VAN DEN BRINK 1966; ROUFS & MEULENBRUGGE 1967; KISHTO & SAUNDERS 1970.

[103] see KISHTO & SAUNDERS 1970; BOUMAN & VAN DEN BRINK 1952 consider that there is no difference in temporal summation between centre and periphery.

[104] see BIERSDORF 1955.

[105] ROUFS 1966.

[106] ROUFS 1966; ROUFS & MEULENBRUGGE 1967.

[107] SPERLING & JOLLIFFE 1963.

[108] COLLIER 1954; FIORENTINI & RADICI 1961; MATIN 1962; BATTERSBY & WAGMANN 1962; BATTERSBY et al. 1964; BATTERSBY & DEFAUBAUGH 1969.

physiological experiments[109]. Very variable reports have been made by different authors on the range of partial temporal summation. Agreement has not been reached as to whether the change is gradual from total temporal summation to no summation, or abrupt with no noticeable area of partial summation. In this matter we shall follow the results of perimetric experiments.[110].

Broca-Sulzer effect.

The relationship described above between the luminance and the presentation time of a stimulus applies to threshold luminances. When the luminance is supraliminal the Broca-Sulzer effect appears[111]. When the brightness of flashes of variable duration is compared with the brightness of a stimulus which is

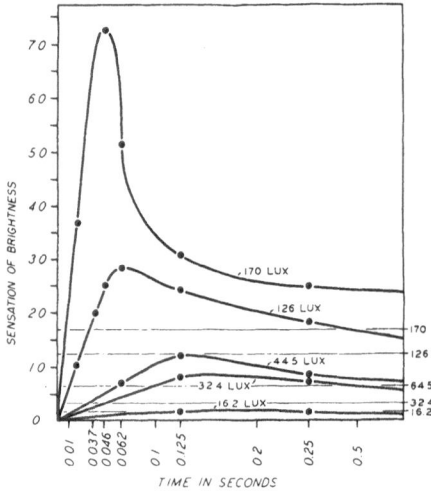

Fig. 13. Broca-Sulzer effect: brightness of flashes having various luminances, as functions of flash duration.
(after Broca and Sulzer 1902; reproduced from Adler, Physiology of the Eye)

presented for 2 seconds, a graph results as shown in Fig. 13. The ordinate gives the luminance which the constant stimulus must have in order to give a sensation of brightness equal to that of the short stimulus. The sensation of brightness on presentation of a supraliminal flash increases up to a certain t_m (time at which the maximum sensation is experienced), after which it decreases asymptomatically to the level of the sensation of brightness produced by a continuously pres-

[109] GRANIT & DAVIS 1931; HARTLINE 1934; STURR et al. 1966; VAN LITH 1966.
[110] see Chapter IV.
[111] BROCA & SULZER 1902, 1903; KATZ 1964.

ented stimulus. As the flash becomes more supraliminal the period t_m becomes shorter. Up to the t_m summation of supraliminal stimuli occurs. After the t_m inhibition occurs[112], so that the sensation of brightness decreases. It appears thus that time is necessary for the appearance of inhibition and that the length of time is dependent upon the degree to which the flash lies above threshold level. The t_m lies somewhere between 0.03 and 0.1 s[113].

Critical fusion frequency.

A property of the visual system, with which temporal factors are also largely concerned, is the frequency at which intermittently presented stimuli are no longer seen separately: the critical fusion frequency: c.f.f. The literature on this subject is extensive but its discussion lies outside the scope of this book. The reasons why the determination of the c.f.f. has not been included in the routine visual field examination are given on page 97.

Local adaptation.

Under steady fixation, visual objects presented continuously in the same place disappear spontaneously after a time. With the help of stabilized images this phenomenon can be demonstrated quite easily, but it also occurs under natural steady fixation[114]. This phenomenon was first demonstrated for the periphery by TROXLER[115]. FERREE[116] suggested that Troxler's phenomenon is caused by a process of local adaptation. The phenomenon can be demonstrated when a stimulus is presented in the periphery of the visual field while the subject is fixating closely on a fixation target. Many examinations have been carried out in this way[117]. The brightness of a continually presented peripheral supraliminal stimulus is compared with a foveal stimulus, the luminance of which can be regulated. After an initial latency of 1–2 seconds the brightness of the peripheral stimulus decreases and in certain circumstances it disappears completely. The length of time between the first perception and the disappearance of the object, the local adaptation time (t_a) decreases from the centre to the periphery and increases

---

[112] BOYNTON 1961. Inhibitive mechanisms are also responsible for the after-images which appear after light stimulation. After-images only occur after supraliminal stimulation.

[113] LEGRAND Optique Physiologique part II, page 296.

[114] RIGGS et al. 1953; YARBUS 1956; DITCHBURN 1963.

[115] TROXLER 1804.

[116] FERREE 1906.

[117] CLARKE 1960, 1961.

as the size and luminance of the stimulus increase. A stimulus at threshold level disappears very quickly. After some time the lost image is usually seen again as the result of blinking or eye movements[118]. The process can then be repeated. The sharpness of the image on the retina also affects the t_a. When the image is not sharply defined the t_a is shorter[119].

It is improbable that local adaptation occurs at receptor level[120]; it is a neural process but 'there is no necessity to think of a more central localization of Troxler's effect than the retinal receptive fields'.[121]

Movement.

A stimulus which is in motion causes a specific reaction in the visual system, which differs from the reaction to an immobile stimulus. A distinction must be made between the detection of movement and the detection of direction.

Detection of movement.

Within certain limits of distance and duration, which correspond to the limits of total temporal and spatial interaction, the threshold for a moving stimulus is the same as the threshold for a static stimulus[122]. When the stimulus is moving at high speed and over a large area, the threshold luminance increases[123]. The sensitivity to movement under photopic conditions decreases from the centre to the periphery[124], a fact which can be explained by the size of the areas of spatial interaction.

Detection of direction.

The perception of movement depends on the direction of movement[125]; the groups which are sensitive to direction are spread evenly over the various directions in the visual field [126]. In man the analysis of movement probably takes place at the cortical level[127]. In electrophysiological experiments units

---

[118] GUILFORD 1927.

[119] FRY & ROBERTSON 1935.

[120] CLARK & BELDER 1962, PIRENNE & MARIOTTE 1962.

[121] LEVELT 1965.

[122] BOUMAN & VAN DEN BRINK 1953; 7° eccentricity.

[123] POLLOCK 1953.

[124] see e.g. MAC GOLGIN 1961.

[125] SEKULAR & GANZ 1963.

[126] ERCOLES 1968.

[127] PANTLE & SEKULAR 1968, 1969; SEKULAR et al. 1968.

which are specifically sensitive to direction have been demonstrated.[128]

We have as yet insufficient information about the processes on which the perception of movement is based to be able to give an adequate explanation[129]. In visual field examination the specific sensitivity to movement at the cortical level should be taken into account.

FIXATION.

Physiological fixation nystagmus

The accuracy of the visual field examination depends entirely upon the accuracy of the fixation. It is a known fact that under physiological conditions completely stable fixation does not exist; there is a physiological fixation nystagmus which can be classified by direction, frequency and amplitude. The direction is subdivided into horizontal, vertical and torsional movements. The following types of fixation nystagmus have been demonstrated:[130]

1. a *tremor* with an irregular high frequency (70–90 Hz) and small amplitude (horizontal and vertical ± 5–30 seconds of arc; torsional up to 45 seconds of arc).
2. slow *drifts* with a frequency of ± 2 Hz and an average amplitude of between 0.8′ and 6.0′. The speed of the drift is ± 6′/second.
3. rapid *micro-saccades* or flicks which occur irregularly and have an average amplitude of between 2.0′ and 50′, although seldom more than 20′[131].

The duration of the micro-saccades is 10-20 ms. The function of these saccades is to correct the deviation of fixation resulting from the drifts. The interval between 2 saccades varies between 0.2 and 25 s. There are considerable differences from subject to subject in the amplitude and frequency of the various forms of physiological nystagmus.

Tremor and drift are probably the result of oculomotor instability. Within

---

[128] Only in animals with an extended inner nuclear layer e.g. frog, Necturus and rabbit the ganglion cells of the retina are sensitive to direction. In these animals no evidence of sensitivity to direction has been found distal to the ganglion cells (NORTON & SPEKREIJSE 1970). In some frog ganglion cells which are sensitive to movement the response is proportional to the speeds of movement (GRÜSSER et al. 1968); this sensitivity to movement is probably determined by the temporal integration properties of the receptive fields of these ganglion cells and not by a special coding (personal communication; SPEKREIJSE).

[129] GRAHAM 1966.

[130] DITCHBURN & GINSBORG 1953; DITCHBURN & FOLEY-FISCHER 1967; YARBUS 1967; ALPERN 1972; CRONE 1973.

[131] MOSES 1970; ALPERN 1972.

a certain foveal area ($\pm$ 6') variations in fixation do not lead to correcting saccades. This area corresponds to the size of the foveal receptive fields.[132] Saccades occur more frequently when the fixation is concentrated than when it is relaxed[133]; saccades can be suppressed.[134] The amplitude of the saccades increases when the fixation object is less bright or the contrast is decreased[135]. The function of the drifts is apparently to prevent fading of targets.[136]

Little is known about torsional movements during fixation.

Fixation and visual field examination.

In perimetry the fixation tremor is of little importance. The drifts and saccades, on the other hand, can affect the results. We investigated the accuracy of fixation under the conditions of the visual field examination, making use of the blind spot. Every shift in fixation results in displacement of the blind spot. This displacement was registered at the nasal and lower margins of the blind spot (Fig.14).

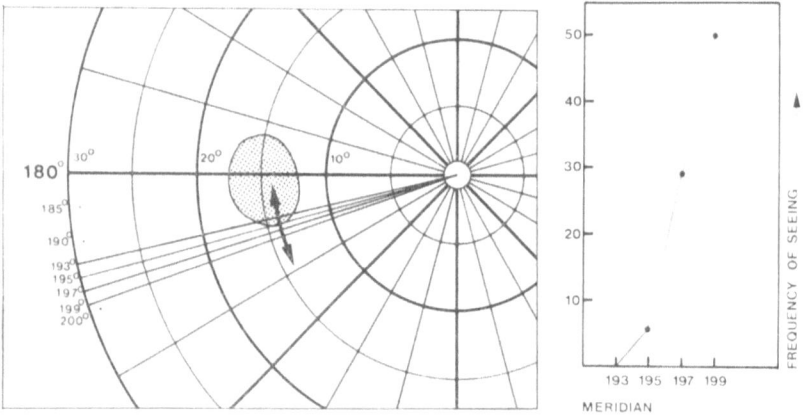

Fig. 14

Measurements of the change of position of the blind spot due to the physiological fixation nystagmus (see text). The meridians in which the measurements were performed are indicated as well as the frequency with which a supraliminal stimulus was seen.

A strong supraliminal stimulus was presented 50 times in various positions within and outside the blind spot at spatial intervals of 15'. If the stimulus falls

---

[132] CORNSWEET 1956; GLEZER 1965.

[133] BARLOW 1952.

[134] STEINMAN et al. 1967.

[135] GLIEM 1967; CARIFA & HEBBARD 1967.

[136] ALPERN 1972.

within the blind spot it will be seen 0 times out of 50: 0%; if it falls completely outside the blind spot it will be seen 50 times out of 50: 100%; if it falls on the margin of the blind spot only a proportion of the presentations will be seen because of the physiological fixation movements. The area in which there is variable perception is a measure of the amplitude of the fixation movement.

The results show that the amplitude in the horizontal direction is small, ± 30′ The amplitude of the vertical or torsional fixation movements is greater: ± 4 degrees of arc, i.e. varying between the 193° meridian (0 out of 50) and the 199° meridian (50 out of 50) .Vertical and torsional fixation movements cannot be differentiated by this method.[137] From the literature also it appears that the vertical components of the fixation nystagmus are larger than the horizontal components.[138] Our experiments were performed on trained subjects; experience shows that fixation is generally less accurate in patients than in trained subjects. The values given here for the amplitude of physiological nystagmus must therefore be regarded as optimum values. The experiments were performed under photopic conditions; under scotopic conditions the fixation amplitude is greater. The consequence of this physiological nystagmus is that a stimulus moves over the retina during its presentation. A stimulus in static perimetry presented for the period of 1 second will move over an area of ± 1° of the retina; the amplitude will be greater in the periphery than in the centre. The effect of this movement becomes greater as the stimulus becomes smaller. For a stimulus of 10′ this is a considerable shift. In normal visual fields this shift has hardly any effect on the height of the difference threshold[139]. On the other hand the physiological nystagmus can influence the examination of physiological angioscotomata and other defects of small diameter[140].

For kinetic perimetry a longer period of constant fixation is necessary than for static perimetry. For fixation under pathological conditions the reader is referred to CRONE[141]. As the visual acuity becomes poorer the chance of bad fixation becomes greater. In the presence of a central scotoma fixation can sometimes be eccentric; the patient fixates on the edge of the scotoma. The position of scotomata changes with the eccentricity of the fixation. The eccentricity of the fixation can be deduced from the displacement of the blind spot.

---

[137] It has been known for a long time (RÖSSLER) that a normal eye makes torsional movements when fixating the fixation object of a perimeter. Torsional movements of 1°–3° have been described. This is ascribed to the absence of any structure in the perimeter background.

[138] DITCHBURN & FOLEY-FISCHER 1967.

[139] BOUMAN & VAN DEN BRINK 1953; see also page 00.

[140] see Chapter VII.

[141] CRONE 1973.

CHAPTER III

THE FUNDAMENTAL PRINCIPLES OF STATIC AND KINETIC PERIMETRY

STATIC PERIMETRY

Visual field examination is the quantitative investigation of the topography of the light sensitivity of the greatest possible number of positions within the absolute limits of the visual field. The simplest way to examine this number of positions is to place an infraliminal stimulus in every position and then to increase the luminance until the stimulus is seen (method of limits). In this way the difference threshold of a well-defined position is measured. The examination starts from the infraliminal level, because the chance of the subject moving his fixation is smaller than when one starts from the supraliminal level and the subject has to indicate when the stimulus disappears; the presentation of a supraliminal stimulus can also give rise to local adaptation at the position to be examined. The level of the threshold measured with the infraliminal approach is not exactly the same as that obtained with the supraliminal approach; in the latter case the threshold has been found to be 0.1 log unit lower.

Static perimetry, which was introduced by SLOAN[1] for clinical visual field examination, has become well known through the work of HARMS[2] and AULHORN.[3] Although the term 'profile perimetry' is often used for this method, we prefer the term 'static perimetry' because this better expresses the essential feature of this method: an immobile, static stimulus.

The threshold measurement in static perimetry is obtained by increasing the luminance of the stimulus in steps of a given magnitude. Increasing the luminance continuously is not to be recommended, because temporal interaction and the reaction time of the subject and the examiner may influence the threshold perception. One of the greatest advantages of static perimetry is the fact that, thanks to the examination of a fixed position and the step-by-step increase in luminance, the level of the difference threshold does not depend on the reaction time of the subject and the examiner.[4] The size of the steps is decided by the intraindividual variation of threshold measurements and the significance one ascribes to defects of slight intensity.[5] After each step a certain amount of time is needed for the presentation of the stimulus. The length of the presentation time is limited by the local adaptation.[6] Between the steps an interval of about 2 s is usual.

The duration of the investigation depends upon the number of positions examined, the presentation time and the number and magnitude of the luminance steps.

The increase of luminance in steps, the intervals between the steps, and the time spent waiting for the patient's reaction after each presentation make the static method a time-consuming procedure.

When one considers the three-dimensional representation of light sensitivity, the 'island of vision' (Fig. 1), static perimetry consists of the measurement of the distance between various positions on the island and a given known level. The topography of the measured light sensitivity can then be recorded on a graph, in which the position is indicated on the abscissa and the threshold luminance on the ordinate, the threshold luminance increasing from above downwards. This means that the light sensitivity increases from below upwards. Although it is possible to investigate any arbitrary succession of positions, as a rule[7] the light

[1] SLOAN, 1939.

[2] HARMS, 1950–1969.

[3] AULHORN & HARMS, 1972.

[4] see page 58.

[5] see chapters VII and XI.

[6] see chapters II and IV.

[7] HARMS & AULHORN, 1967.

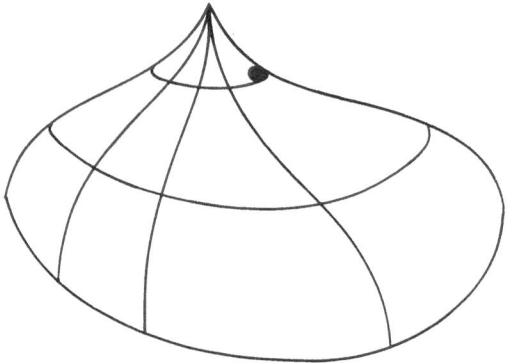

Fig. 1
Island of vision.

sensitivity in a meridian of the visual field is recorded. This means that a vertical section (profile) of the 'island of vision' is made, in which the increase in stimulation runs parallel to the ordinate (Fig. 2). The curve thus produced reflects how

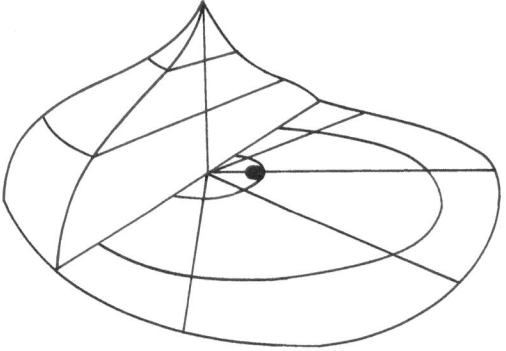

Fig. 2
Meridional section through the island of vision.

the *light sensitivity varies as function of the position* on the meridian. There is a gradual decrease in sensitivity from the centre to the periphery at the photopic level of adaptation. We have called this curve the sensitivity-gradient curve, or in short *sensitivity curve*, after BAIR[8] and SLOAN.[9] The investigation of the difference threshold, as performed by means of static perimetry, is the examination of one of the most fundamental functions of the visual system. There is only one

---

[8] BAIR, 1940.
[9] SLOAN, 1961.

variable: the luminance. All other factors which influence the level of the differ-ence threshold[11] position, level of adaptation, stimulus size, presentation time and colour are kept constant. Because there is only one variable, static perimetry is a relatively simple method of examination with little variation of measurements.[10] As has been clearly pointed out by AULHORN & HARMS[11], the light sensitivity forms the starting point for many other methods of examination (CFF, local adaptation, colour perimetry, visual acuity).

KINETIC PERIMETRY

Kinetic perimetry is the oldest and best-known method of visual field examina-tion[12]. From the historical point of view a description of kinetic perimetry should be given first. The fundamental principles of perimetry, however, can be most easily explained with the help of static perimetry. If we take more space for the description of kinetic perimetry, this is not because it is superior to static perime-try, but because it is more complicated. Measurement of the light sensitivity is also the object of kinetic perimetry. As in static perimetry the difference thresh-old is measured at a number of positions in the visual field.

The method of measurement, however, is different: in kinetic perimetry an extra variable is introduced: *the movement*. Using a stimulus of known luminance positions in the visual field are searched for where this stimulus is only just perceptible. As in static perimetry the threshold is approached from the infra-liminal level. One takes advantage of the fact that photopic light sensitivity decreases from the centre to the periphery of the visual field. A stimulus which is moved centripetally from the periphery will be infraliminal at first and will be seen at a certain degree of eccentricity, dependent upon the intensity of the stimu-lus. The light sensitivity of the position where the stimulus is seen is the reciprocal of the luminance of the stimulus. In kinetic perimetry, therefore, *the position is a variable;* various positions are recorded with different stimulus luminances under photopic conditions. The position at which the stimulus will be seen is not known beforehand, whereas in static perimetry a well-defined position is exam-ined. Kinetic perimetry produces a horizontal section through the 'island of vision'. A stimulus of given luminance is moved from the infraliminal level parallel to 'sea level' until 'the island of vision' is reached. This procedure is repeated in a number of meridians so that a series of points with equal light

---

[10] see chapter VII.

[11] AULHORN & HARMS, 1972.

[12] VON GRAEFE, 1856.

sensitivity are obtained. By linking these points a graphic representation of iso-liminal points, the *isopter*, is obtained.

The approach of a kinetic stimulus to the photopic 'island of vision' is shown in Fig. 3.

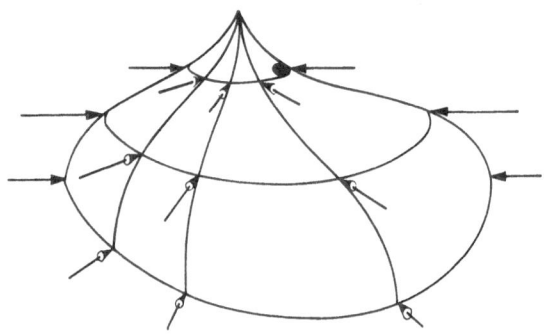

Fig. 3
Kinetic approach of the island of vision.

THE FUNDAMENTAL DIFFERENCE BETWEEN KINETIC AND STATIC PERIMETRY

In kinetic perimetry the *luminance of the stimulus* is constant and the threshold is approached in spatial steps: with each step the stimulus comes closer to threshold level. In static perimetry the *position* of examination is constant and the luminance is variable: with each step of luminance the stimulus comes closer to threshold level. In Fig. 4 the kinetic stimulation proceeds along a

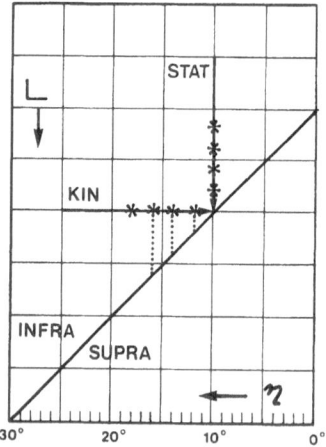

Fig. 4
Horizontal and vertical method to examination.

50

horizontal line parallel to the abscissa, the static stimulation proceeds along a vertical line parallel to the ordinate.

In static perimetry the stimulus is presented for a short time, which is followed by an interval of 2 s. In this interval the luminance is brought one step closer to the threshold, until the subject indicates perception of the stimulus. In principle the same procedure can be followed in the position-variable (horizontal) method.[13] An infraliminal stimulus is presented at a given position for a short time, followed by an interval of 2 s. In this interval the stimulus is moved one spatial step nearer to threshold level.

The only difference between these two methods is that in the horizontal method various *positions* are examined (though infraliminally) whereas in the vertical method one well-defined position is examined. In the vertical method the position is known at the outset. In the horizontal method the position is not known at the outset. If a position B is to be examined, in the vertical method the luminance must be altered and in the horizontal method the position is changed by a proportional number of spatial steps.

The procedures described above are *equivalent* to each other. As the presentations are short and there are intervals between them, interaction between the stimuli does not occur and the reaction time of the patient is not important. The horizontal method described here, however, is not kinetic perimetry.

If the intervals between the separate presentations and the spatial steps are steadily decreased, so that a series of flashes close together is presented, at a given moment the visual system will experience this train of flashes as a continuous movement. The horizontal method has now become kinetic perimetry.

A similar procedure could also be followed for static perimetry. By shortening the intervals and the luminance steps a stimulus of continuously increasing luminance is produced. The difference between the two methods, however, is now much greater; they are no longer equivalent as far as the final threshold is concerned. Infraliminal stimulation in rapid succession of positions lying close together results, in the horizontal method, in *spatial* interaction: successive lateral summation. In both procedures the reaction time now becomes important. The vertical method described above, however, is not static perimetry.

Static perimetry is performed according to the procedure which was described first: in steps and with intervals between the presentations. In this way temporal

---

[13] The term 'kinetic method' has been avoided intentionally as there is now no question of movement.

interaction does not occur between the presentations and the reaction time does not affect the result.

The fundamental difference between kinetic and static perimetry is to be found in the continuous presentation, the movement of the stimulus in kinetic perimetry, on account of which interaction and reaction time influence the threshold measurements.

The short duration of the kinetic examination is the result of this continuous presentation. If the same method were to be followed in static perimetry the duration of the examination would be just as short. The quickness of the kinetic examination is thus deceptive because it is achieved by making concessions which affect the accuracy of the examination.

FUNDAMENTAL LIMITS OF THE ACCURACY OF KINETIC PERIMETRY

The price which has to be paid for the quickness of kinetic perimetry is the inaccuracy of the method. This inaccuracy is the result of the movement: the speed of the movement, the acceleration and the direction. The difference threshold for a moving stimulus is arrived at in a different way from the threshold for a static stimulus and it depends upon the reaction time of the patient and the examiner.

Movement; successive lateral spatial summation

It has already been explained that the visual system is specifically sensitive to movement[14]. Certain cortical units give an optimum reaction to movement in a certain direction and do not react at all to movement in the opposite direction. The speed and acceleration of the movement influence the response of specific units.

When a stimulus is moved centripetally, the stimulation will at first not be strong enough to produce a sensation (dotted line, Fig. 5). The closer the stimulus approaches the 'island of vision', i.e. the smaller the difference between the luminance of the stimulus and the threshold luminance, the less infraliminal the stimulation will be; when the stimulation is only just infraliminal a series of receptors in succession will be stimulated infraliminally. In the periphery where, even under photopic conditions, good spatial summation is possible, summation of the successive infraliminal stimuli can occur, so that a kinetic stimulus will be seen more peripherally than a static stimulus. We have called

---

[14] see chapter II.

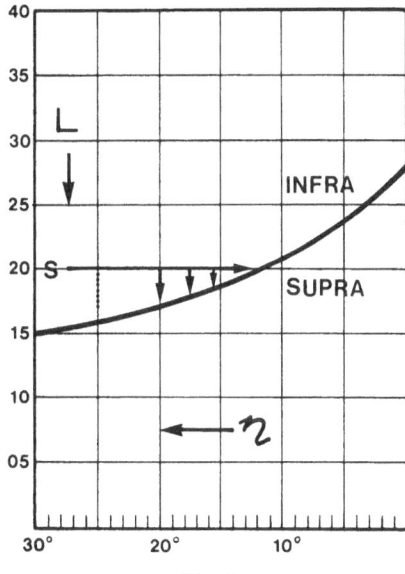

Fig. 5
Successive lateral spatial summation.

this form of interaction 'successive lateral spatial summation'[15]. The diagram in Fig. 5 represents the radial centripetal movement of a stimulus.

Gradient of sensitivity

The degree of successive lateral spatial summation (SLSS) depends upon the *position* in the visual field and also upon the sensitivity *gradient* of the path along which the stimulus moves. When the gradient is flat the stimulus will be close to threshold level in a large area, so that each successive stimulation will form an important contribution to the achievement of a sensation (Fig. 6a.). When, on the other hand, the gradient is steep, the stimulation is far below the threshold in a large area and only little spatial summation takes place (Fig. 6b.). Because of this the threshold values in kinetic perimetry are dependent on the gradient of sensitivity.

The gradient affects the result not only through the degree of successive lateral spatial summation, but also through the zone of uncertain perception which the kinetic stimulus traverses. The threshold value for every position is subject to a certain intra-individual variation.[16] The individual sensitivity curve

---

[15] GREVE & VERRIEST, 1971.
[16] see chapter VII.

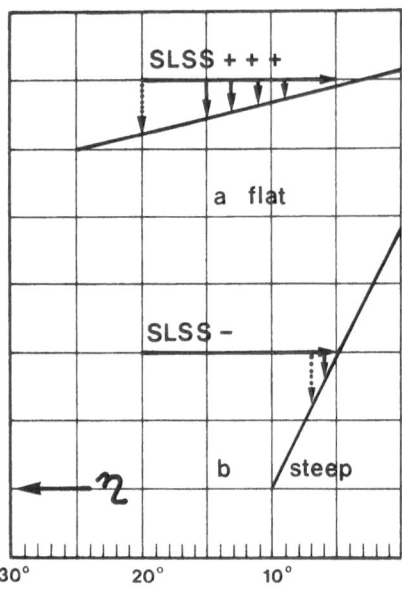

Fig. 6

Successive lateral spatial summation in case of a flat (a) and steep (b) gradient.

is the average of a number of slightly different measurements. This is shown in Fig. 7; the average curve varies between the 0% curve and the 100% curve. The 0% curve represents the highest luminance at which the stimulus is never seen; the 100% curve represents the lowest luminance at which the stimulus is seen at every presentation. Between these two curves lies an area of uncertain perception, in which the chance that the stimulus will be seen varies from 1%

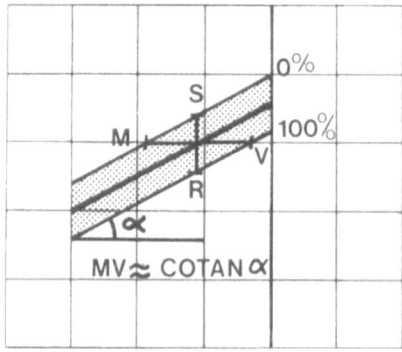

Fig. 7

Zone of varying chance of perception around the mean (50%) sensitivity curve.

to 99%. The height (SR) of this area is the same for every gradient; the width (MV), i.e. the number of degrees covered, is determined by the gradient. The area of uncertain perception SR is in static perimetry the same for every gradient. The area of uncertain perception traversed by the kinetic stimulus (MV) becomes larger as the gradient becomes less steep.

The variation in the measurements is proportional to the co-tangent of the angle α, which the sensitivity curve forms with the abscissa. If α is large (steep gradient) the variation is small. When the gradient is 45°, SR and MV are equal. When the gradient is less steep the kinetic stimulus traverses a much larger area of uncertainty than the static stimulus. In this case the influence of the successive lateral spatial summation on the threshold measurements is also maximum. When the gradient is steeper than 45°, MV < SR. The successive lateral spatial summation is in this case also of less significance. The variation in the kinetic threshold measurements is then minimum. The influence of the reaction time is of course undiminished.

When the gradient is very steep the physiological fixation movements exert influence, although only in a very small area. When the position of the static stimulus shifts from S to S′ as the result of fixation movements or other causes (head movements, altered position relative to the correcting lens, inaccurate positioning), apparently a great variation in the threshold measurements (Fig. 8) will occur. This pseudo-variation only appears at the edge of a scotoma, within an area of $\pm$ 1–2°. In kinetic perimetry this only means that the edge of the scotoma shifts 1°; this falls within the normal variation and is of no significance.

As the gradient becomes steeper more stimuli are needed in order to be able

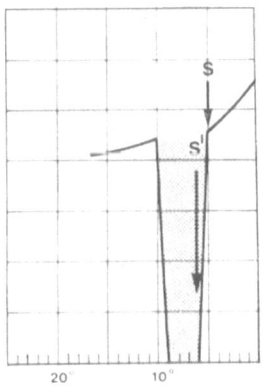

Fig. 8
Variation of threshold measurements due to very steep gradient in combination with physiological fixation-nystagmus.

55

to carry out the examination at approximately threshold level. If position B is to be examined at threshold level, a different stimulus (S′) will have to be chosen from the stimulus (S) which was seen at position A (Fig. 9). When the gradient is steep a stimulus moved centripetally, after perception at threshold level, diverges rapidly from this threshold level and becomes steadily more supraliminal.

At the two extremes which are possible for the gradient, horizontal and vertical, the relationship between the isopters for stimuli of different luminances can be well demonstrated.[17] When the gradient is horizontal, only one stimulus

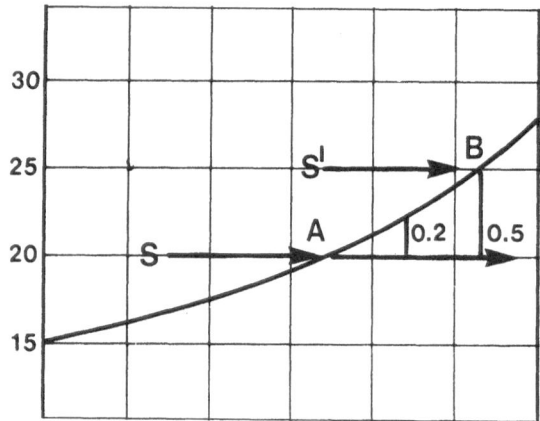

Fig. 9

A centripetally moved kinetic stimulus (s) becomes continuously more supraliminal after perception at threshold level.
To examine location B a second stimulus (s) is needed.

is at threshold level throughout the whole area and there is in fact no isopter but a complete surface of equal sensitivity. When the gradient is vertical the isopters for stimuli of different strengths are seen at the same place; thus the isopters of stimuli of different strengths overlap each other. As the gradient becomes less steep the isopters separate from each other. Finally, when the gradient is horizontal, the isopters are infinitely far removed from each other.

The gradient of sensitivity is dependent on the *adaptation level*. By definition[18] the gradient is horizontal at the mesopic level; this means that there is no gradient. The whole central and intermediate visual field is then isoliminal (Fig. 10).

---

[17] see also AULHORN & HARMS, 1967.
[18] see chapter II.

56

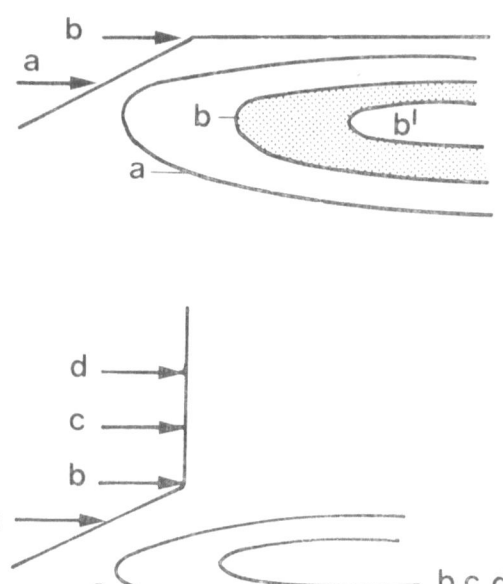

Fig. 10. Horizontal and vertical sensitivity curves and their relation to isopters.

Sensitivity curves for static and kinetic stimuli

The difference in the sensitivity for a kinetic or a static stimulus becomes apparent in the difference threshold. In Fig. 11 the sensitivity curves for static perimetry (0°/s) and for kinetic perimetry at a speed of 1°/s are given.

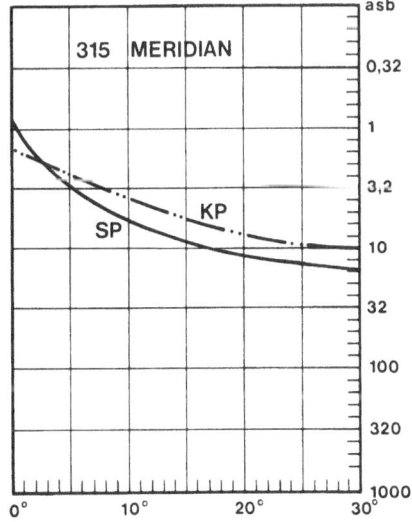

Fig. 11. Sensitivity curves for static perimetry (SP) and kinetic perimetry (KP 1°/s).

It appears (Fig. 11) that for normal subjects the discrepancy in the difference threshold between static and kinetic (1°/s) perimetry is demonstrable but small: for object I of the Goldmann perimeter not more than 0.2 log unit. The difference threshold in the periphery is lower for a kinetic stimulus and in the central visual field it is lower for a static stimulus. This means that under photopic conditions a static stimulus in the periphery which is 0.2 log unit infraliminal will be seen when it is moved. Only a slight difference in threshold can be demonstrated between speeds of 1°/s and 5°/s. The variation of the measurements, however, increases with increasing speed.[19]

Influence of reaction time

In practice, as we all know, kinetic visual field examination is usually performed at higher speeds than those mentioned above (5°/s–20°/s)[20]. The speed of kinetic visual field examination is not standardized.[21] The reaction times of the subject and the examiner become steadily more important as the speed of movement increases. The differences in threshold for a stimulus moved by hand at speeds of 1°/s, 5°/s and 15°/s are given below (Table I).

TABLE I

Position and variation of isopters in the infero-temporal (315°) meridian in 3 parts of the visual field and for 3 different speeds of movement (1°/sec., 5°/sec. and 15°/sec.). Goldmann perimeter, 5 measurements, object I.

	I/4/f	I/1	I/3
1°/s	5–6°	31–34°	65–72°
5°/s	1.5–4°	27–30°	62–68°
15°/s	–	20–27°	56–65°

It appears that the point at which the stimulus is seen is closer to the centre when the speed of movement is higher. This means that the level of the threshold varies as function of the speed and movement. The variation of the measurements also increases with the speed of movement. These results apply to a normal subject with a normal reaction time and a normal visual field. The combined reaction time of the patient and the examiner varies normally between 0.4 and 1 s.

---

[19] FANKHAUSER & SCHMIDT, 1959 and next page.

[20] see also page 13.

[21] SCHMIDT (1971) has recently described an instrument which can be mounted on the pantograph of the Goldmann perimeter, by means of which constant speed of movement can be obtained.

The fact that, in kinetic perimetry, the ability to detect defects depends on the *speed* of movement is of fundamental importance. The slower the movement is, the smaller the defects which can be detected. The optimum speed for the detection of defects is 0, i.e. static perimetry. FANKHAUSER[23] has pointed out the restrictions of kinetic perimetry for the detection of defects and has illustrated this as shown in Fig. 12. In this figure the cumulative effect of the speed of movement and the reaction times of the patient and the examiner is clearly shown. In favourable circumstances e.g. speed of movement 2.5°/s and combined patient-examiner reaction time of 0.5 s – the diameter of the smallest detectable defect is ± 2.5°. In less favourable circumstances, which are far from

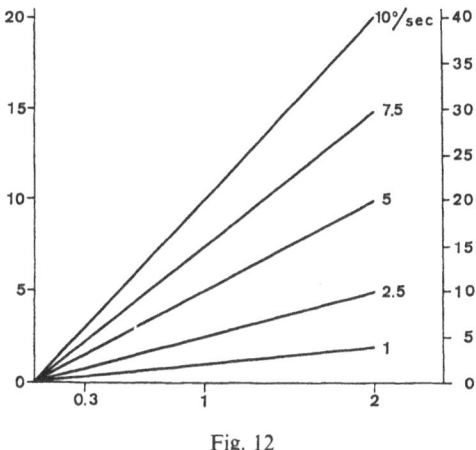

Fig. 12

The relation between speed of movement, reaction time and defect detection.
abscissa: reaction time in s
ordinate (right): smallest detectable diameter of defect in degrees

uncommon in practice, e.g. speed of movement 10°/s and reaction time of 1 s, a defect will have to have a diameter of at least 20° in order to be detected.

Everyone who regularly compares the results of kinetic and static visual field examination recognizes this limitation of the defect-detecting capacity of kinetic perimetry. Consequently static perimetry is to be preferred for the detection of defects.

The variation of the measurements as function of the speed of movement also affects the registration of the topography of the defects. Defects will appear

---

[23] FANKHAUSER, 1969.

larger at higher speeds, because the patient cannot indicate the perception of the stimulus quickly enough. This can be demonstrated at the blind spot; when a stimulus is moved rapidly outwards from the centre of the blind spot, pseudo-enlargement of the blind spot is easily produced.

The *reproducibility of defects* decreases as the speed increases. In order to obtain reproducible results and acceptable defect detection with kinetic perimetry, the speed of movement must be *constant* and moderate. The speed of 5°/s recommended by GOLDMANN can be taken as a guide for the periphery; this is slower than the speeds used in practice. In the central visual field the speed should be still lower (2°/s). Static perimetry is to be preferred for patients who react slowly.

Influence of the direction of movement

Another factor which causes variation in the kinetic measurements is the direction of movement of the stimulus. For the normal visual field this is no problem. Examination is always carried out in a standard direction: radial, i.e. following the meridians. It is well known that the normal isopters are round or egg-shaped

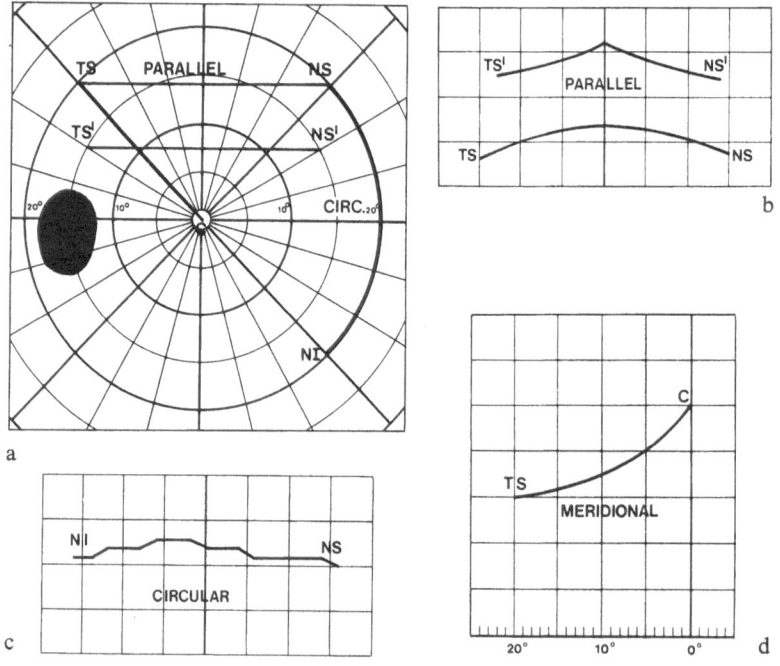

Fig. 13
Gradient in relation to direction of movement.

with an almost uniform degree of curvature. It is justified, in normal cases, to join two positions of equal light sensitivity by a line and thus give an impression of the sensitivity of the area between these two points. Only the physiological blind spot is examined in various directions. The rule which applies for the blind spot and for pathological visual field defects is that the direction of movement must be perpendicular to the edge of the defect. The supposition is made that the contour of the defect is known. This is in fact true of the normal blind spot, but in pathological defects the contour of the defect is not known. The degree of curvature of the edge of a defect can vary markedly in a very small area. This means in practice that a defect has to be examined from many different directions. The gradient of sensitivity is different for every direction of movement. As the direction of movement diverges further from the radial direction the gradient becomes more and more flat. In Fig. 13 these gradients are shown for 3 different directions.

The visual system is specifically sensitive to movement and each different direction of movement results in a kinetic stimulus of different strength. Several different examiners will be unable to examine a defect in exactly the same direction and also the same examiner at different times will not be able to carry out an exactly similar examination. The more irregular the outline of a defect is, the greater will be the variation of the measurements.

CONCLUSION

The factor movement, on account of which the duration of the examination with kinetic perimetry is relatively short, is associated with inaccuracy, which is expressed as a limited capacity to detect defects and poor reproducibility of results. Kinetic perimetry is much more dependent than static perimetry on the knowledge and skill of the examiner and the co-operation of the patient. GOLDMANN has rightly said: 'Schliesslich möchte ich betonen, dass Perimetrie, besonders kinetische Perimetrie, eine Kunst ist'.

The function of kinetic perimetry in the practice of visual field examination will be discussed in chapter V.

CHAPTER IV

CHOICE OF THE CONDITIONS OF EXAMINATION

Choice of adaptation level

Selective detection of disturbances in the photopic or the scotopic system
Visual field examination at mesopic adaptation levels
Threshold examination at mesopic and photopic levels
Intra-individual variation at various adaptation levels
Influence of preretinal factors
Scotopic perimetry
High-photopic adaptation levels
Conclusion

Choice of stimulus size; spatial interaction and visual field examination

Spatial interaction in the normal visual field
Constant size of stimulus
Dubois-Poulsen's work; spatial interaction and visual field defects
Problems of kinetic perimetry
Inter-individual variation of the summation exponent
Results obtained by other authors
Inhibition in perimetric examinations
Conclusion: Choice of stimulus size
    The significance of the examination of spatial summation in visual field
    defects

Choice of presentation time; temporal interaction and visual field

Temporal interaction in the normal visual field
    Position
    Adaptation
    Stimulus size

Arguments for the use of a short presentation time
  intra- and inter-individual variation
  total duration of the examination
  latent period for eye movements
  normal fixation movements and temporal summation
  subjective experience
  abnormal temporal summation in visual field defects
  technical possibilities
  kinetic perimetry
Conclusion

Local adaptation and visual field examination

  Local adaptation in the normal visual field
  Local adaptation and visual field defects
  Conclusion
Some remarks about critical fusion frequency (C.F.F.) and colour in visual field
examination.

CHOICE OF ADAPTATION LEVEL.

In Chapter II a number of fundamental concepts about adaptation have been
dealt with. In a large range of adaptation levels the difference threshold is
probably produced by a combined action of the rod system and the cone system
(except in the centre of the visual field). When the visual system is more adapted
to light the cone system dominates, and when it is more adapted to darkness
the rod system dominates. This is associated with a change in the topography of
the light sensitivity. These and other conclusions which are given on page 30,
raise the question at which adaptation level visual field examination can best
be performed. It is of course theoretically possible to carry out the examination
at three different levels of adaptation[1], but in practice this is generally not possible because it takes too much time. The routine examination is performed at a
certain adaptation level and, only if time, apparatus and personnel allow it,
additional examination can be performed at other levels of adaptation.

Selective detection of disturbances in the photopic or the scotopic system.

The reason for an examination at different adaptation levels is the possibility
that one of the two projector systems will show a larger defect than the other.
If one of the receptor systems should be selectively affected, examination at an
adaptation level at which this receptor system is dominant would be more

---

[1] adaptoperimetry.

sensitive. At this adaptation level the defects would be easier to detect. As an example may serve juvenile macular degeneration, in which the cone system is mainly affected. The question now arises, at which level of adaptation visual field examination is most sensitive, in particular for glaucomatous defects[2].

The choice of adaptation level also depends on the variation of measurements at different adaptation levels, and at which level the least problems arise regarding the technique and duration of the examination. On this last point, arguments against scotopic visual field examination are that an adaptation time of at least 30 minutes is necessary and that the exclusion of light from the apparatus and examination room requires special provisions. It is also very difficult, to check the fixation at scotopic levels.

Routine visual field examination is usually performed at photopic levels of adaptation. Over the years repeated pleas for mesopic visual field examination have appeared in the literature.

Visual field examination at mesopic adaptation levels.

The choice of the adaptation level was determined for a long time by the limited technique of examination. Examination using 'reduced illumination' was regarded as a sensitive method. This older literature will not be considered here[3].

BAIR[4] proposed the use of 'a selected low level of adaptational background brightness'. He considered that this method 'was more delicate and accurate than the ordinary method of examination at relatively high levels of adaptation and minimised certain technical difficulties in refined examination'. The adaptation level used by BAIR was mesopic according to our standards. He chose that level in which the 'meridional gradient of sensibility has a minimal average value'.

In order to follow BAIR's train of thought it should be realized that he had no knowledge of modern quantitative kinetic and static perimetry with the Goldmann (or Tübinger) perimeter. His preference for the mesopic level of adaptation was largely based on technical considerations. For visual field examination at that time projected stimuli, the luminance of which could be altered at will, were generally not available. Round white objects on black wands were used, usually against the dull black background of a Bjerrum screen. The sensitivity of the method was increased by using small objects and by carrying out the examination at a greater distance. These problems do not exist any more.

---

[2] SLOAN 1947; 1950.

[3] An example of the way of thinking then current is MARLOW's article (1932).

[4] BAIR 1940.

BAIR defended the use of the mesopic adaptation level with the following arguments:

1. the 'reduced illumination' applied to both the background luminance and the luminance of the stimulus. As the ratio $\dfrac{L}{\Delta L}$ is larger at the mesopic level than at the photopic level the same object luminance will be nearer to the threshold at the mesopic level than at the photopic level.

2. at this adaptation level the sensitivity curve is relatively flat, i.e. the central area is approximately isoliminal. For the methods of examination in use at that time, the fact that the central and intermediate visual fields are isoliminal had the advantage that a stimulus which was (juxta)liminal at 30° remained so at all other positions within the 30° parallel. This part of the visual field could thus be examined with only one kinetic stimulus[5].

3. at this adaptation level the effect of ametropia on the light difference sensitivity is less marked than at higher adaptation levels.

4. in a comparative study of photopic and mesopic campimetry BAIR considered that he had shown that the latter was more sensitive.

The argument that perimetric objects come closer to the threshold under mesopic than under photopic conditions does not apply to modern techniques. It would appear to be desirable technically to be able to examine the whole 30° visual field with one stimulus. The flattened sensitivity curve which makes this possible, however, has disadvantages for the kinetic examination method.[6] The flatter the curve, the greater the variation of measurements in kinetic campimetry. In view of the flattened curve the static method is to be recommended.

The argument that ametropia has less influence on the mesopic light sensitivity than on the photopic sensitivity is correct. Ametropia however, can easily be corrected and a correction scotoma[7] can easily be differentiated from a glaucomatous defect.

WEEKERS & ROUSSEL[8] consider that 'la campimétrie en lumière atténuée continue, dans l'état actuel de la question, est la méthode de choix pour déceler des scotomes de faible densité'. These authors examined the position of the 2/2000 isopter on a Bjerrum screen with an illumination of 3 lux. Assuming that the reflection coefficient of this screen is 0.01–0.04 the luminance used

---

[5] see next page.

[6] see Chapter III.

[7] see Chapter X.

[8] WEEKERS & ROUSSELL (1945), quoted by DUKE ELDER, etc. It is not known if these authors are still of the same opinion, but as this article is used as an argument for mesopic campimetry a short analysis is necessary here.

becomes 0.03–0.12 asb. Pre-adaptation of the subjects was first carried out for 10 minutes with an illumination of 3000 lux. The isopter was then determined after varying lengths of time; the examination was thus more a form of *adaptometry*. They also demonstrated that, in cases of night blindness, adaptocampimetry is more sensitive than photopic campimetry. This can be readily understood considering the specific disturbance of the rod system which underlies night blindness. These findings form a better argument for scotopic perimetry than for mesopic campimetry. The authors also considered that angioscotomata and the centrocecal defects of tobacco amblyopia can be examined better at mesopic adaptation levels. This may perhaps be explained by the different approach to the threshold in the mesopic and the photopic examinations, as will be considered later?[9]. Glaucomatous visual field defects were not included in this study.

GOLDMANN[10] pointed out that the sensitivity curve is nearly flat at 0.05 asb. He introduced the term 'equivalent isopters'. These are isopters which have the same position when the background luminance is 30 asb as when it is 0.05 asb. GOLDMANN proposed kinetic perimetry at two adaptation levels. He considered that mesopic campimetry was particularly important for the early diagnosis of glaucoma. In this he followed BAIR's line of thought, which has already been considered.

JAYLE & AUBERT[11] also agree that the sensitivity of the mesopic kinetic examination is superior to that of the photopic examination. These authors are of the opinion that certain defects can be discovered earlier by mesopic examination, have a greater intensity and remain demonstrable longer, than on photopic examination. Also, according to the authors, the variation of the measurements is less at lower adaptation levels. JAYLE & AUBERT consider a background luminance of 6.36 UL psb (0.06 asb) to be mesopic. In addition to mesopic campimetry these authors recommend adaptoperimetry. Most of JAYLE & AUBERT's investigations were performed with the Acui-campimètre of JAYLE-MOSSE; a Bjerrum screen is illuminated in such a way that the background luminance given above is obtained. The isopter which runs at 23.5° is first determined[12]. This means that the size of stimulus chosen depends on the patient's sensitivity

---

[9] see page 67.

[10] GOLDMANN 1952, 1954.

[11] JAYLE & AUBERT, 1958; JAYLE, 1971 and personal communication.

These publications are also quoted by other authors as evidence of the sensitivity of mesopic campimetry (DUKE ELDER, BEDWELL). JAYLE & AUBERT's theories were supported in 1962 by OURGAUD & ETIENNE in their report on the investigation of glaucoma.

[12] 'isoptère périphérique'

level; the larger the stimulus the flatter is the curve[13]. Here again the disadvantage of kinetic mesopic campimetry is apparent: a flat curve gives greater variation. The isopter which runs at 23.5° lies close to the temporal edge of the blind spot. Examination with a stimulus which gives an isopter in this area may easily result in pseudo-defects.[14] An enlarged blind spot, or 'baring of the blind spot', can then be found when no pathological process is present.

The above mentioned objections do not apply when static perimetry is used instead of kinetic perimetry. The examples given by JAYLE et al.,[11] to demonstrate the superior sensitivity of the mesopic examination only prove that defects can be more readily detected by the mesopic examination employed by JAYLE than by the photopic technique employed by JAYLE. The supposed superior mesopic sensitivity given by these authors can be attributed to the incomparability of the measurements made during mesopic examination with those made during photopic examination.[15] JAYLE et al. mainly used the object 1/2 of the Goldmann perimeter for photopic perimetry. If this object reaches threshold level at 23.5°, at 5° the examination is being performed more than a half log unit above threshold level and relative defects will either be missed or appear less intense than at mesopic levels. (In normal young subjects the 1/2 isopter runs at 36° nasal and 56° temporal and at 5° this object is 1 log unit supraliminal).

Threshold examination at mesopic and photopic levels.

If it were proved that mesopic examination is more sensitive, that would settle the argument. But objections can be raised to the comparative studies made by a number of authors between mesopic and photopic kinetic campimetry.

Visual field examination is a threshold investigation. In order to compare mesopic and photopic campimetry the difference threshold in *both* cases must be determined for the whole 30° visual field, or at the very least the examination must be juxtaliminal in both cases. In all the comparative kinetic studies known to us however, a juxtaliminal stimulus is presented over the whole 30° visual field in the mesopic examination, but not in the photopic examination. This may be explained by the different shape of the sensitivity curve at mesopic and photopic adaptation levels.

In Fig. 1 these curves are reproduced schematically. A stimulus which is juxtaliminal on both curves at 20° in the periphery and is moved centripetally, remains juxtaliminal with respect to the mesopic curve. However, the luminance

---

[13] FANKHAUSER & SCHMIDT, 1958.

[14] AULHORN & HARMS 1967, DRANCE 1967.

[15] see also fig. 1.

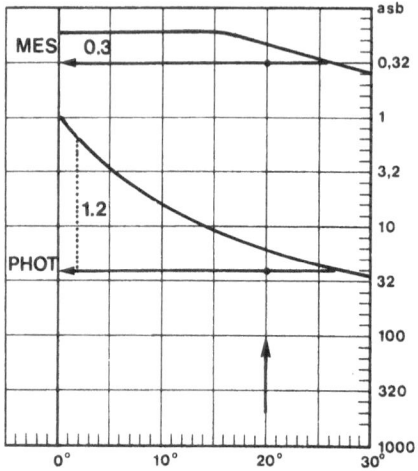

Fig. 1

Photopic and mesopic sensitivity curve and juxtaliminal stimuli at 20° eccentricity (see text).

abscissa: eccentricity
ordinate: luminance in log units

gap between the stimulus and the photopic liminal level increases steadily. In other words: the examination becomes increasingly less sensitive. At the photopic adaptation level therefore, the stimuli chosen must be progressively weaker in order to examine more centrally localized positions. If one stimulus luminance is used both at mesopic and photopic levels, this only shows that more defects are revealed by mesopic kinetic examination with one stimulus than by photopic examination with one stimulus. It does not follow that the intensity of visual field defects is greater at mesopic adaptation levels. A conclusion like this can only be drawn if a threshold examination is performed in both cases, preferably with the help of static perimetry. It is certainly true that in some diseases mesopic static perimetry gives clearer evidence of a defect than photopic static perimetry.[16] In the case of glaucoma, however, this has not been convincingly proved. DANNHEIM & DRANCE[17] have examined glaucomatous defects by means of static perimetry at photopic and mesopic levels of adaptation. They concluded that there was no difference in the intensity of the glaucomatous defects at the two levels of adaptation.

From the data in the literature it may be concluded that there is no reason to

[16] GREVE, BOS, MESKER & LEDEBOER 1972.

[17] DANNHEIM & DRANCE, personal communication.

suppose that the sensitivity of mesopic visual field examination is greater for glaucomatous defects.

Intra-individual variation at various adaptation levels

The variation of the measurements at various levels of adaptation has given rise to widely divergent views.

FANKHAUSER & SCHMIDT[18] found no statistically significant difference in the variation at mesopic (0.04 asb) and photopic (40 asb) levels. AULHORN & HARMS[19] concluded that the variation increases as the background luminance decreases (Fig.2).

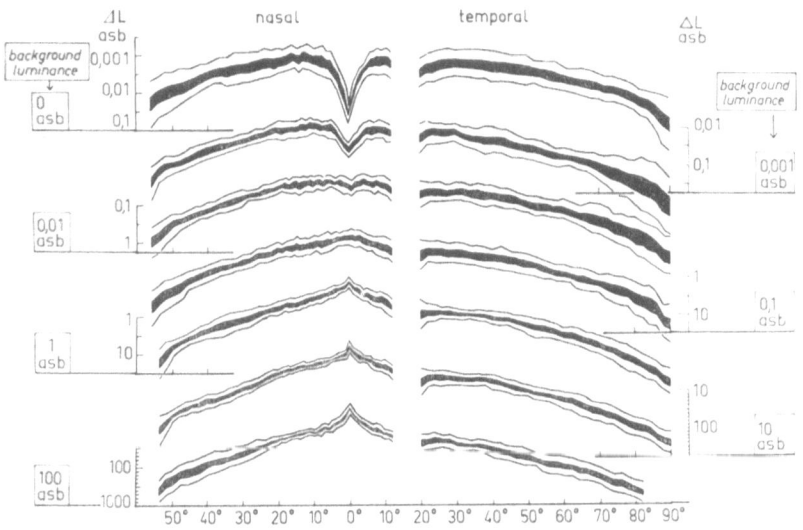

Fig. 2

Increase of inter-individual variation with decreasing background luminance; horizontal meridian; mean and standard deviation of 10 normal subjects.

abscissa: eccentricity

ordinate: luminance in log units

JAYLE et al. also studied the scotopic, mesopic and photopic variation. Their early publications were concerned with the variations in the position of the isopter. The 23.5° isopter, however, is not representative for the variations

---

18 FANKHAUSER & SCHMIDT, 1961.

19 AULHORN & HARMS, 1967.

which occur in the mesopic area, because the greatest changes take place in the central visual field.

JAYLE et al.[20] investigated this variation in later experiments with static methods. They concluded that the variation decreased as the background illumination decreased.

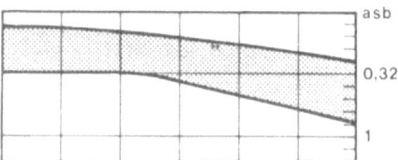

Fig. 3
Range of mesopic (0.01 asb background luminance) sensitivity curves of 20 normal subjects. The 20 curves fall within the two indicated extremes.

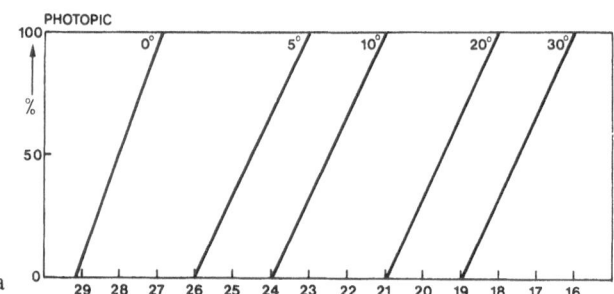

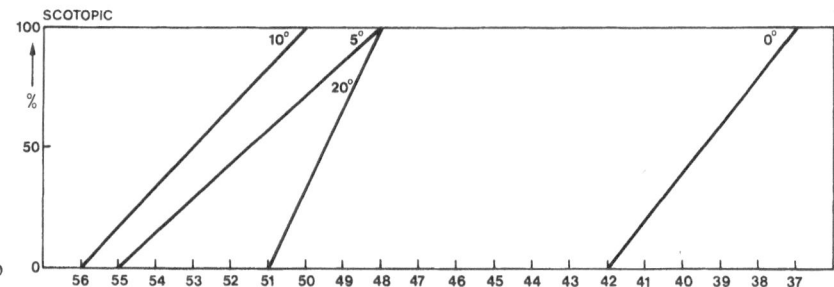

Fig. 4
Intra-individual variation at 0°, 5°, 10°, 20° and 30° eccentricity in scotopic and photopic perimetry as expressed in modified frequency-of-seeing curves. The slope of the straight line indicates the size of the variation.
abscissa: luminance in steps of 0.1 log unit
ordinate: frequency-of-seeing in percent

---

[20] JAYLE, VOLA, AUBERT & BRACCINI, 1965; see also MEUR 1965.

From our own experiments it appears that there is no significant difference in the inter-individual and intra-individual variation of measurements made by means of static perimetry at photopic (10 asb) and mesopic (0.01 asb) adaptation levels. The results of the examination of 20 normal subjects are given in Fig. 3. In the case of scotopic static perimetry we only investigated the intra-individual variation. This was found to be significantly greater than the variation found for photopic perimetry (Fig. 4).

Influence of preretinal factors.

DUBOIS-POULSEN & MAGIS[21] have raised objections to the mesopic adaptation level on the grounds of the graph shown in Fig. 5. A slight change in the objective or subjective background gives rise to a large change in the central light

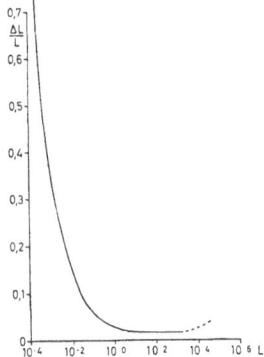

Fig. 5

Relation between $\dfrac{\Delta L}{L}$ (ordinate) and L (abscissa).

difference sensitivity at the mesopic level. In this way a change in the background luminance can give rise to a relative central scotoma without a lesion of the visual system being present. Fig. 6 shows the sensitivity curve of a patient with lens opacity without other disorders[22]. A central scotoma appears on mesopic examination (scotopization). The inassessible influence of preretinal factors becomes more apparent at the mesopic level than at the photopic level.

---

[21] DUBOIS-POULSEN & MAGIS 1960, 1967. This graph can be compared with the graph in Fig. 7 on page 24 of AULHORN, HARMS & RAABE. From this graph, which applies to the central visual field, it appears that at the level where the background luminance is less than 1 cd/m² the term ΔL is no longer constant when L becomes smaller.
[22] Tübinger perimeter.

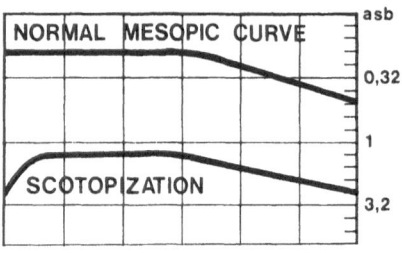

Fig. 6

Scotopization of a mesopic sensitivity curve due to cataract. The normal mesopic curve
is also indicated.

abscissa: eccentricity

ordinate: luminance in log units

Conclusions about the intensity of central scotomata must be drawn very guardedly in mesopic perimetry if there is any opacity of the media.

Scotopic perimetry

At the beginning of this chapter some technical disadvantages of scotopic perimetry were mentioned. The only instruments[23] on the market which are suitable for scotopic examination are the Tübinger perimeter and the perimeter of JAYLE-BLET. Kinetic perimetry or campimetry at the scotopic level meets with practical problems[24]. The only acceptable possibility for scotopic examination is static perimetry[25].

The reaction time is prolonged when examination is carried out in the scotopic area[26]. Fixation under scotopic conditions is difficult and it is usually impossible to check it. Furthermore the examination is unpleasant and tiring. In our opinion scotopic static perimetry only serves a useful purpose when it forms part of an adaptoperimetric examination.

JAYLE, OURGAUD and co-workers[27] consider that *circular* scotopic static examination is the ideal method for the investigation of glaucomatous visual fields. They perform this examination after kinetic photopic or mesopic perimetry.

---

[23] see Chapter VI.

[24] FRANCOIS & VERRIEST (1956) published a series of articles on scotopic campimetry using LIVINGSTON's method. Although they concluded that scotopic campimetry incurs a number of technical problems, they list a number of conditions in which scotopic examination is more sensitive than photopic examination.

[25] see also MCMARTIN & DIMMICK 1949.

[26] LEMMON & GEISINGER 1936.

[27] OURGAUD, SARACCO, METGE & MARTIN 1968; JAYLE, OURGAUD & METGE, 1969.
In circular static perimetry a number of positions on a parallel are investigated.

We have not been able to find a comparative study by these authors showing that static visual field examination in the scotopic range is more sensitive than in the mesopic range[28]. With regard to the choice of one parallel (in this case the 15° parallel) for examination, we refer to the discussion on the detection phase in glaucoma and the localization of defects.[30]

High-photopic adaptation levels

SHIGA's theory[29] that visual field examination with high-photopic background luminance is more sensitive than the usual low-photopic luminances has, as far as we know, not been confirmed. It is possible that this method may yield more interesting results in the future. The variation of the measurements will probably be greater at such high levels of background luminance.[31]

Conclusion

The conclusion presents itself that the choice of adaptation level in the usual instruments for visual field examination is very reasonable. Background luminances of 31 asb (Goldmann perimeter) and 10 asb (Tübinger perimeter) are photopic, be it low-photopic according to our standards. For this level of adaptation only a short adaptation time is needed, changes in the retinal illumination due to preretinal factors cause no changes in the shape of the sensitivity curve that cannot be recognized as such. At this level of adaptation the difference threshold probably depends on both the rod and the cone systems.

At present there is no reason to assume that routine visual field examination of glaucoma patients would be better performed at a different level of adaptation.

---

[28] ZUEGE & DRANCE (1967) performed adaptometric examinations at 5°, 15° and 20° eccentricity in two oblique temporal meridians on normal subjects and on glaucoma patients. The results were expressed in the ratio: threshold at 15°/threshold at 30°. This threshold is the rod threshold after 30 minutes. In patients with raised ocular pressure, but without excavations or visual field defects the rod threshold ultimately found was normal. This means that scotopic examination in these cases produces no new information. The ratio 15°/30° threshold was found to be abnormal in 4 of the 16 cases. The significance of this is uncertain. The Bjerrum area in the intact half of the visual field was examined in 8 patients with bundle scotomata. In 6 cases an abnormal ratio was found in the absence of static and kinetic photopic defects. This is one of the few cases in which a comparative study has indicated that a defect may perhaps be detected earlier by means of scotopic examination. These indications are still too limited to justify the use of such a cumbersome method.

[29] SHIGA, 1968.

[30] see chapters V and XI.

[31] KISHTO, 1970.

Knowledge of the various degrees of spatial interaction in the visual system and the resulting variable relationship between the luminance and the stimulus size enables us to answer the following questions, which are important for the practice of perimetry:

1. a. What is the relationship between the degree of stimulation produced by stimuli of different sizes?
   b. Should the size or the luminance of the stimulus be variable?
2. If one stimulus size is decided upon, what is the optimum size?
3. Does the study of spatial interaction provide additional information about the nature and the site of lesions of the visual system?

Spatial interaction in the normal visual field.

Although FERREE & RAND[1] studied the relationship between the size and contrast of a perimetric stimulus, it was not until the Goldmann perimeter was introduced that the investigators' attention was really directed towards spatial summation. GOLDMANN[2] concluded from a few experiments on a limited number of subjects that a fourfold increase (0.6 log units) in the surface area of a stimulus allows a threefold decrease (0.5 log units) of luminance at threshold level.

This indicates that partial summation of light stimuli occurs at the adaptation level of the Goldmann perimeter (background luminance = 31.5 asb). Goldmann also recorded the limits within which this partial spatial summation was valid and constant. With the stimulus combination I-II[3] Goldmann's law applied from 5° eccentricity outwards; with the combination I-III[4] it applied from 15° to 25° eccentricity and with the stimulus combination I-IV[5] it only began to apply at 45° eccentricity temporal and 30° nasal. With the largest stimulus of the Goldmann perimeter the law did not apply at all.

In his first publications GOLDMANN already raised the question of possible changes in spatial summation under pathological conditions; he suggested that the investigation of spatial summation might be of diagnostic significance.

GOLDMANN's results have stimulated many authors to a more detailed study of

---

[1] FERREE & RAND, 1931.

[2] GOLDMANN 1945a, b, c.

[3] 0.25 mm² and 1.0 mm² at 30 cm, i.e. ± 7' and ± 10'.

[4] III = 4 mm², i.e. ± 30'.

[5] IV = 16 mm², i.e. ± 60'.

spatial interaction in the normal visual field[6]. The results can be expressed in the form of a summation curve for one position in the visual field (see Chapter II, Fig. 11) or in the form of sensitivity curves for different stimulus sizes (Fig. 7).

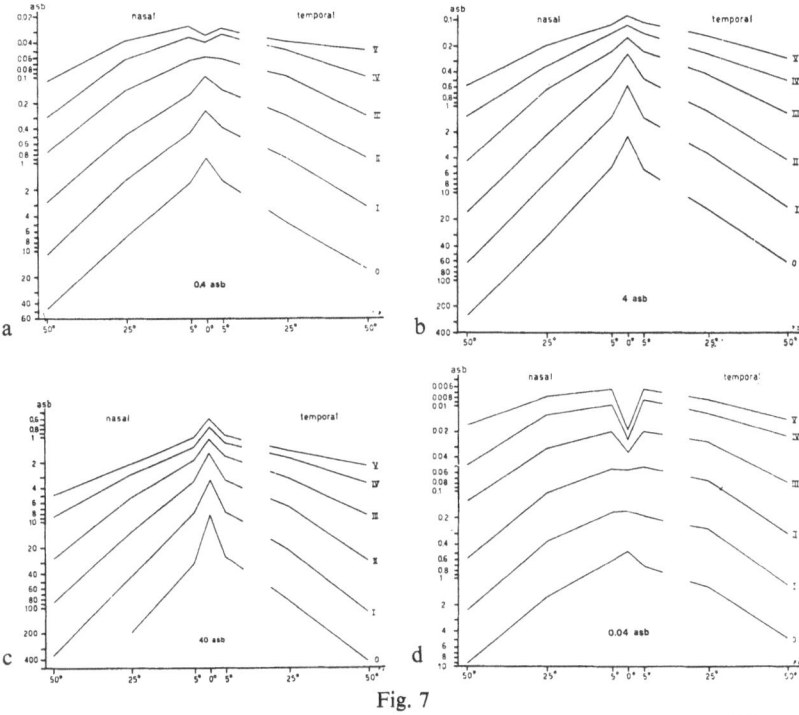

Fig. 7

Sensitivity curves of normal subjects for 6 different sizes of stimulus and 4 different levels of adaptation (indicated in each figure in asb; Goldmann perimeter,

FRANKHAUSER & SCHMIDT; 1958).

abscissa: eccentricity
ordinate: luminance in asb.

---

[6] The degree of spatial summation in most perimetric experiments is examined by determining the threshold luminance at one position for two stimuli of different sizes (static perimetry). For stimulus I and stimulus II: $L_I \times S_I K = C$ and $L_{II} \times S_{II} K = C$, where L is the threshold luminance and S the surface area of the stimulus. For both stimuli K, the summation exponent and C, a constant, are the same. Thus:

$L_I \times S_I K = L_{II} \times S_{II} K$

$\text{Log } L_I + K \log S_I = \log L_{II} + K \log S_{II}.$

$$K = \frac{\log L_I - \log L_{II}}{\log S_{II} - \log S_I}$$

From this formula K can be calculated. The graphical representation of the formula $L \times SK = C$ would be a straight line if K was not dependent on S. ($\log L = -K \log S + C$; cf. $y = ax + B$). The slope of the straight line is determined by ($-K$).

The data from the psychophysical literature were confirmed in perimetric experiments and some specific perimetric problems were elucidated:

1. As the stimulus becomes larger the value found for spatial summation becomes smaller[7];

2. Under photopic conditions the spatial summation for white stimuli increases from the centre to the periphery[8];

3. Spatial summation increases on dark adaptation[9]. This increase in spatial summation is larger in the centre than in the periphery of the visual field. As the eye becomes more adapted to darkness the difference in spatial summation between the centre and the periphery becomes smaller[10];

4. If the above experiments 2 and 3 are performed with coloured stimuli it appears that[11]:
   a. spatial summation is greater for colours with less spectral brightness.
   b. the degree of spatial summation for red and blue stimuli is almost independent of the eccentricity and adaptation. For stimuli from the yellow and green part of the spectrum the spatial summation increases with the eccentricity and the dark adaptation.

5. Agreement has not been reached about the relationship between spatial summation and age. A slight increase in the value of K with age has been reported[12], but others have found no age effect[13].

In all the experiments mentioned above relatively long presentation times were used. Points 1, 2 and 3 were also found to apply for very short presentation times (flashes of $\pm$ 300 µs) and white stimuli[14]. The values found for the summation exponent with short presentations are somewhat higher than the values for longer presentation times.[15] This is in agreement with data from the psychophysical literature[16].

---

[7] FANKHAUSER & SCHMIDT 1958, GOUGNARD 1961, SLOAN 1961.

[8] FANKHAUSER & SCHMIDT 1958, 1960; GOUGNARD 1961; SLOAN 1961; WILSON 1967; VERRIEST & ORTIZ-OLMEDO 1969; DANNHEIM & DRANCE 1971.

[9] FANKHAUSER & SCHMIDT 1960; MEUR 1965; AULHORN & HARMS 1966.

[10] With a background of 0.5 asb K at the fovea is 0.35 and at 20° 0.85; with a background of 0.000005 asb K is at the fovea 0.83 and at 20° 1.0.

[11] CONREUR & MEUR 1966.

[12] ASPINALL, 1967.

[13] DANNHEIM & DRANCE, 1971.

[14] OBSTFELD 1971.

[15] Compare results of OBSTFELD with those of MEUR (background of 0.5 asb).

[16] GLEZER 1965; BARLOW 1958, chapter II.

In Fig. 8 some of GOUGNARD's findings are represented graphically[17]. The summation exponent, determined with stimuli of various sizes, was plotted against the eccentricity. The dependence of the summation exponent on the tismulus size and the eccentricity can be clearly seen. In these figures the varia-

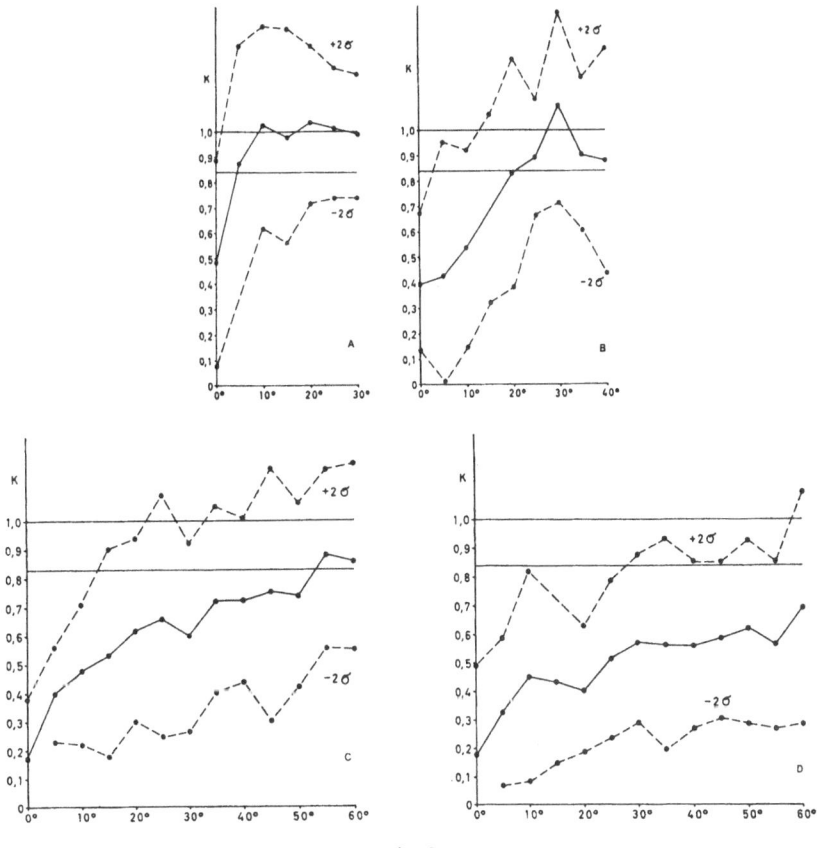

Fig. 8

Interindividual variation of the coefficient of spatial summation (K) with eccentricity (Goldmann perimeter).

    A) stimulus size 0 and   I

    B) stimulus size   I and II

    C) stimulus size II and III

    D) stimulus size III and IV

abscissa: eccentricity (nasal part of horizontal meridian)

ordinate: value of K

           mean value of K

           2 × standard deviation of K

---

[17] GOUGNARD 1960.

tion of the summation exponent is represented as twice the standard deviation. The degree to which the real spatial summation departs from Goldmann's law also becomes apparent (K = 0.83).

Constant size of stimulus.

Visual field examination can best be performed with a stimulus of constant size. If stimuli of various sizes are used the differences in strength of the stimuli depends upon spatial summation. This in turn depends on many factors and varies from case to case, so that the increase in stimulation on increasing the size of the object is not really known.

The examination is therefore carried out with a stimulus of constant size and variable luminance, so that the light sensitivity of every position can be expressed in the same way as the reciprocal of the luminance threshold.

The results of perimetry with small stimuli, and thus also of the investigation of spatial summation, are very sensitive to the use of the proper correction. The sharpest possible image of the object on the retina is essential for the correct interpretation of the investigation of spatial summation.

Dubois-Poulsen's work: spatial interaction and visual field defects.

Following GOLDMANN's suggestions, DUBOIS-POULSEN[18] has undertaken the study of spatial summation in the presence of visual field defects. He described the anomalies which he found primarily as 'troubles de sommation' and later as 'dysharmonie photométrique.' The last term avoids giving the impression that disturbances of spatial summation are the only mechanism involved in the anomalies he described. If disorders of spatial summation or inhibition exist, this has consequences for the choice of stimulus size in visual field examination. Increase in summation would mean that examination with small stimuli is more sentitive than with large stimuli, and increase in inhibition would have the opposite effect. For this reason it is important to study DUBOIS-POULSEN's findings more closely.

DUBOIS-POULSEN made use of the principle of equivalent isopters. The stimulus sizes and luminances of the Goldmann perimeter are chosen so that one step increase in stimulus size produces approximately the same increase in stimulation as one step increase in luminance. The isopter obtained with a given stimulus size-luminance combination (e.g. I/4) will therefore be in more

---

[18] DUBOIS-POULSEN 1952–1967.

78

or less the same position as the isopter obtained with a combination which is four times as large but three times as weak (e.g. II/3). This is based on the laws of partial spatial summation given above.[19]

DUBOIS-POULSEN examined visual field defects with two equivalent stimulus size-luminance combinations and discovered disharmony when the equivalent isopters diverged more than 5°. At a later stage he determined which isopters were equivalent with the help of additional grey filters. All DUBOIS-POULSEN'S results, of which a large number are given in his report[20], were obtained with kinetic perimetry.

Problems of kinetic perimetry.

Kinetic perimetry has a number of disadvantages, which have already been discussed. During the movement of the stimulus a number of receptors are stimulated in succession: successive lateral spatial summation. The interaction which takes place differs from the interaction when using static stimuli. The degree of spatial summation is greater when the speed of movement is 5°/s than when it is 2°/s.[21]

The variation of the results also increases with the speed of movement. Another disadvantage is that the divergence of equivalent isopters is dependent on the gradient of sensitivity.[22]

When the curve is steep all the isopters lie close together, when it is flat they are far apart. Especially in defects where the gradient is not known, this can give rise to problems. For these and other reasons, which have already been mentioned, conclusions about divergence from normal spatial summation obtained by means of kinetic perimetry must be regarded with caution. A number of authors have pointed out that static perimetry is more suitable for the investigation of spatial summation.[23]

DUBOIS-POULSEN, in later publications, has pointed out that divergence of the equivalent isopters over the whole line is not as important as local divergence.

According to this author 'dysharmonie photométrique' only occurs in lesions

---

[19] In the graph of stimulus size and luminance on the perimetric chart of the Goldmann perimeter the stimulus combinations of equivalent isopters are found on the diagonals running from the left top corner to the right bottom corner, with the limitations given by GOLDMANN.

[20] DUBOIS-POULSEN 1952.

[21] FANKHAUSER & SCHMIDT 1958.

[22] see Chapter III.

[23] FANKHAUSER & SCHMIDT 1958; AULHORN & HARMS 1972.

of the visual system situated distal to the lateral geniculate body. He considers that conditions which are associated with oedema in particular are responsible for disharmony. In a long list of disorders in which disharmony was found, glaucomatous visual field defects are also included ('glaucome chronique en periode évolutive, glaucome vasculaire, glaucome chronique irritatif et glaucome simple').

In the great majority of cases DUBOIS-POULSEN found increased spatial summation (or decreased inhibition), from which follows that the visual field defects were larger with small stimuli.

Inter-individual variation of the summation exponent.

An important matter, which complicates the study of spatial summation in the presence of visual field defects, is the fact that the inter-individual variation in the summation exponent K in normal subjects is very great. The limits given by Goldmann for constant partial spatial summation have been found only to apply to a very small concentric area; outside this area the partial summation increases and inside it decreases[24]. This means that values of K can only be regarded as pathological if they differ markedly from the average value of K. The equivalence of some isopters in the Goldmann perimeter (based on K = 0.83) is thus only a pseudo-equivalence. For this reason DUBOIS-POULSEN laid down the criterion for disharmony as $10°$ divergence of the isopters in his later publications. GOLDMANN considers that conclusions about pathological summation are only justified if measurements have been made before, during and after the development of a defect. The problem of inter-individual variation can be avoided when the spatial summation of defective parts of the visual field is compared with that of comparable normal parts of the visual field of the same or the other eye.

Results obtained by other authors.

DUBOIS-POULSEN'S conclusions on the occurrence of 'dysharmonie photométrique' in various disorders have been disputed by some authors.

SLOAN & BROWN concluded that disharmony occurs in several different types of visual field defects and that there is no clear relationship with specific conditions (including retinal oedema).[25]

---

[24] FANKHAUSER & SCHMIDT 1958; GOUGNARD 1961; MEUR 1965; see also GOLDMANN 1969.
[25] SLOAN & BROWN 1962.

WILSON[26] considered that a change in the spatial summation occurs in all

[26] WILSON, 1967. The patients examined by WILSON were divided into 4 groups: in the first group the lesion was anterior to the lateral geniculate body; in the second group the lesion was posterior to the lateral geniculate body; the third group consisted of patients with neurological disorders but without visual field defects; the fourth group was made up of normal subjects. The composition of the groups was not further specified. Data from individual patients in each group were combined. The average curves thus obtained show a difference in spatial summation between the groups with defective and the groups with normal visual fields, but careful study of these defects reveals that:
1. there is enormous inter-individual variation in spatial summation between the normal subjects (the slope of the summation curve varies between –0.2 and –0.8).
2. there is even more marked inter-individual variation between the summation measurements in the visual field defects.

This means that a number of the patients examined by WILSON must have had normal spatial summation curves.

WILSON's conclusion should have been that a number of patients with lesions anterior to the lateral geniculate body and a number with lesions posterior to the lateral geniculate body had disturbances of spatial summation. For the purposes of diagnosis it is only important to know whether anomalies of summation found in the individual patient (and not in a group) are of significance for the localization of a lesion.

visual field defects. As the intensity of the defects increased the spatial summation also increased, according to his findings. His conclusions were based on average values from a group of patients; the application of this conclusion to individual patients does not seem to be justified.

DANNHEIM & DRANCE[27] found no change in spatial summation in patients with glaucomatous visual field defects.

Another important problem in the study of spatial summation, which is not mentioned in the literature, however, is that the topography of the sensitivity in visual field defects sometimes shows marked variations. Areas of relatively good and of poor light sensitivity may exist side by side. When the spatial summation is examined with stimuli of various sizes, the larger stimuli fall in part on other portions of the defect than the small stimuli. This may give rise to a pseudo-'dysharmonie photométrique'. In such cases a greater defect intensity will be found with small stimuli than with larger ones.

This is probably the most important argument for the use of small stimuli. In practice it has been found that the finer details of a defect can be more easily recorded with small stimuli than with large stimuli.

---

[27] personal communication.

In the perimetric experiments described above only total and partial summation have been considered. From the psychophysical and electrophysiological literature it appears that partial summation is probably the result of summative and inhibitive interaction.

The theory has been expressed that the 'dysharmonie photométrique' in the sense of an increase in the summation exponent K, is the result of reduction in the cone inhibition. This hypothesis is based on the fact that, when the visual field defects present are caused by disorders which mainly affect the rod system, disharmony cannot be demonstrated[28].

VERRIEST & ORTIZ-OLMEDO[29] have made the existence of inhibition plausible by means of experiments on spatial interaction using ring-shaped objects. The summation coefficient K, determined on the one hand for a normal object I and a normal object II of the Goldmann perimeter and on the other hand for a ring-shaped object with the same surface area as object II, is in some cases more than 1 for the combination of object II with the ring-shaped object (Fig. 9). This is explained by the high threshold for the ring-shaped object.

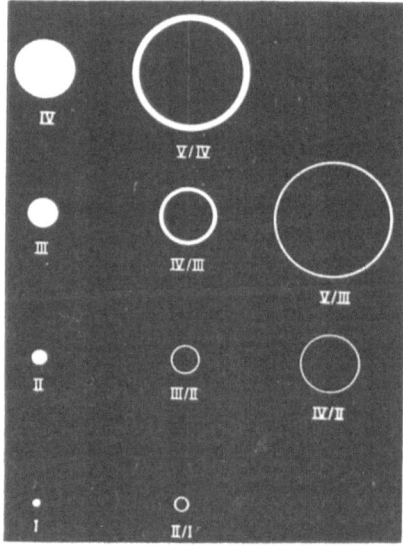

Fig. 9
Objects used by VERRIEST & ORTIZ-OLMEDO to investigate inhibition in spatial interaction.

---

[28] Congenital nightblindness; 'pigmentary degeneration of the retina'; SLOAN & BROWN, 1962.

[29] VERRIEST & ORTIZ-OLMEDO 1969; FRANCOIS, VERRIEST & ORTIZ-OLMEDO 1970.

This high threshold could be caused by inhibition at the periphery of the receptive field, which is not compensated in the case of ring-shaped stimuli by summation at the centre of the receptive field. It was found that the threshold luminance for ring-shaped stimuli is always higher than for normal stimuli of the same surface area, except for small stimuli in the periphery (total spatial summation) and large stimuli at the centre of the visual field (no summation). The same authors also investigated spatial interaction by means of ring-shaped objects in the presence of visual field defects (kinetic perimetry). In a glaucoma patient they found no change in the spatial interaction.

ENOCH and co-workers[30] introduced a psychophysical method of examining spatial summation into perimetry. This long-standing method was used by WESTHEIMER[31] for the comparison of electrophysiological[32] and psychophysical results. In the experimental set-up of these authors the size and luminance of an 'adapting field' can be varied in such a way that a small stimulus in the centre of the adapting field is always at threshold level (Fig. 10).[33] The underlying

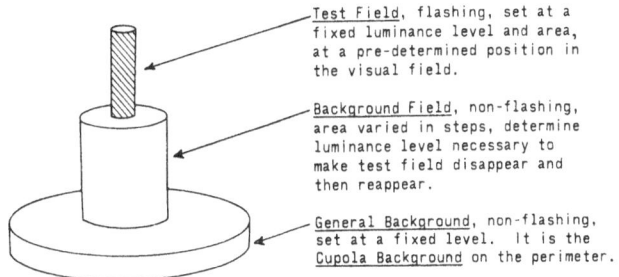

Test Field, flashing, set at a fixed luminance level and area, at a pre-determined position in the visual field.

Background Field, non-flashing, area varied in steps, determine luminance level necessary to make test field disappear and then reappear.

General Background, non-flashing, set at a fixed level. It is the Cupola Background on the perimeter.

Fig. 10

Relationship between stimulus, variable adapting field and background in the investigation of ENOCH & SUNGA.

theory is the justifiable assumption that the different adapting field conditions are equivalent as regards their stimulating effect on the visual system.

The difference between this method and the customary techniques described above is that the adapting field with which the spatial summation and inhibition are examined can be chosen at any supraliminal level. By this method it has been possible to demonstrate peripheral inhibition in interaction experiments. In the usual summation curves obtained with liminal stimuli, only total, partial,

[30] ENOCH & SUNGA 1969; SUNGA & ENOCH 1970a en b, ENOCH, SUNGA & BACHMAN 1970.
[31] WESTHEIMER 1965, 1966, 1967 and 1968.
[32] according to BARLOW, FITZHUGH & KUFFLER 1957.
[33] after ENOCH & SUNGA 1969.

or absence of summation can be expressed. The value of this method for perimetry was investigated by means of a Goldmann perimeter adapted for the purpose. The results obtained by these authors are expressed in summation curves, in which the luminance and size plotted are those of the adapting field and not of the stimulus.

In the curves three parts are distinguished: a descending part (negative slope), an ascending part and a horizontal part. The first part is regarded by ENOCH et al. as the summation arm and the second as the inhibition arm. The horizontal part indicates that no more interaction occurs and thus that the boundaries of the receptive field have been passed. The conclusions of these authors agree in general with the psychophysical characteristics of spatial summation already given. An important difference is, however, that now a peripheral ring of inhibition has been demonstrated, like that known from electro-physiological experiments. Inhibition can only be demonstrated when the constant stimulus has a distinctly supraliminal luminance. With a luminance of 0.5 log unit above the difference threshold only slight inhibition could be demonstrated. The total interaction zone (summation + inhibition), as revealed by these experiments, is larger than the summation zone found in the usual experiments at threshold level.

This is illustrated in Fig. 11 and Fig. 12[34]. The terms 'minimum value' and 'limit of interaction zone' appear in these figures. The latter term is self-evident, the former indicates the transition from summation-arm to inhibition-arm. The

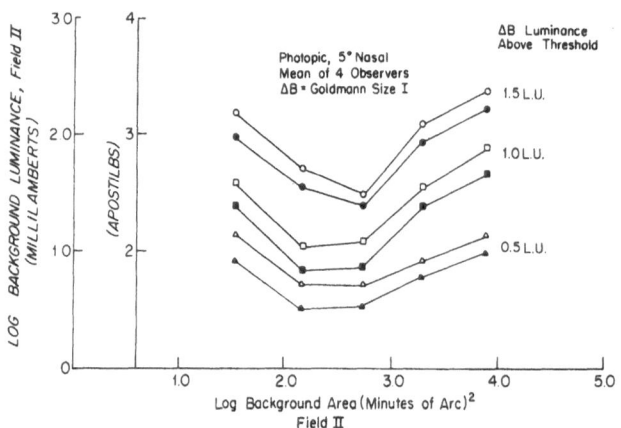

Fig. 11
Curves indicating spatial interaction; results of ENOCH et al.

---

[34] after ENOCH & SUNGA, 1969.

84

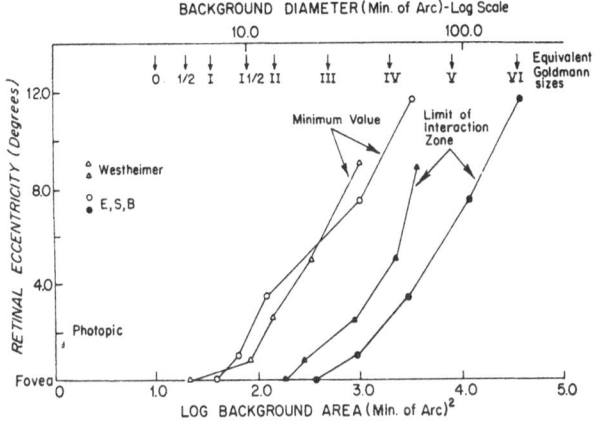

Fig. 12

Derived dimensions of areas of neural interaction (photopic) are presented as a function of eccentricity. In addition, minima falling between the summation and inhibition arms of these functions are plotted. As an aid to the reader, the log diameter (in minutes of visual angle) of the backgrounds are presented across the top of the figure.

For comparison purposes WESTHEIMER's findings are presented.

'minimum value' for the fovea was found at 7′, which is in agreement with the usual value for the summation zone. However, the zone of total interaction appears to be much larger ($\pm$ 25′). As expected, these values increase towards the periphery: at $\pm$12° the zone of total interaction has already increased to nearly 3°. In the vicinity of the blind spot strangely enough, no inhibition-arm was found.

A number of patients with visual field defects were also examined by this method. It was concluded that the 'Westheimer type functions' were unaltered in visual field defects caused by lesions in the outer parts of the retina. On the other hand, in visual field defects caused by lesions in the inner parts of the retina reduced inhibition was found. In neuritis, chiasmal lesions and disorders of the post-chiasmal visual system complicated variables appeared, which made a definite conclusion impossible. Decreased summation means that small stimuli are more sensitive than large stimuli.

Conclusion. Choice of stimulus size.

From the above survey it appears that nearly all authors agree that, if spatial interaction is disturbed in visual field defects, this is expressed as reduced inhibition.

The chances for spatial summation are thus increased. This means that the luminance threshold for large stimuli will be relatively lower. For small stimuli spatial summation is good under normal conditions and increase in summation will not affect the threshold noticeably. The intensity of a defect measured with a small stimulus will thus be greater than when it is measured with a large stimulus. By small stimuli we mean stimuli in which there is summation of all impulses. As the examination is performed with only one size of stimulus, the choice will be based on the size of the zone of total summation in the central visual field. This is approximately the size of the Goldmann perimeter stimulus I ($\pm$ 6'50")[35].

The choice of the object size is also influenced by some other factors:

1. The accuracy with which a defect can be recorded becomes greater as the stimulus becomes smaller.
2. The minimum stimulus size is limited by the 'contrast transfer function' of the eye, which is approximately 6 minutes at the fovea.[36]
3. The intra- and inter-individual variation is not much affected by differences in stimulus size.
4. Large stimuli are less affected by refractional anomalies than small stimuli. The influence of refractional anomalies is discussed under 'Preretinal factors'. This influence is eliminated by adequate correction.

Small objects (6'–10') are to be preferred to larger objects for visual field examination.

The significance of the examination of spatial summation in visual field defects. For this examination static perimetry is the best method. Either the usual procedure can be followed, with the determination of the threshold luminance for stimuli of different sizes, or ENOCH & SUNGA's method of examination with supraliminal luminances can be employed.

The findings of several authors with static perimetry are conflicting. Conclusions about the significance of the results can therefore not be drawn. Spatial summation in glaucomatous defects is probably not disturbed. There are as yet too few particulars available to judge the significance of ENOCH & SUNGA's promising method.

CHOICE OF PRESENTATION TIME;

TEMPORAL INTERACTION AND VISUAL FIELD EXAMINATION

Unlike spatial interaction, temporal interaction has not received much attention from perimetric investigators. On the basis of information about temporal

---

[35] ENOCH, SUNGA & BACHMANN 1970.

[36] FANKHAUSER 1969, quoting CAMPBELL & GREEN, 1965.

interaction the best presentation time for static perimetry could be chosen. As with spatial summation, the results of the perimetric measurements of temporal summation can be expressed in a summation curve or as a sensitivity curve for different presentation times.

Temporal interaction in the normal visual field.

The data from the psychophysical literature have been confirmed in the few perimetric studies on temporal summation which have been performed: temporal summation is dependent upon the eccentricity, the adaptive state and the size of the stimulus. As far as we know, the influence of the wavelength of the stimulus has not been investigated.

Position

Temporal summation is slightly greater in the periphery of the visual field than in the centre, as appears from a longer critical duration and from the shape of the sensitivity curves for various presentation times.[37] Fig. 13 shows how the

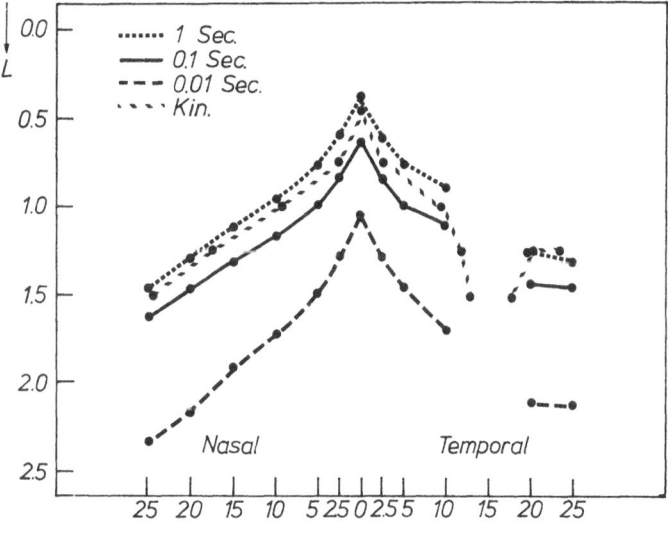

Fig. 13

Sensitivity curves of static perimetry measured with 3 different durations of presentation. For comparison purposes the kinetic sensitivity curve is added.

abscissa: eccentricity

ordinate: log luminance of the stimulus

[37] DANNHEIM & DRANCE, 1971.

sensitivity curves for a presentation time of 0.01 s on the one hand and of 0.1 and 1 s on the other hand diverge slightly as the eccentricity increases[38]. The sensitivity curve for the short presentation time is steeper than for the long presentation time.

Fig. 14 shows the summation curves for a stimulus in the centre and at 25° in the periphery of the visual field. It appears again that temporal summation in the periphery is better than in the centre[39]. In our experiments the critical duration was found to be ± 0.06 s at 25°.[40]

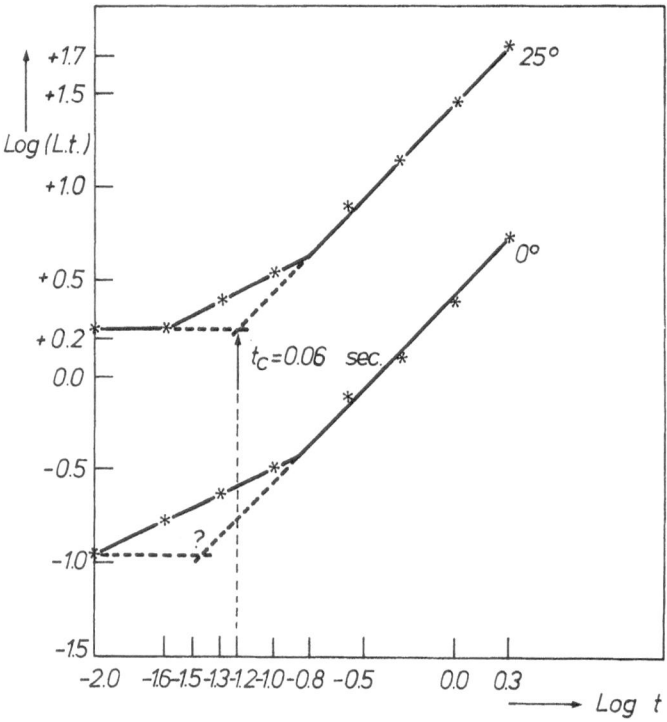

Fig. 14
Temporal summation curve of a normal subject at the fovea and 25° eccentricity.
abscissa: log t
ordinate: log L.G

---

[38] stimulus size: 11′; background luminance: 31 asb.

[39] the differences in temporal summation at various positions is slight compared with the differences in spatial summation.

[40] DANNHEIM & DRANCE found a t_c of 0.1 s for a stimulus of 45′ in the periphery. As there are considerable inter-individual variations in the t_c and DANNHEIM & DRANCE did not specify their interpretation of the t_c further, this difference is not significant.

88

Adaptation

Temporal summation is better under mesopic than under photopic conditions.[41]

Stimulus size

In our own experiments we found that the temporal summation was greater for an 11′ stimulus than for a stimulus of 30′ or 1° diameter. For larger stimuli the difference in temporal summation between the centre and the periphery is negligible.

It may be concluded that a presentation time of 0.01 s or less is certainly shorter than the critical duration and thus falls within the zone of total temporal summation, and that a presentation time of 1 s almost certainly lies within the zone of no summation.

Arguments for the use of a short presentation time.

The question is now: which presentation time should be chosen for routine visual field examination? It should be remembered that in the previous chapters it was decided to use relatively small stimuli at the photopic level of adaptation. The following considerations must be taken into account:

1. intra- and inter-individual variation of measurements with different presentation times;
2. total duration of the examination;
3. latent period for eye movements;
4. normal fixation movements;
5. disturbed temporal interaction in visual field defects;
6. technical possibilities;
7. subjective experience;
8. relationship of static perimetry results using different presentation times with kinetic perimetry.

Intra- and inter-individual variation.

In the past, an argument which was used for long presentation times (0.5 s – 1.0 s) was that in the zone without temporal summation, variations in the presentation time have no more influence on the level of the threshold. By using

---

When DANNHEIM & DRANCE's curves are compared with ours it appears that in both cases the total temporal summation ceases at ± 0.03 s. Between the zones of total summation and no summation there appears to be a transitional zone of partial summation which, dependent upon the position, extends from 0.01 s to 0.2s.

[41] HARMS 1969; DANNHEIM & DRANCE, 1971.

long presentation times one variation factor could be eliminated. This argument would apply if it were true that the variation (either intra- or inter-individual) was greater with short than with longer presentation times.

In our study of 20 normal subjects, however, it was found that there was no difference in the variation whether the presentation times were long or short[42]. The variation can therefore not be used as an argument against short presentation times.[43]

From these experiments it also appeared that the variation in the values for temporal summation in different subjects is fairly large (variation of K). This has consequences for the significance one may attach to changes in temporal summation in visual field defects (cf. spatial summation).

Total duration of the examination.

It is obvious that the total duration of the examination will be shorter when the presentation times are short than when they are long. If 150 positions are examined by means of static perimetry, the total duration of the examination with a presentation time of 1 s will theoretically be about 30 minutes, as compared to 20 minutes with presentations of 0.01 s. As the length of the examination is one of the few disadvantages of static perimetry, the time saved by using short presentation times increases the efficiency of this method.[44]

Latent period for eye movements.

If a short presentation time is chosen it is not possible for the patient to direct his gaze to the place where the stimulus appears, as the latent period for eye movements is 150 ms[45]. When the presentation time is 1 s this possibility certainly exists, as every visual field examiner knows from experience.

---

[42] KISHTO (1970) even reported that the variation increases with longer presentation times.

[43] see also: technical possibilities.

[44] If one assumes that every threshold perception is proceded by an average of 3 negative perceptions, 4 determinations are necessary for each threshold value. There is at least 2 s interval between each determination. With a presentation time of 1 s the total duration of the investigation of 150 positions is thus $150 \times 4 \times 3 \text{ s} = 1800 \text{ s} = 30$ minutes.

With a presentation time of 0.01 s the duration is $150 \times 4 \times 2 \text{ s} = 20$ minutes. This is a gain in time of 30%. In practice both examinations take rather longer on account of technical and other factors.

[45] WESTHEIMER, 1954.

Normal fixation movements and temporal summation.

Under the conditions of visual field examination the normal fixation movements can have an amplitude of $\pm 1°$, dependent on the eccentricity at which the amplitude is measured[46]. With a presentation time of 1 s this means that the stimulus moves over a number of receptors. When a short presentation time, such as 0.01 s is used, the position being examined in the visual field is more circumscribed.

As long as the movement over the retina is smaller than the area in which complete spatial summation takes place, the movement will have no influence on the threshold. If the limits of the summation area are passed it is possible that the threshold for longer presentation times will be lower[47]. The extent of the influence of fixation movements on the threshold when long presentation times are used has, as far as we know, not been investigated. Experience shows that small defects can often be recorded better with short presentation times. Angioscotomata form an example. One may imagine that, when the presentation time is long and the defect is small, the stimulus falls for part of the time in the defect and for part of the time outside of it.

When an area outside the defect is stimulated for longer than 0.3–0.5 s a normal threshold will be recorded; 0.3 s is approximately the limit of the time in which temporal summation occurs. A stimulus of 1 s, for example, can easily stimulate for 0.7 s an area within a small defect and for 0.3 s an area outside it.

Our hypothesis is thus that with a long presentation time a surplus of energy is offered which can stimulate a normal portion of the visual field as the result of the physiological fixation movements.

Support for this hypothesis is the fact that the edges of defects can often not be registered accurately to a half degree.

Subjective experience.

In our experience a short presentation time is found to be more agreeable for the subject than a long presentation time.

Abnormal temporal summation in visual field defects.

Presentation of a stimulus for a length of time which exceeds the critical duration means that a surplus of time is presented.

We have already pointed out the consequences of this surplus in connection with the fixation movements. If temporal summation were to take place more

---

[46] see chapter II: Fixation.
[47] see chapter II: Movement.

slowly in a visual field defect (i.e. if more time were needed to reach the threshold) it is theoretically possible that the abnormal summation would not be expressed with long presentation times, because the 'lack of time' to reach the threshold would be compensated by the surplus time of the long presentation. The result could be that, in this sort of abnormal temporal summation, the threshold for short presentations would be higher than for long presentations. This would be expressed as a pseudo-increase in temporal summation. If increased temporal summation is found in visual field defects, this argues in favour of short presentation times.

Very little is known about the pathology of temporal summation. It is probable that there are no changes in temporal summation in glaucomatous defects[48]. WILSON considers that temporal summation is only disturbed in lesions posterior to the geniculate body[49]. As the threshold becomes higher the temporal summation becomes greater. The objections to these findings are the same as those already given under 'spatial summation'.

The most interesting fact which emerges from WILSON's investigations is that, when a change in temporal interaction does occur, this is always expressed as

---

[48] DANNHEIM & DRANCE; these authors have also observed, however, that defects can be recorded better with short presentation times; personal communication.

[49] WILSON, 1967. Wilson's investigations were carried out at the photopic level with an object of 80.8'. This is a very large stimulus, so that relatively poor temporal summation may be expected. This does appear to be the case, as the curve for normal subjects never reaches a slope of –1 (45°) (shortest time: 5.1 ms). A stimulus like this will also fall, in a number of cases, on positions of different light sensitivity. The measurements at 3 positions (5°, 15° and 30° on one of the oblique meridians) from all the patients in one group were averaged (Fig. 6).

From this figure it appears that the temporal summation curve for lesions situated anterior to the geniculate body have the same shape as the normal curve. The curve for the lesions posterior to the geniculate body, however, diverges from the normal curve: the difference for the shortest time is ± 0.4 log unit in the direction of temporal summation. The threshold luminance is relatively higher for shorter presentation times, this is expressed by a steeper curve. The zone of partial summation also extends further, between 317 msec. and 950 msec. the curve is still not horizontal.

Careful inspection of Fig. 7 shows that, of the 20 lesions posterior to the geniculate body, 12 fall within the normal zone of temporal summation (2 × sd for the slope of the temporal summation curve). Eight fall outside this zone; of these eight, three have a threshold which is higher than that found in lesions anterior to the geniculate body. As differential diagnostic procedure, the examination of the temporal summation could, in 40% of the cases, give an indication of the localization of the lesion anterior or posterior to the geniculate body. More often than not, however, this will already be obvious from the shape of the defect.

increased summation. This is also an argument in favour of short presentation times.

Technical possibilities.

One of the arguments brought against short presentation times is that, in the zone of complete temporal summation, every variation in the presentation time leads to a variation in the threshold. The electro-magnetic shutters now available, however, are so reliable that this technical argument no longer applies. An accurate time of 0.01 s can generally be obtained with electro-magnetic shutters. On the basis of the above considerations this time is short enough. Gas-filled flash lamps (e.g. Xenon flash lamps) produce very short flashes (1 ms). The variation in the presentation time of these flash lamps is also very small.[50]

Kinetic perimetry.

Not only in static perimetry is temporal summation a factor to be considered. When a stimulus is moved over the visual field in kinetic perimetry, a series of receptors will be excited consecutively for a certain length of time. The duration of the stimulation depends on the speed with which the stimulus is moved. When a stimulus is moved at a speed of 10°/s, an area of 1° will be stimulated for 0.1 s.

The sensitivity curve for kinetic campimetry (5°/s) lies between the sensitivity curves for static perimetry with presentation times of 0.1 s and 1 s.

Conclusion

For the above reasons the use of short presentation times appears to be advisable.

'Short' means in this case: a period of time which is shorter than the critical time, e.g. 0.01 s.

The shorter the time is, the less influence normal fixation movements will have.

The upper limit of the presentation time is curtailed by local adaptation.

LOCAL ADAPTATION AND VISUAL FIELD EXAMINATION

In kinetic perimetry it is improbable that local adaptation plays any part, unless the movement is very slow.

In static perimetry local adaptation can be involved in the perception of a stimulus. With long presentation times (1 s) in the periphery of the visual

---

[50] see Chapter VIII.

field, the length of time that a stimulus is perceived is restricted by local adaptation, especially when the stimulus is at threshold level.

Local adaptation in the normal visual field

The variation in local adaptation has been studied recently with the Goldmann perimeter in normal subjects.[51]

The t_a was measured at 2°, 5°, 20° and 40° eccentricity with stimuli of various luminances (but always supraliminal), of various sizes and with various wavelengths. For each position the difference threshold was first determined, and then the stimulus luminance was set at a level that was by the same amount above threshold for every position. It was found that the t_a for normal subjects is variable; particularly measurements made on different days varied greatly. In general the t_a increased with increasing luminance (Fig. 15).

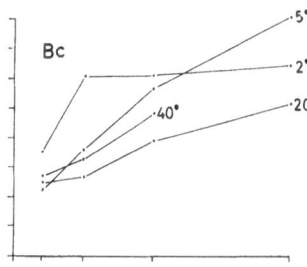

Fig. 15
Influence of luminance on the duration of the local adaptation time t_a: at 4 different eccentricities.
abscissa: number of log. units that the stimulus is above threshold
ordinate: log t_a

The t_a for 20° and 40° eccentricity increased with the size of the stimulus. For 2° and 5°, on the other hand, the t_a decreased slightly as the stimulus became larger.

The wave-length of the stimulus had no effect on the t_a. The influence of the eccentricity was found to be complex. The 15 normal subjects exhibited marked variation in the t_a, with a tendency towards a shorter t_a in the periphery. Between 20° and 40° the variations were not significant. Dependent upon the factors given, the t_a varied from 1 to 30 s.

---

[51] VERRIEST & LAVALLEE, 1966.

Local adaptation and visual field defects.

In the presence of lesions in the visual system changes in the local adaptation time (t_a) can occur.

A number of patients with various visual field defects were examined by CIBIS & MULLER[52]. They reported in general shortening of the t_a, and found a close connection between light sensitivity and local adaptation. The shortening of the t_a discovered by these authors can probably be explained by the fact that in many cases they used the same stimulus for the normal and the pathological parts of the visual field. This means that the stimuli in the visual field defects were much less supraliminal, thus giving rise to a shorter t_a. As these authors used old-fashioned methods of visual field examination, there is no information about the nature and extent of the defects.

In a number of neurological visual field defects shortening of the t_a has been described[53]. Although the results given in the older literature are difficult to

[53] BAY, 1954; this author considered that the examination of the local adaptation time was more accurate than the (in 1954) usual visual field examination. BAY writes: 'Size, shape, even type of field defect depend largely on the stimulus employed in perimetry and therefore are not significant for the extension and location of the cerebral lesions. In opposition to the unreliable findings of perimetry the examination methods pertaining to the Functionswandel (local adaptation) allow a more exact and constant evaluation of impediments of the visual functions and consequently a reliable localization within the visual system'.

The first part of this quotation shows that BAY was not familiar with the essentials of quantitative visual field examination, which is not suprising considering the date of the publication.

The same objection can be made to BAY's investigations as to those of CIBIS: the degree to which the stimulus is supraliminal is not constant, but varies with the intensity of the defect.

BAY's conclusions on the comparative merits of local adaptation examination and perimetry must, in the light of more recent investigations, be handled with caution.

interpret, we must take the possibility into account that the t_a may be shortened in some visual field defects, particularly in those of patients with a neurological disease.[54]

In a series of patients with visual field defects FRANÇOIS et al.[55] found no shortening of the t_a but in many cases a lengthening. In this group of patients only a few had neurological conditions and none had glaucoma.

---

[52] CIBIS 1948; CIBIS & MULLER, 1948.

[54] see also SUNGA & ENOCH, 1970.

[55] FRANÇOIS, VERRIEST, LAVALLÉE & LEBRUN, 1969.

95

The method used by these authors, with very short minimum t_a values, makes it difficult to detect pathological shortening of the t_a. Experience also shows that the examination of the t_a meets with many problems in practice (including fixation problems when vision is poor, patients' failure to grasp the methods of examination, technical limitations of the apparatus). VERRIEST et al. do not advocate this method of local adaptation examination for practical purposes.

From a recent study it appears probable that shortening of the t_a does occur in a number of neurological visual field defects (diseases of optic nerve and optic pathways).[56] In this study a 'time-related response anomaly' was also described: visual fatigue. As opposed to the pathological shortening of the t_a on continuous presentation, visual fatigue is a decrease in sensitivity on repeated presentation of short stimuli in the same position.

We have found no reliable information in the literature about changes in local adaptation in glaucomatous visual field defects.

Conclusion.

The length of the presentation time in visual field examination is limited by local adaptation.

As a preference for short presentation times has already been expressed local adaptation will not affect the normal difference threshold.

The investigation of changes in local adaptation in patients with visual field defects is difficult and appears to be limited to a few patients who are able to fixate and react well[57].

The investigations which have been performed up to now do not give a clear picture of the pathology of local adaptation. Both lengthening and shortening of the t_a have been found. No useful information has been obtained about changes in the local adaptation time in glaucomatous visual field defects.

SOME REMARKS ABOUT CRITICAL FUSION FREQUENCY AND COLOUR
IN VISUAL FIELD EXAMINATION.

Critical fusion frequency (C.F.F.).

We shall only deal shortly with these time-dependent measurements of the sensitivity of the visual system.

It has been found that the inter-individual variation in the CFF measurements is greater than in the normal measurements of the difference threshold by means

---

[56] SUNGA & ENOCH, 1970.

[57] VERRIEST and AULHORN; personal communications.

of static perimetry[58]. As the CFF method has not been shown to be more sensitive than the usual techniques, from the point of view of visual field pathology there are no arguments in favour of introducing this method into routine visual field examination.

A discussion of this subject can be found in DUBOIS-POULSEN's report. Recent perimetric studies on normal subjects were performed by DE CORTE & LAVERGNE[59], who consider that the CFF method does not belong to routine visual field examination.

GOLDMANN's[60] recent conclusions about the value of the CFF for visual field examination are the following:

1. many contradictory results appear in the literature, from which it is clear that this method of examination is very variable, particularly when small changes in luminance occur;
2. the size of the stimuli must be 1° or larger;
3. the method is only suitable for the examination of the central visual field;
4. the demands made on the patient are heavy.

It is possible that special situations, in which this examination method will be applicable, may be found in the future.

Colour

A survey of visual field examination with coloured stimuli and/or coloured backgrounds would alone be enough to fill a book. The descriptions in this study will be limited to visual field examination with white stimuli on a white background.

For recent studies on this subject see VERRIEST and co-workers[61], and the findings reported at the Symposia of the International Research Group on Colour Vision Deficiencies.[62]

---

[58] HARMS & AULHORN, 1959.

[59] DE CORTE & LAVERGNE, 1968, 1969, 1970.

[60] GOLDMANN, 1969.

[61] VERRIEST & ISRAEL, 1965; FRANÇOIS, VERRIEST & ISRAEL, 1966.

[62] Ghent, 1971; Edinburgh, 1973.

CHAPTER V

THE PLACE OF STATIC AND KINETIC PERIMETRY
IN THE TWO PHASES OF VISUAL FIELD EXAMINATION

Detection phase
   present-day kinetic perimetry
   number and position
   size of stimulus
   size of defect
   conclusion about number and position
   static and kinetic perimetry in the detection phase
   subdivision of detection phase
   two separate halves of the visual field
   repeat examination
   static and kinetic perimetry in visual field defects
Assessment phase

In Chapter III a preliminary survey is given of the possibilities and limitations of kinetic and static perimetry. In Chapter IV conclusions are drawn about the optimum level of adaptation, the optimum size of stimulus, the velocity of movement and the duration of presentation. The present chapter deals with the most suitable method of performing routine visual field examination.

In addition to the routine examination several variations are possible, e.g. investigation of spatial and temporal interaction, examination using coloured stimuli and coloured backgrounds, and adaptoperimetry. Some of these methods may provide additional information either for the differential diagnosis or the prognosis of a disease. If possible and where necessary these methods have been described in more detail. Generally speaking their significance is not yet fully understood. Although they hold promise for the future these methods are at present of secondary importance. The necessity of carrying out routine visual field examination effectively is of primary importance. Until this has been achieved there is little point in describing further differentiation of visual field examination.

The purpose of routine visual field examination is the early and efficient detection, the assessment and the follow-up of functional loss of the visual system, i.e. visual field defects. The efficiency must be judged in the light of our increased knowledge of the theory and technique of visual field examination and the types of visual field defects, and the recent introduction of sensitive and standardized instruments. The time needed for this earlier detection of defects and greater accuracy of the examination has increased proportionally. It is always perilous to increase the length of time necessary for established methods of a routine investigation. This is only acceptable when the extra time needed results in more and better information about the disease and is thus directly to the patient's advantage.

The average duration of a complete visual field examination in both eyes of a glaucoma patient is $1\frac{1}{2}$ hours[1]. The visual field examination must be as efficient as possible within the limits set by accuracy on the one hand and the longest permissible duration of the examination on the other. The relative value of kinetic and static perimetry has been the subject of long discussions in the literature.[2] Some aspects of these discussions have already been mentioned in former chapters. In general the differences between the detection phase and the assessment phase are not stressed.

From the literature one may conclude that either kinetic perimetry is used alone or that a combination of kinetic and static perimetry is preferred. For DUBOIS-POULSEN & MAGIS kinetic perimetry includes the examination of the equivalent isopters. For AULHORN & HARMS the detection phase consists of a combination of kinetic perimetry and static perimetry in the two oblique meridians.

Other authors prefer the examination of the 15° parallel by means of scotopic static perimetry[3]. Two further detection procedures will be discussed later[4].

Visual field examination should be subdivided into 2 phases:
I. The detection phase.
II. The assessment phase.

---

[1] see Chapter XI.
[2] see HARMS, 1950; 1969; AULHORN & HARMS, 1960; AULHORN, 1969; DUBOIS-POULSEN & MAGIS, 1959; 1966; DUBOIS-POULSEN, 1966; GOLDMANN, 1969; SCHMIDT, 1965; FANKHAUSER, 1969; JAYLE et al. 1969.
[3] JAYLE et al. 1969.
[4] see Chapter VIII.

This distinction is important because the demands made on the investigation procedure are totally different in the two phases. The purpose of the detection phase is to determine whether there is a defect in the visual field and where this defect is. In addition one tries to get an impression of the shape and extent of the defect. The detection of a defect means that a significant reduction of sensitivity has been demonstrated in part of the visual field.

The purpose of the assessment phase is to obtain a general view of the topography of the defect, and to determine with great accuracy the topography and intensity of the defect at selected locations, using the data provided in the detection phase.

In this way the details of the type of defect are assessed and a basis is laid for repeat examination by means of a reproducible delimitation of the defect.

DETECTION PHASE

In the detection phase it is important to know if there is any information from other sources about the localization of the defect. For instance, if a patient with macular degeneration is examined one knows that the defect will be localized in the central visual field. Because of this knowledge the detection phase can be shortened. In many cases, however, there is no previous information about the localization of a defect and the object of the detection phase is to look for a defect which may in theory be anywhere in the visual field.

Present-day kinetic perimetry.

In the majority of standard procedures for kinetic perimetry only a small number of positions are investigated. The instructions for these standard procedures vary from author to author but usually the examination is limited to 4 isopters (Fig. 1). Two of these are outside the 30° parallel. The reason that only 2 isopters are within the 30° visual field is that the customary steps of luminance in kinetic perimetry are 0.5 log unit. One step of 0.5 log unit in a normal photopic gradient is equal to a distance of 15–20 degrees between two isopters.

If 16 positions per isopter are examined a total of 32 positions are situated within the 30° parallel. Furthermore, the blind spot is examined in 8 different directions, which brings the total to 40 positions. It may be pointed out that 32 positions represent too small a number for the reliable detection of defects.

The fundamental limitations of kinetic perimetry for detection have already

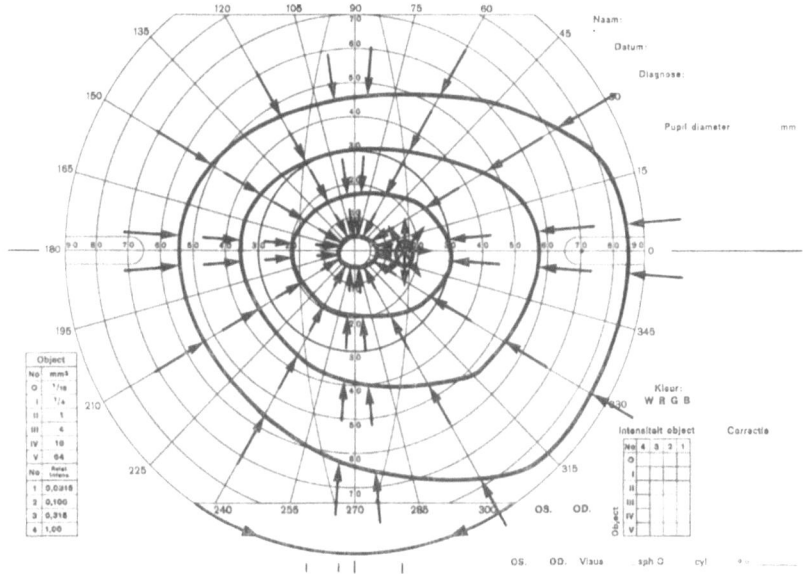

Fig. 1

The four isopters of the standard procedure in kinetic perimetry.

been discussed[5]. This limited capacity to detect defects is accentuated in practice because usually too few positions are examined. We have therefore tried to find a better procedure for the detection phase.

Number and position.

In the first place one should know which requirements must be met in the detection phase regarding the number and distribution of the positions to be examined. From data in the literature[6] as well as from our own results the conclusion may be drawn that the vast majority of glaucomatous defects are detected by an examination limited to the visual field within the 30° parallel. The examination of the peripheral visual field only contributes information of secondary importance. A further limitation within the 30° parallel based on a preferential localization of glaucomatous defects is not possible. This means that in an area of approximately 2826 square degrees the detection should be as efficient as possible. The positions to be examined should be distributed more

---

[5] Chapter III.

[6] BLUM et al., 1959; AULHORN & HARMS, 1967.

CHANCE OF DETECTION OF VISUAL FIELD DEFECTS		
NUMBER OF LOCATIONS IN 30° FIELD	DIAMETER OF DEFECT	CHANCE IN %
50	$9.0°$	95
100	$7.5°$	100
100	$6.4°$	95
100	$6.0°$	91
100	$5.0°$	69
100	$4.0°$	44
100	$3.0°$	25
452	$3.0°$	95

TABLE I

Chance of detection of visual field defects depending on number of stimulus positions

or less evenly in this area. The spatial accuracy of the investigation is then determined by the number of positions (see Table I). If 150 positions are examined in an area of 2826 square degrees there is one examined position per 18 square

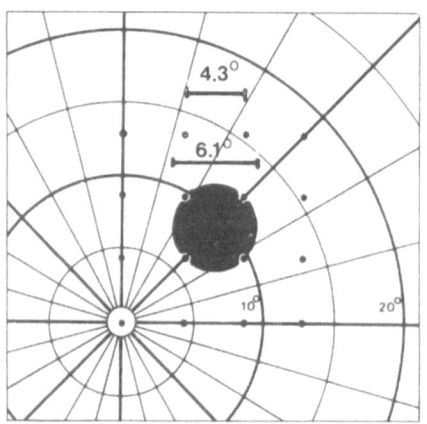

Fig. 2
Grid of stimulus positions with a mutual distance of 4.3° (150 positions in 30° field); a defect of 6.4° diameter has a 100% chance of detection.

degrees (4.3° × 4.3°) if the stimuli are punctate; if 100 positions are examined there is one examined position per 26 square degrees (5.3° × 5.3°) and if 50 positions are examined there is one examined position per 56 square degrees

102

(7.5° × 7.5°). In a grid with meshes of 4.3° × 4.3° the chance of detecting a defect with a diameter of 6.1° is 100%; this is the case if 150 positions are examined (see Fig. 2). As the diameter of the defect becomes smaller the chance of detection decreases, as shown in Tables I and II.

TABLE II

Chance of detection (in %) of visual field defects in the 30°-field if 150 locations are examined (depending on stimulus-diameter).

defect diameter ↓	stimulus-diameter			
	0	1′	10′	30′
6°	99.9	99.9	100	100
5°	92.5	92.7	92.7	92.7
4°	66.7	67.2	72.3	83.0
3°	37.5	37.9	41.8	51.0
2°	16.7	16.9	19.6	27.0
1°	4.2	4.3	5.7	9.4

Size of stimulus.

The chance of detection depends not only upon the number and distribution of the examination positions but also upon the size of the stimulus. As has already been shown limitations are set to the size of the stimulus by the size of the area of spatial summation. Table II shows how the chance of detection increases with the size of the stimulus. If 150 positions are examined with a stimulus diameter of 10′ the chance of detecting a circular defect of 3° diameter is 41.8%. A choice must be made between the increased chance of detection resulting from the increased diameter of the stimulus (i.e. smaller meshes in the grid), and the decreased chance of detection because the diameter of the stimulus exceeds the area of spatial summation. As the data from the detection phase should be comparable with the data from the assessment phase the size of the stimulus should preferably be the same in both phases. The size of stimulus used is thus limited by the assessment phase, for which a diameter of 10 minutes has been chosen.

The probability of missing a defect is further diminished by the fact that an area of decreased sensitivity is often found round a small defect of great intensity. The detection of part of this surrounding relative defect leads to the discovery of the smaller nucleus with greater intensity.

103

Size of defect.

When deciding upon the necessary spatial accuracy in perimetry the size of the defect which one is trying to detect is an important factor. If all defects had a diameter of 10° it would be senseless to place 150 stimuli within the 30° parallel. As the information about spatial interaction in an around small visual field defects is rather limited, it is on theoretical grounds difficult to decide upon the minimum diameter of a defect. Nor is it known whether functional loss occurs in one single nerve fibre in glaucoma, or whether a group of nerve fibres is always involved. In practice it appears that in glaucoma the smallest visual field defects usually have a diameter of at least 3°, when the examination is accurate to 1 degree. Smaller defects may be found, mainly in the paracentral area, but these defects are difficult to reproduce (partly on account of the physiological fixation nystagmus).[7] We shall therefore confine ourselves to defects with a minimum diameter of 3°.

Conclusion about number and position.

From Table I it appears that, in order to have a 100% chance of detecting a defect with a diameter of 3°, 452 positions would have to be examined in the 30° visual field, using punctate stimuli. In a routine examination it is difficult to put such a large number into practice. As an acceptable compromise which gives a good chance of detection we have chosen 150 positions with a stimulus diameter of 10 minutes. Taking into consideration the increasing size of the areas of spatial summation when moving from the centre to the periphery under photopic conditions, we decided to distribute the 150 positions as shown in Fig. 3.

Static and kinetic perimetry in the detection phase.

Because of the fundamental limitations of kinetic perimetry for the detection of visual field defects, static perimetry is to be preferred for the visual field within the 30° parallel. The problem is then to investigate 150 positions, either in one or in two phases, by means of static perimetry.

If the number of examination positions is not reduced and the principle of threshold measurement is maintained, there are only two possible ways to reduce the length of time needed for this part of the detection phase. Either the steps of luminance can be enlarged or a number of stimuli can be presented

---

[7] see example in Chapter XI.

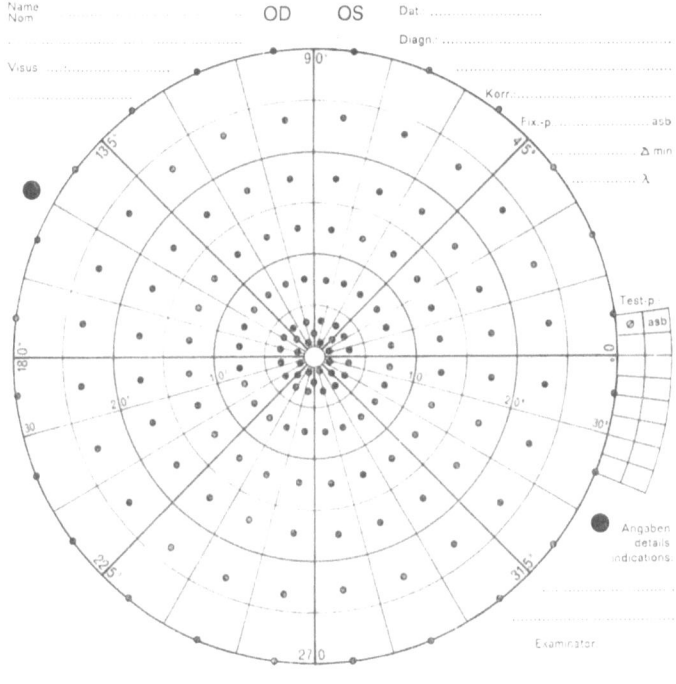

Fig. 3
150 stimulus positions in 30° visual field.

simultaneously. These two possibilities will be discussed later and a conclusion will be drawn with respect to the detection phase in the 30° visual field.[8]

The detection phase, as carried out in our clinic, also includes the kinetic examination of the periphery and the kinetic examination of the blind spot (Fig. 4). An isopter is drawn at the extreme periphery and another between the extreme periphery and the 30° parallel. In the temporal visual field a partial intermediate isopter may be added between these two. For the periphery kinetic perimetry is chosen because the most important early glaucomatous defects are seldom found in the periphery and because the optics of the eye and the structure of the peripheral visual system make accurate perimetry there less essential. Kinetic perimetry is by far the most suitable method for the examination of the extreme periphery.

In the detection phase the blind spot is also better examined kinetically. As is well known the examination of the blind spot gives information about the

---

[8] Chapter VIII.

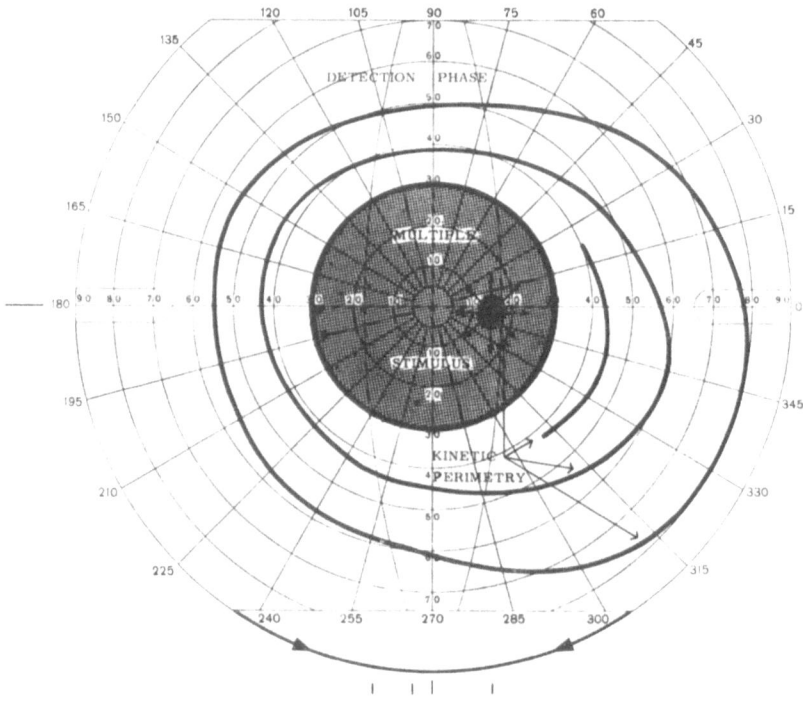

Fig. 4

Detection phase: multiple stimulus perimetry in the 30° visual field; kinetic perimetry of the periphery and the blind spot.

reliability of the patient's reactions and his ability to fixate. The position of the blind spot indicates whether the fixation is central or not.

Our detection phase does not differ from the procedures described in the literature as far as the periphery and the blind spot are concerned. The difference between our detection procedure and others (as far as these have a separate detection phase) lies in the number and position of the stimuli in the 30° visual field, and in the actual use of static threshold measurements for the examination.

Subdivision of detection phase.

In the interests of efficiency subdivision of the detection phase into two phases has been found helpful. In phase IA 50 stimuli distributed over the visual field are presented. Obviously the spatial accuracy of phase IA is limited. The great advantage of this separation is that, if large visual field defects are found in phase IA, further extension of the detection phase is not necessary. This saves 60% of the examination time. If few or no defects are found in phase IA the examination is completed by phase IB (100 stimuli), by means of which spatial accuracy is increased and the chance of missing a small defect is decreased proportionally.

Two separate halves of the visual field.

When examining the visual fields of glaucoma patients one does well to remember that two separate halves of the visual field are to be investigated: the upper and the lower half, separated by the horizontal meridian. Often the extent of the defects in the two halves is markedly different. If a large defect is found in one half of the visual field phase IA will be sufficient for this half, while in the other half a complete detection phase will be needed. The reason for carrying out the complete detection phase when a large defect has already been found in phase IA is as follows: to follow the progression in glaucomatous visual field defects, large defects of maximum intensity are less informative than the smaller, isolated or fragmented fibre bundle defects. The follow-up of early, small and relative defects gives us more information on progression or regression of the disease and thus on the effect of therapy. It is therefore important to look for them.

Repeat examination.

Many authors distinguish between the first visual field examination and subsequent ones. In a repeat examination it should be sufficient to investigate whether the known defects have changed. It is advisable, however, not to omit the detection phase, as new defects may have developed in the period between two examinations. If only the known defects are re-examined at the repeat examination, these new defects will be overlooked. The duration of the repeat examination, both in the detection and the assessment phase, will be shorter than in the first examination, because on the basis of the known facts the examination can be more efficient.

Static and kinetic perimetry in visual field defects.

As it is probable that the perception of static stimuli in the occipital cortex involves other units than the perception of kinetic stimuli, one may wonder if visual field defects exist in which one of these functions is specifically affected. This phenomenon has been described by RIDDOCH: in a number of patients

107

with occipital lesions he found that the visual field defects appeared to be larger for static stimuli than for kinetic stimuli; in an area where a static stimulus was not observed a kinetic stimulus could be seen[9]. RIDDOCH considered that this dissociation of functions was mainly associated with occipital lesions.

The existence of RIDDOCH's phenomenon has recently been confirmed, but the two patients described had lesions of the optic tract and chiasma[10]. It was suggested that a relationship exists between this phenomenon and disturbances in local adaptation. In some patients with neurological disorders we have also observed a discrepancy between the static and kinetic results. As far as we know this discrepancy does not occur in glaucomatous visual fields, unless it is the fundamental discrepancy between static and kinetic perimetry, which we have already pointed out[11].

Assessment phase.

If no defects have been found by the detection procedure described above further examination is not necessary. If, however, there is an indication in the detection phase that a visual field defect exists, this is followed by the assessment phase.

Visual field examination is the *quantitative* investigation of the *topography* of the light sensitivity of the visual system. The light sensitivity is expressed quantitatively in logarithmic units of luminance. The reduction of light sensitivity, i.e. the intensity of a defect, is also expressed in logarithmic units of luminance[12]. In addition to the intensity of the defects the topography should also be recorded, i.e. the position, shape and extent.

In order to register both topography and intensity accurately, static and kinetic perimetry must be combined, as was originally advised by AULHORN & HARMS[13]. The reason for not using kinetic perimetry alone has already been given in previous chapters. In addition, the accurate assessment of a defect using steps of 0.5 log unit is not really possible. The small details of some types of defects cannot be registered accurately by means of kinetic perimetry, even if steps of 0.1 log unit are used. In the second phase kinetic perimetry is mainly useful as the method which provides a relatively rapid survey of the topography of the defects for a given stimulus. It should be realized, however, that the data

---

[9] RIDDOCH, 1917.

[10] ZAPPIA et al., 1971.

[11] see also example in Chapter XI.

[12] see Chapter X.

[13] AULHORN & HARMS, 1967.

108

from kinetic perimetry do not provide direct information about the intensity of a defect; this intensity depends not only on the luminance of the stimulus but also on the position of the isopter traced with this stimulus.

In the literature so far attention has mainly been paid to the topography of defects. Little is known about the intensity of defects, or about the character- istic distribution of the intensity at various points on a meridian. The main reason for this is the limited use of static perimetry. Publications in which the examination of glaucomatous defects by means of static perimetry are described have only appeared in the last few years.

The accuracy of static perimetry, which is fundamentally greater than that of kinetic perimetry, is further accentuated in practice. The use of small steps of luminance (0.1 log unit) and small spatial steps results in accurate registration of the intensity of a defect. With static perimetry the intensity of a defect can be examined degree by degree. This examination is usually carried out along a meridian, along a parallel or parts of a parallel, or parallel to a meridian (Fig. 5)[14]. In this way a vertical section through the defect is obtained. This method

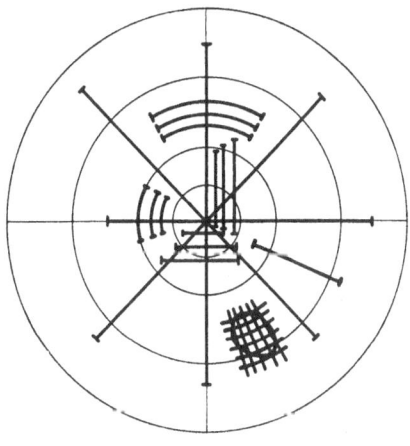

Fig. 5
Possible static perimetric examinations in phase II.

of examination gives a completely different picture of the defects from that obtained with kinetic perimetry[15]. For accurate assessment of regression or pro- gression of a defect static perimetry is the method of choice. For the investiga-

---

[14] after HARMS, 1969.
[15] see Chapter XI.

tion of the central visual field kinetic perimetry is not satisfactory. Reduction in light sensitivity, especially in the central visual field, can be restricted to a very small area. Small defects can hardly be detected without the help of static perimetry. In the assessment phase static perimetry is indispensable in cases of[16]:

1. defects in which areas of very different intensity are found close to each other (sieve-like defects);
2. small defects;
3. paracentral defects;
4. slowly progressing defects;
5. defects of slight intensity.

All these defects may occur in glaucomatous visual fields. Static perimetry does not replace kinetic perimetry in the assessment phase; the two methods supplement each other.

In practice, from the data obtained in the detection phase a meridian or part of a meridian is chosen, along which static perimetry is performed.

It should be emphasized that the choice of the positions to be examined in this phase is completely different from the choice in the detection phase. The spatial accuracy at the site of the defect is much greater than in the detection phase. The selected area is examined degree by degree, while in the detection phase the stimuli are evenly distributed over the whole visual field within the 30° parallel.

Depending upon the intensity of the defect which has been found in the static examination, a suitable stimulus luminance is chosen for kinetic perimetry. In Chapter XI this point will be illustrated. As a rule the use of a maximum luminance and a 'critical luminance' is sufficient; the results represent the maximum extent and the relative extent of the defect. If necessary a second critical luminance may be added. In this way kinetic perimetry provides a general picture of the topography and static perimetry supplies accurate registration of the intensity.

---

[16] see also AULHORN & HARMS, 1967.

CHAPTER VI

THREE INSTRUMENTS FOR SINGLE STIMULUS VISUAL FIELD
EXAMINATION

The Goldmann perimeter
The Tübinger perimeter
The Double Projection Campimeter

In this chapter a short description and critical discussion will be given of the three instruments for kinetic and static visual field examination used in our department: the Goldmann perimeter (GP); the Tübinger perimeter (TP); and the Double Projection Campimeter (DPC).

The Goldmann perimeter is well known and is used all over the world. The Tübinger perimeter is becoming better known but its use is mainly restricted to specialized ophthalmological and neurological centres. The DPC is a modification of SCHOBER's[1] projector devised by HAGEDOORN & VAN DEN BOSCH[2].

The DPC is not on the market, but as a number of patients have been examined with this instrument it will also be described here. The descriptions given are not intended as instructions for the use of the three instruments, but as a survey of their specific advantages, disadvantages and practical application[3].

The physical properties of the stimuli and their standardization are determined by the instrument which is used for the visual field examination. The instrument will be judged on the accuracy with which the stimulation takes place, on the

---

[1] SCHOBER, 1949.

[2] HAGEDOORN & VAN DEN BOSCH, 1955.

[3] For the Netherlands and the Flemish-speaking part of Belgium we have published detailed instructions for the use of the Goldmann perimeter (GREVE & VERRIEST, 1971).

choice of the parameters which determine the stimulation, on the ease of operation of the instrument and the length of time needed for the examination.

The three instruments will be discussed on the basis of the physical properties of the stimulation[4].

THE GOLDMANN PERIMETER.

The Goldmann perimeter was originally built for kinetic perimetry and has

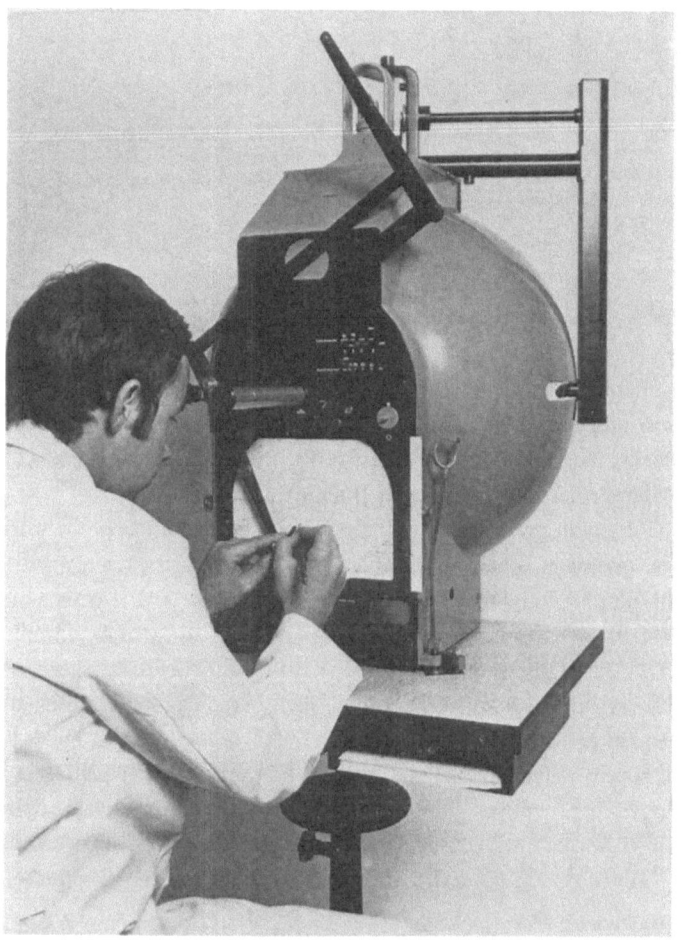

Fig. 1
Goldmann perimeter.

---

[4] see Chapter II.

been adapted for static perimetry (Fig. 1)[5]. The GP consists of a hemisphere of radius 30 cm, on to which a stimulus can be projected at any desired point. The position of the stimulus in the hemisphere is registered by means of an ingenious transmission mechanism on the perimetric chart. The stability of the transmission mechanism and the size of the chart determine the precision of the positioning. The GP is less stable than the TP and the DPC but its stability is sufficient for the requirements of kinetic perimetry. For static perimetry the positioning and, more especially, the stability are not ideal. Slight movements of the subject or of the investigator result in movements of the projector.

Chart: the GP has one chart for kinetic perimetry which covers nearly the whole of the visual field[6]. 90 degrees are spread over 108 mm. One degree of eccentricity in the visual field is thus represented by 1.2 mm on the chart. This is sufficient for the peripheral visual field (outside the 30° parallel) but not for the 30° visual field. Exact positioning in this part of the visual field is desirable and modifications for this purpose have been described but are not generally available[7].

The chart of the GP for static perimetry covers a total area of 60° on both sides of the centre[8]. The abscissa gives the eccentricity and the ordinate the threshold luminance (ΔL) in log units decreasing from below upwards, so that in fact the light sensitivity ($\frac{L}{\Delta L}$; increasing from below upwards) is recorded. A difference of 0.1 log unit (one step) on the ordinate corresponds with 2 degrees on the abscissa (1:2). On the TP chart one luminance step corresponds with one degree (1:1); the result of this is that the sensitivity curve on the GP chart is steeper than on the TP chart, even when the gradient of sensitivity in the two cases is more or less the same. The difference is in the graphical representation because the ratio between the luminance steps and the spatial steps is different in the two cases.

Background: The inside of the hemisphere, which forms the perimetric background, is sprayed in a neutral off-white tint with a coefficient of reflection of approximately 0.7[9]. The background is illuminated using the principle of Ulbricht's sphere, by the lamp which also serves as the source of light for the

[5] HAAG-STREIT, Bern, see for description also GOLDMANN, 1945, 1946; FANKHAUSER & RÖHLER, 1967; VERRIEST & ISRAEL, 1965.

[6] see fig. 7, Chapter VII.

[7] SCHMIDT et al., 1961.

[8] see fig. 3, Chapter VII.

[9] see for spectral reflection curve: VERRIEST & ISRAEL, 1965.

stimuli. This light source is an Osram lamp[10]. The luminance of the background does not vary more than 1% over the whole surface.

Stimulus: The luminance of the stimuli can be regulated by means of neutral density filters. These filters are neither entirely neutral nor completely uniform, but these variations are not significant for perimetry.

The maximum luminance of the stimuli is standardized at 1000 asb (316 cd.m^{-2}). The standard GP for kinetic perimetry has 3 neutral density filters which reduce the luminance by 0.5, 1.0 and 1.5 log units respectively. The modification of the GP for static perimetry is supplied with an additional series of four neutral density filters, which allow luminance steps of 0.1, 0.2, 0.3 and 0.4 log units. The resulting luminance values, expressed in apostilb, are given in Table I.

TABLE I

Luminance values of the Goldmann perimeter

	4	3	2	1	steps
lux	1430	450	143	45	3,1
asb	1000	315	100	31,5	3,1
cd/m²	315	100	31,5	10	3,1
$\dfrac{\Delta L}{L}$	±30	10	3	1	3,1
log L asb	3	2,5	2 2	1,5	0,5

Background: 31,5 asb. = 10 cd/m².
Coëfficient of reflection 0,7.

$(1 \text{ asb} = \dfrac{1}{\pi} \text{ cd/m}^2)$.

The GP has stimuli of 6 different sizes, with normal values of: 1/16 mm² (stim 0), 1/4 mm² (stim I), 1 mm² (stim II), 4 mm² (stim III), 16 mm² (stim IV) and 64 mm² (stim V). The stimuli are projected at an angle of 45° so that the lengths of the axes are in the ratio of $1/\sqrt{2}$ (1/1.414). Measurements of the real size of the stimuli are recorded in Table II[11].

---

[10] the Osram lamp has a spectral energy distribution corresponding to a black body of 2885° K (at 5.3V) or 2850° K (at 6V). If a different lamp is used this figure may rise to 3025° K (VERRIEST & ISRAEL, 1965).

[11] according to FANKHAUSER & RÖHLER, 1967.

TABLE II

Real values of the sizes of the stimuli of the Goldmann perimeter

Target	Nominal area	Measured dimensions on cupola		Measure area
		long axis	short axis	
0	0.0625 mm²	0.33 mm	0.23 mm	0.059 mm²
I	0.25	0.67	0.47	0.249
II	1.0	1.34	0.94	0.97
III	4.0	2.68	1.89	3.89
IV	16.0	5.35	3.78	16.0
V	64.0	10.70	7.56	63.2

The GP is standardized by means of a luxmeter (Metrawatt AG). The graduated scale of the luxmeter is adapted to the largest size of stimulus of the GP. The maximum luminance of the stimulus is set at 1000 asb by means of a variable resistance.

The background luminance is standardized by visual comparison with a stimulus luminance of 31.5 asb. If desired the background luminance can be reduced to 0.01 asb.

The steps of luminance and size of the stimuli, 0.5 and 0.6 log units respectively, were chosen by GOLDMANN because he thought that, within certain limits and under the conditions of his perimeter, a value of 0.83 (0.5/0.6) held for the coefficient of spatial summation.

An increase in size from stimulus I to stimulus II, etc., represented the same increase in stimulation as an increase in luminance of one step (0.5 lu).

It has become apparent however, that the value of 0.83 for the coefficient of spatial summation is subject to great individual variation[12]. In any particular case the increase in stimulation on enlargement of the stimulus cannot be deducted from this value.

For static perimetry the stimulus is presented by hand for 1 second. The luminance is increased by means of two handles, a rather complicated manoeuvre, especially in comparison with the semi-automatic luminance control of the TP.

The examiner alone determines speed and direction of movement. The problems in this connection have already been extensively discussed.[13] The pantograph of the GP has excellent motility in all directions. To change from kinetic to static perimetry with the GP, reconstruction of the pantograph is necessary, and a different perimetric chart is required (Fig. 2).

---

[12] see Chapter IV; Spatial interaction and visual field examination.
[13] see Chapter IV.

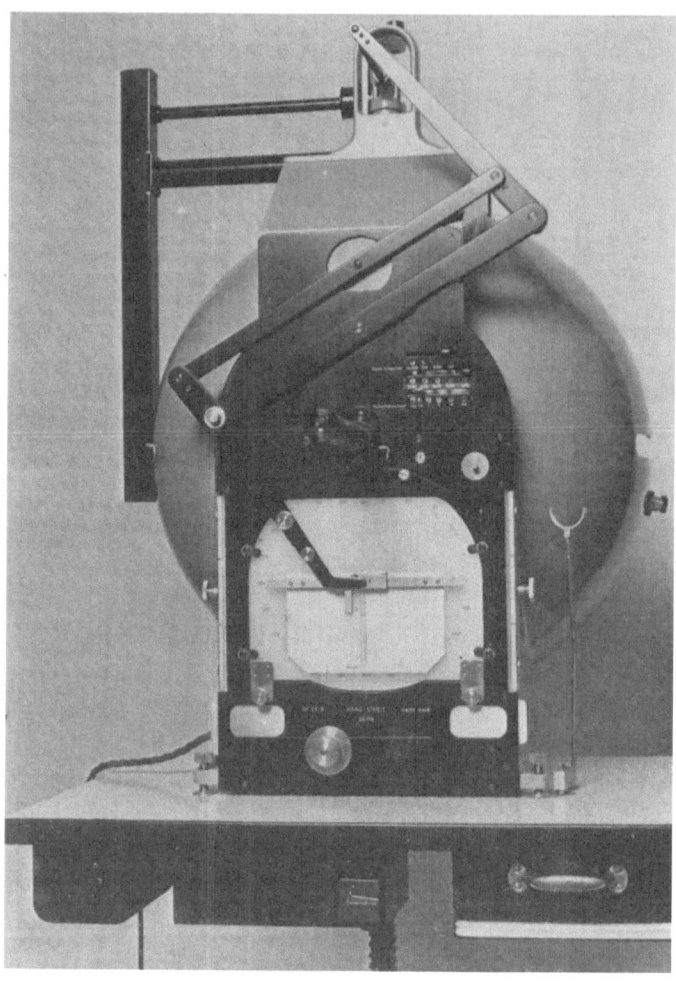

Fig. 2
Goldmann perimeter equipped for static perimetry.

Fixation control: The GP is equipped with a good telescope for control of fixation. This telescope perforates the dome at the centre. At the same point the fixation target, in two different sizes, is situated. This construction makes it impossible to examine an area of 2° round the fixation point. In order to examine the central and paracentral light sensitivity an accessory fixation object projector must be used.

Conclusion: the Goldmann perimeter is a standardized instrument, preeminently suitable for kinetic visual field examination. A greater cartographic accuracy in the 30° visual field would be preferable. It is quite possible to carry out static perimetry with the Goldmann perimeter, but it is a fairly circumstantial procedure and therefore time-consuming. Static visual field examination can be carried out more easily with the TP or the DPC. For further comparison of the three instruments see Table III.

THE TÜBINGER PERIMETER.

The TP was specially developed for static perimetry (Fig.3)[14]. In its original form the TP could be used for several other investigations besides kinetic and static perimetry: adaptometry, adaptoperimetry, investigation of the c.f.f., peripheral visual acuity, sensitivity to glare, colour perimetry[15].

In the TP, as in the GP, the background is formed by a hemisphere which is evenly illuminated according to the principle of Ulbricht's sphere. A stimulus can be projected anywhere in this hemisphere. The transmission mechanism is extremely stable, as is the whole construction of the perimeter. Positioning is carried out by means of a small light which is projected onto the back of the chart.

Chart: One of the great advantages of the TP is that two different charts can be used with this instrument[16]. One chart covers the whole 90° (radius) visual field and there is a separate chart for the 30° visual field. Both charts have a radius of 20 mm. This means that on the 90° chart one degree is represented by 1 mm and on the 30° chart one degree is represented by 3 mm. The latter chart allows great cartographic accuracy in the important central and intermediate visual field and is of particular significance for static perimetry. The change from 90° chart to 30° can be made, by simple transposition of the transmission ratio projector-chart.

Background: The background luminance of the TP is 10 asb (3.15 cd.m^{-2}). The background, as in the GP, is sprayed with off-white diffusely reflecting paint. The reflection coefficient is 0.8 for 425 nm and rises evenly throughout the spectrum up to 0.93 for 800 nm. By means of neutral density filters[17] any desired

---

[14] Firm Oculus, Dutenhofen, HARMS 1960.

[15] see also SLOAN, 1971.

[16] see fig. 4, Chapter VII.

[17] the results of measurements of the transmission of these filters will be published in the Proceedings of the 2nd Symposium of the Int. Research Group on Colour Vision Deficiences (VERRIEST, PADMOS, GREVE, 1973).

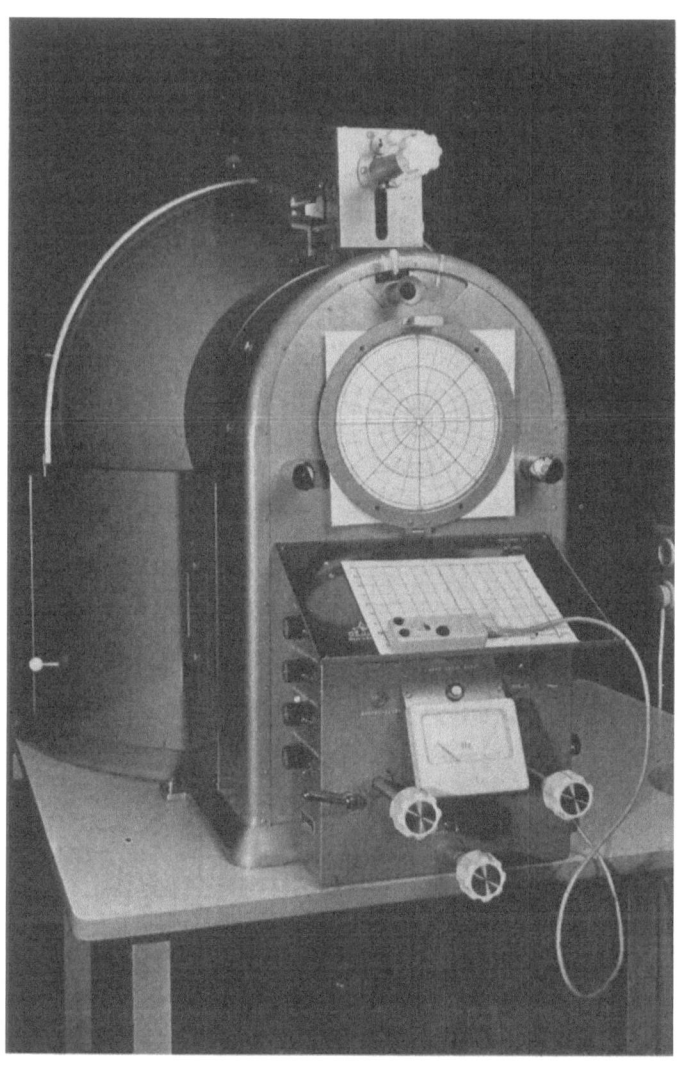

Fig. 3
Tübinger perimeter

level of the background luminance from 10 to 0 asb can be obtained. In the standard model filters of 1 log unit are included. (In the GP the background luminance cannot be reduced to less than 0.01 asb). The light source for the background luminance is an incandescent lamp.

Stimulus: Unlike the GP the TP has separate light sources for background

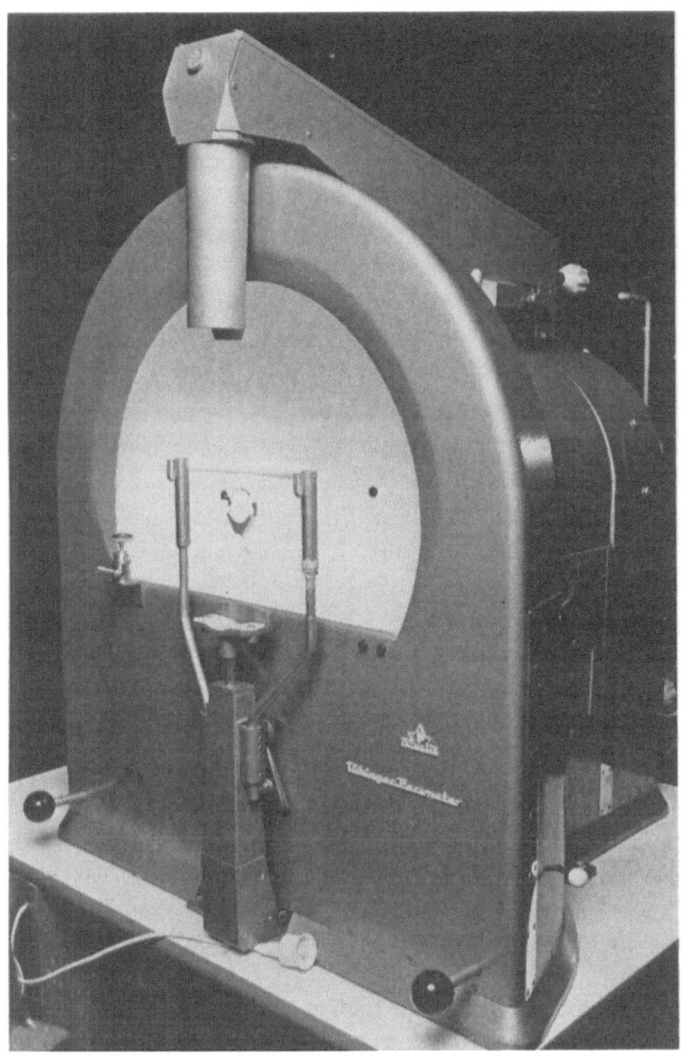

Fig. 3
Tübinger perimeter; patients side

and stimulus. Both sources are stabilized. The maximum luminance of the
stimuli is 1000 asb and this can be reduced by means of two series of neutral
filters through 8 log units. The discs in which these filters are mounted are
electrically driven, so that the luminance can be changed by merely flicking
over two switches, the movement of a finger.

These switches, together with a button for stimulus presentation, are mounted on a small switchboard, which can be held in the hand. This semi-automatic remote control makes static perimetry easier and quicker. Standardization of the luminance of the background and the stimulus is performed with a luminancemeter, specially developed for the TP, by means of visual comparison with a standard luminance of 10 asb.

The TP has stimuli of 8 different sizes, which subtend angles of 7′, 10′, 12′, 18′, 27′, 44′, 69′ and 116′. The size of the steps between these stimuli (with the exception of the 10′ stimulus) is approximately 0.2 log unit, i.e. a surface increase of 0.4 log unit (the steps vary between 0.34 and 0.46). Unlike the GP the TP stimuli are round.

The presentation time is regulated by an electromagnetic shutter and can be varied from 0.1 to 1 second. The stimulus time can also be regulated by hand.

Movement of the stimulus, in kinetic perimetry, is obtained by turning a knob. The TP is constructed in such a way that turning the knob produces movement of the stimulus in a radial direction. If circular movement of the stimulus is desired, i.e. movement along a parallel, the whole (heavy) arm must be turned. All other directions of movement must be built up from a combination of these radial and circular movements. These combined movements are not as easy to perform as with the GP. It is again apparent that the two perimeters were not developed with the same object in view: the TP was constructed for static perimetry and emphasis is laid on accurate stable stimulus presentation on one meridian; the GP was constructed for kinetic perimetry and its strong point is easy movement of the stimulus in all directions.

It may be emphasized once more that both instruments can be used for kinetic as well as for static perimetry. The only differences are the accuracy and the ease with which the two methods of examination can be performed with the TP and the GP.

Fixation control: In the TP the fixation is controlled through a hole in the hemisphere, which is placed at the site of the blind spot in the visual field. By rotating the hemisphere through 180° the hole is changed from the right hand side to the left hand side. The centre of the hemisphere is thus available for measurements of the central and paracentral light sensitivity. The TP possesses a series of fixation lights varying in size and luminance, which are projected onto the centre of the hemisphere. The luminance of the fixation light can be altered in steps of 0.2 log unit and its colour may also be altered by means of coloured filters. We always use a red fixation light. The size of the fixation light varies between 10′, 30′, 1°, 2° and 4°; for the examination of the central light sensitivity four lights with a mutual distance of 2° or 5° can be chosen.

The DPC was developed by HAGEDOORN & VAN DEN BOSCH[18] on the basis of Schober's projector[19] and modified by CRONE and GREVE[20] (Fig. 4).

The purpose was to construct a standardized projection campimeter for accurate examination of the central and intermediate visual fild. The advantages of the DPC are the simple, stable mechanism for the transmission of the position of the stimulus on the background to the chart, and the greater distance between the eye and the background.

In the system of double projection, one projector projects the stimulus onto the background of the campimeter and a second projector projects a ray of light onto the chart. The two projectors are connected by a construction without hinges.

The DPC combines the advantages of the standardized conditions of the GP with the accurate registration of a 2-metre campimeter. The DPC cannot be used to examine the peripheral visual field.

Chart: As well as the simple and stable transmission mechanism the size of the chart contributes to the accuracy of the registration. One degree covers an area of approximately 2.5 mm. This means that the position can be determined accurately to a half degree. Greater cartographic accuracy than this has no significance in visual field examination.

Background: The patient's eye is at a distance of 185 cm from the background, which is formed by a flat screen of 230×230 cm. The coefficient of reflection of the white screen is 0.8. Uniform illumination of the background is provided by fluorescent tubes, fitted at the sides of the projector; illumination is regulated by altering the openings in front of the fluorescent tubes. The illumination is standardized at 40 lux, the background luminance is then 32 asb. The fixation light is projected onto this background.

Stimulus: The stimulus projector is above the patient's head. The source of light is a Philips lamp, which gives a maximum luminance of 315 asb ($100\ cd.m^{-2}$). Standardization is carried out with an AEG luxmeter. The luminance can be regulated in steps of 0.05 log unit by means of a neutral wedge; in routine practice steps of 0.1 log unit are used. There are three different sizes of stimulus: 10', 30' and 60'. The 10' stimulus is used for routine examination with both the kinetic and the static methods. The stimulus can be moved freely in all direc-

---

[18] HAGEDOORN & VAN DEN BOSCH, 1955.

[19] SCHOBER, 1949.

[20] unpublished modifications.

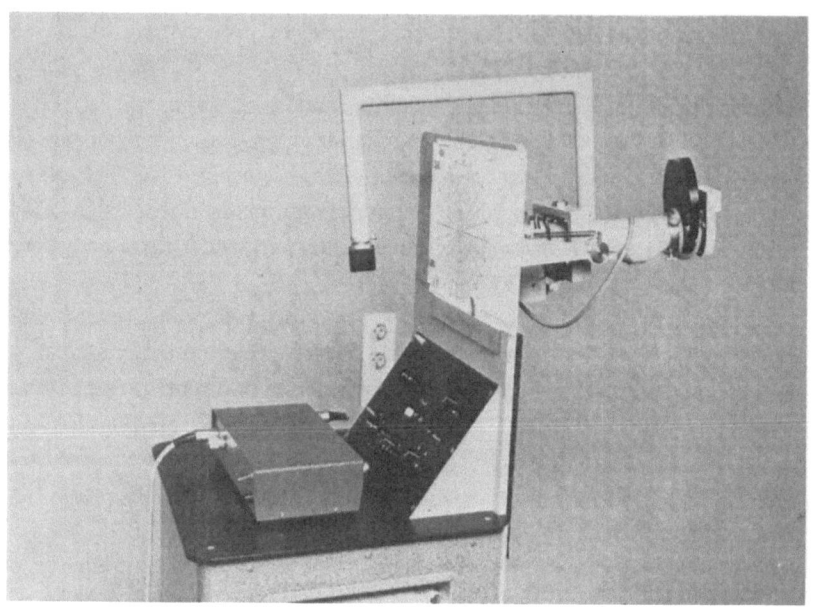

Fig. 4a
Double Projection Campimeter.

tions, so that kinetic campimetry is easy and quick. For static campimetry the stimulus is presented for 0.5 second by means of a Compur shutter. The switch from static to kinetic campimetry requires no adjustments.

Fixation control: The fixationlight (or lights) is projected onto the background. The construction of the DPC, whereby the examiner stands behind the patient, makes control of the patient's fixation rather difficult; this is a disadvantage in comparison with the GP and TP.

Our conclusion is that the DPC is a well standardized projection campimeter for kinetic and static perimetry. The instrument is as accurate as the 2-metre campimeter: movement of the eye backwards and forwards has little effect on the results; there is less accommodation strain and less correction necessary than with the perimeters. We mainly use the DPC to supplement the results obtained with the Goldmann perimeter from the central and intermediate visual field. The normal kinetic and static visual fields obtained with these instruments will be described in Chapter VII.

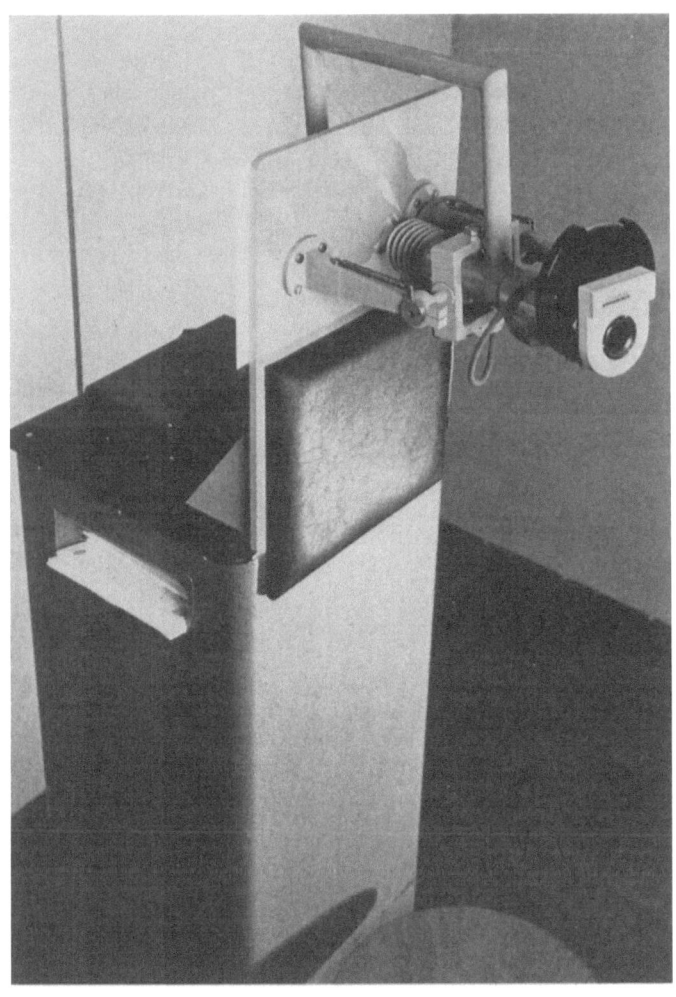

Fig. 4b
Double Projection Campimeter

TABLE III

Comparison of data of Goldmann perimeter, Tübinger perimeter, Double Projection Campimeter and Visual Field Analyser.

	Goldmann perimeter radius 90°	Tübinger perimeter radius 90°	Double Projection Campimeter radius 30°	Visual Field Analyser* radius 25°
distance eye-background	30 cm	33 cm	185 cm	33 cm
projection mechanism	not very stable	very stable	very stable	
possible positions	all within 90° (60° for static perimetry)	all within 90°	all within 30°	46 fixed positions within 25°
cartographic exactness	1° = 1.2 mm	periphery 1°= 1 mm central: 1°= 3 mm	1° = 2.5 mm	maximum; no positioning
background luminance	31.5 asb = 10 cd/m²	10 asb = 3.15 cd/m²	31.5 asb = 10 cd/m²	0.5 asb = 0.16 cd/m²
maximum stimulus luminance	1000 asb = 315 cd/m²	1000 asb = 315 cd/m²	315 asb = 100 cd/m²	2.4 log unit above normal threshold level
possible luminance steps	0.1 log unit	0.1 log unit	0.05 log unit	0.2 log unit
changing stimulus luminance	circumstantial; two handles	easy; semi-automatic	relatively easy; non-automatic neutral wedge	circumstantial; two switches
standardization apparatus	good	good	good	difficult
standard stimulus size	ellipse 7.6′–5.4′	10′	10′	increasing from 15′30″
examination central light sensitivity	circumstantial; accessory fixation projector; change of registration mechanism	easy; only change of fixation light necessary	easy	easy
fixation control	good; telescope through centre	good; telescope through blind spot	difficult	difficult
method of examination	kinetic and static; especially kinetic	kinetic and static; especially static	kinetic and static; both methods	static
presentation time static perimetry	1 s by hand	0.5 s shutter	0.1 s shutter	± 380 μ s flash tube

* see for description of Visual Field Analyser: Chapter VIII.

CHAPTER VII

NORMAL VALUES AND NORMAL VARIATION OF THRESHOLD MEASUREMENTS

Normal values and inter-individual variation
  Kinetic perimetry with the Goldmann perimeter
  Static perimetry with the Goldmann perimeter
  Kinetic perimetry with the Tübinger perimeter
  Static perimetry with the Tübinger perimeter
  Kinetic campimetry with the Double Projection Campimeter
  Static campimetry with the Double Projection Campimeter
Intra-individual variation
  Causes of intra-individual variation
  Size of intra-individual variation
  Size of luminance steps and intra-individual variation
  Significance of defects
  Variations between successive examinations
Influence of age
  Reaction time
  Position of the eye in the orbit
  Senile miosis
  Senile lens opacities
  Senile degeneration of the visual system
  Oxygen shortage
Blind spot
  Optic disc and blind spot
  Pericecal visual field
  Size and position of the blind spot
Angioscotomata
  Normal angioscotomata
  Variation in the size of angioscotomata
  Conclusion
Cartography and visual field

As rule of thumb the absolute limits of the visual field are taken to be: 50° superior; 60° nasal; 70° inferior; 100° temporal.[1] The temporal limit of 100° is not of practical importance as 90° is the limit of the measurable area in the perimeters available. These absolute limits show individual variation.

Kinetic perimetry with the Goldmann perimeter.

The standard isopters are the I/4, I/3, I/2 and I/1 isopters. These isopters are supplied with the Goldmann perimeter on a transparent sheet of plastic and are the mean of measurements on 26 normal subjects of 20–30 years of age[2].

In Table I[3] the position of the standard isopters in eight meridians is shown in degrees (average and standard deviation).

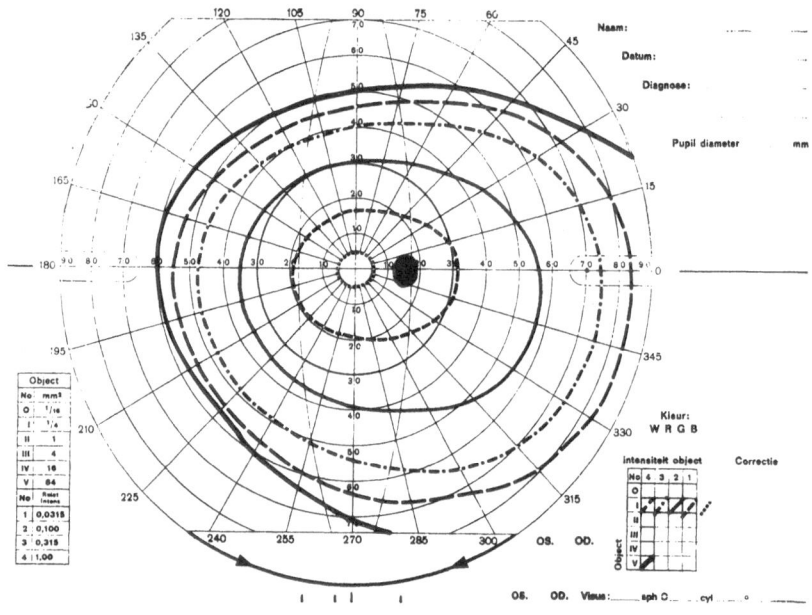

Fig. 1

Normal isopters of subjects of 20–30 years of age as measured with the Goldmann perimeter.

---

[1] The smaller extent of the nasal visual field can possibly be partly ascribed to peripheral 'amblyopia ex anopsia' (nose), SCHMIDT et al; 1971.

[2] ZEHNDER-ALBRECHT, 1950; see also VERRIEST, 1969; GALAN, 1968.

[3] ZEHNDER-ALBRECHT, 1950.

126

TABLE I
Positions of the normal isopters of the Goldmann perimeter in 8 meridians

		T 0°	TS 45°	S 90°	NS 135°	N 180°	NI 225°	I 270°	TI 315°
I/4	M	85.0	60	44.5	46.5	54.5	53.0	63.0	80.5
	sd	2.5	5.6	5.8	5.3	3.8	3.1	3.6	3.6
I/3	M	76	52.5	39	41.5	48.5	48	54	70
	sd	3.8	4.4	5.5	5.9	2.4	3.4	4.9	4.5
I/2	M	58.5	38	28.5	32	36	36	37.5	51.5
	sd	6.3	3.9	5.4	4.4	4.6	5.0	5.0	6.2
I/1	M	31.5	20	16.5	17	19.5	18.5	18.5	24.5
	sd	6.6	3.4	3.4	3.2	2.8	2.9	3.3	5.0

The greatest inter-individual variation is found in the temporal meridian where the gradient is flattest. Four times the standard deviation, i.e. 26.4°, is in this position equal to a variation of 0.5 log unit. The value of the 95% tolerance limit (2.6 × sd for 26 subjects) lies 0.3–0.4 log unit below the average kinetic sensitivity curve.

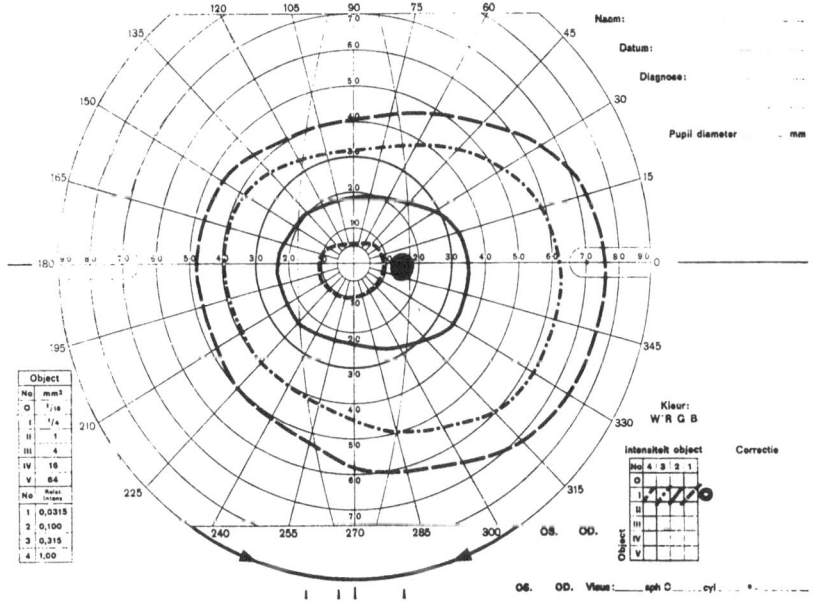

Fig. 2

Normal isopters of subjects of 60–70 years of age as measured with the Goldmann perimeter.

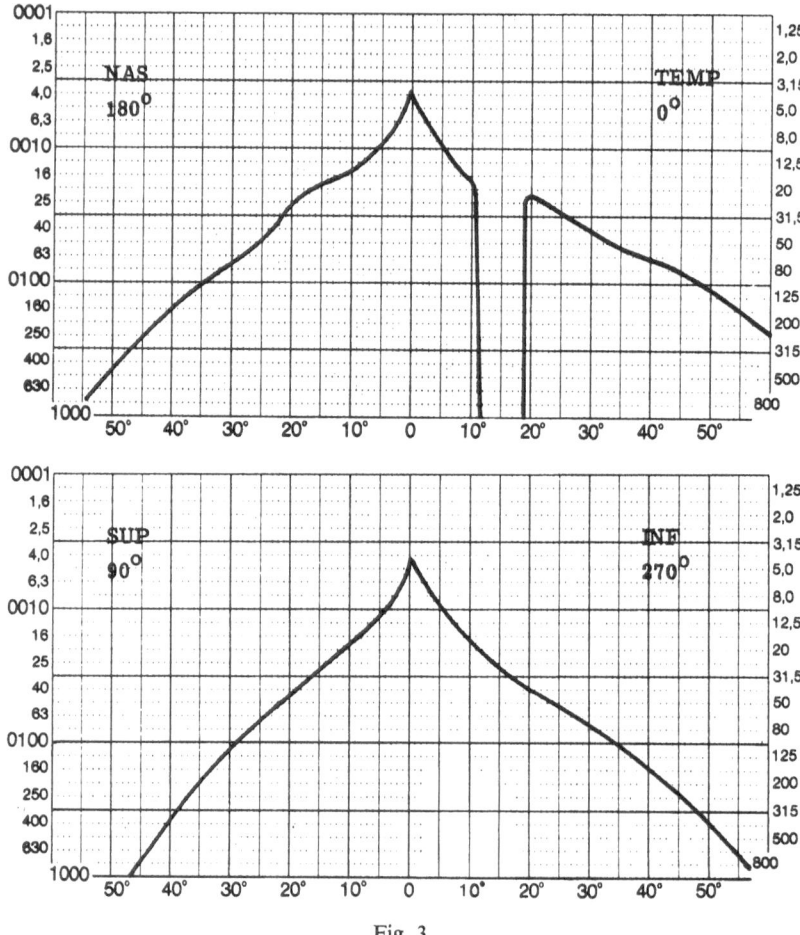

Fig. 3

Normal sensitivity curves of subjects of 20–30 years of age as measured with the Gold-mann perimeter.

The average isopters for 60–70-year-old subjects have shifted their position centripetally by ± 0.5 log unit (Fig. 2). This means that the I/3 isopter takes the place of the I/2 isopter, etc.[4].

The inter-individual variation in this older age group was found to be much greater than in the younger age group. In the older age group the position of the isopters can differ by nearly 1.0 log unit. This means that the I/4 isopter of one subject can be in the same position as the I/2 isopter of another subject. From Table I it can be seen that the variation for the I/4 and the I/3 isopter is

---

[4] see also MAZZANTINI, 1963.

128

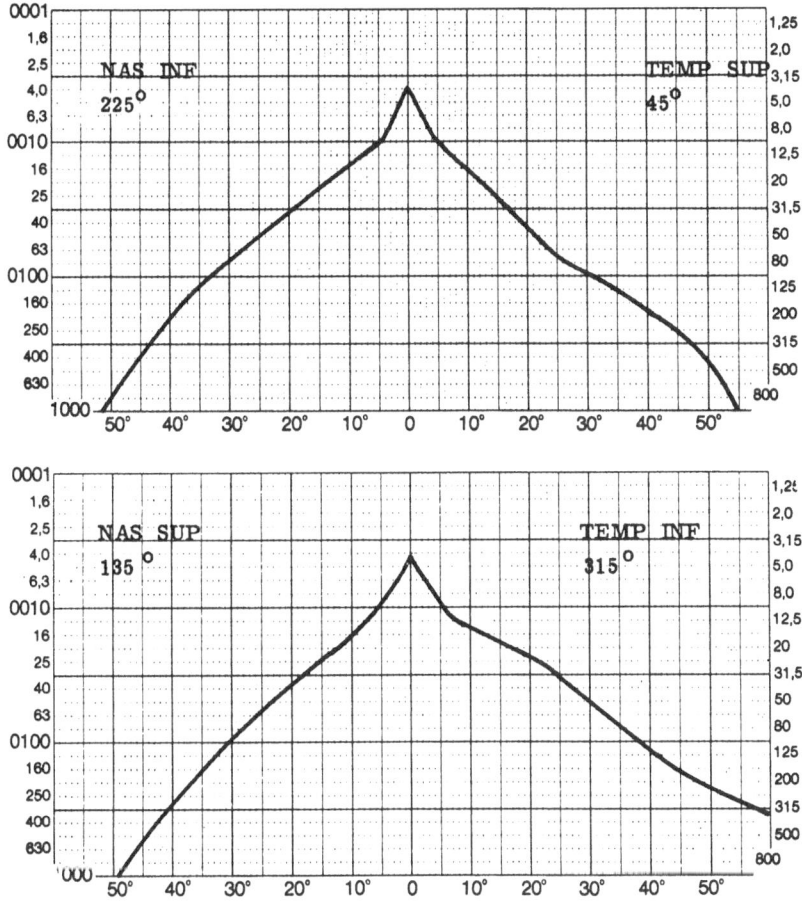

about equal, that the I/2 isopter show the greatest variation and the I/1 isopter the least variation. The I/1 isopter, which usually lies at ± 20° eccentricity, thus shows less variation than the peripheral isopters. This is in agreement with the findings in static perimetry of the central and intermediate visual field, that the variation of the threshold measurements increases towards the periphery.

Static perimetry with the Goldmann perimeter.

In Fig. 3 the average static sensitivity curves are shown on 4 meridians[5]. The

---

[5] The data on the horizontal meridian have been compiled from FANKHAUSER & SCHMIDT's results.

TABLE 1

Normal values for static threshold measurements with the Goldmann

		nasal												
		55°	50°	45°	40°	35°	30°	25°	20°	15°	10°	5°	3°	2°
19-30 years N = 25	Lowest value	2,6	2,3	2,1	2,0	1,8	1,6	1,5	1,3	1,2	1,0	0,9	0,8	0,7
	Highest value	—	—	2,8	2,5	2,4	2,3	2,0	1,9	1,9	1,8	1,6	1,3	1,2
	Mean			2,40	2,24	2,10	1,94	1,77	1,58	1,42	1,31	1,19	0,99	0,8
	Standard deviation	—	—	0,16	0,16	0,17	0,17	0,21	0,21	0,19	0,19	0,15	0,13	0,1
32-48 years N = 20	Lowest value	2,7	2,5	2,4	2,2	2,0	1,8	1,5	1,4	1,2	1,1	0,9	0,8	0,6
	Highest value	—	—	2,9	2,7	2,5	2,3	2,1	2,0	1,7	1,5	1,4	1,2	1,1
	Mean	—	—	2,66	2,47	2,29	2,10	1,87	1,67	1,46	1,32	1,19	1,01	0,9(
	Standard deviation	—	—	0,15	0,15	0,15	0,17	0,18	0,16	0,14	0,11	0,13	0,11	0,1
50-71 years N = 23	Lowest value	2,7	2,5	2,5	2,4	2,2	2,0	1,6	1,5	1,3	1,3	1,1	1,0	0,8
	Highest value	—	—	—	—	2,9	2,6	2,4	2,0	1,9	1,8	1,5	1,3	1,2
	Mean	—	—	—	—	2,48	2,27	2,03	1,82	1,56	1,39	1,23	1,06	0,9(
	Standard deviation	—	—	—	—	0,19	0,18	0,23	0,16	0,15	0,13	0,12	0,10	0,1

problem with the normal curves of older subjects is that the condition of the media cannot be assessed quantitatively. From the slit-lamp appearance of the lens the general reduction of sensitivity cannot be determined. The method of selection of the group of older subjects for static perimetry can be one of the reasons for the smaller difference between the young and old age groups as compared with the kinetic results. If the standard deviation of the old age group does not differ from the standard deviation of the young age group, this indicates that the selection of the older age group was very strict.

The difference in the position of the sensitivity curve between the young and the old age group increases from the centre to the periphery. This means that the average gradient in the older age group is steeper. The differences, however, are slight. In our experience, as soon as there is any significant lens opacity the

perimeter in three age groups; horizontal meridian; stimulus size 0.275 mm²

						temporal								
1°	0°	1°	2°	3°	5°	10°	20°	25°	30°	35°	40°	45°	50°	55°
),6	0,3	0,6	0,7	0,8	1,0	1,1	1,2	1,3	1,3	1,6	1,7	1,7	1,7	1,8
1,0	0,8	1,0	1,1	1,3	1,5	1,8	2,5	1,9	1,9	2,0	2,1	2,2	2,4	2,6
),78	0,56	0,79	0,90	0,98	1,22	1,38	1,62	1,53	1,64	1,77	1,81	1,99	2,12	2,27
),13	0,14	0,10	0,10	0,13	0,14	0,19	0,27	0,17	0,15	0,13	0,14	0,13	0,14	0,15
),5	0,5	0,7	0,8	0,8	1,0	1,2	1,4	1,4	1,5	1,6	1,7	1,8	1,9	2,2
1,0	0,8	0,9	1,0	1,1	1,4	1,5	2,7	1,8	2,0	2,2	2,3	2,4	2,6	3,0
),79	0,63	0,80	0,91	1,00	1,22	1,36	1,80	1,59	1,74	1,88	2,02	2,16	2,31	2,50
),11	0,10	0,09	0,08	0,09	0,10	0,09	0,23	0,12	0,15	0,13	0,15	0,17	0,17	0,19
),8	0,5	0,8	0,8	1,0	1,1	1,2	1,4	1,4	1,5	1,6	1,7	1,9	2,0	2,2
1,1	0,9	1,1	1,3	1,3	1,6	1,7	1,9	2,0	2,1	2,2	2,3	2,5	2,6	—
),88	0,69	0,88	0,97	1,07	1,25	1,46	1,66	1,69	1,83	1,96	2,09	2,24	2,36	—
),10	0,12	0,10	0,12	0,09	0,12	0,13	0,17	0,17	0,16	0,16	0,16	0,17	0,16	—

sensitivity curve becomes less steep. In Table II the average values for the threshold measurements on the horizontal meridian and their standard deviation are given for the young and the old age groups[6]. In the periphery the difference (0.4 log unit at 35° nasal) is in good agreement with ZEHNDER-ALBRECHT'S results. The standard deviation is seldom larger than 0.2 log unit and increases from the centre to the periphery.

Kinetic perimetry with the Tübinger perimeter.

The standard isopters for the Tübinger perimeter apply to the 10′ stimulus and luminances of 1000 asb, 100 asb, 32 asb, 10 asb, (5.0 asb) and 3.2 asb. In Table III

---

[6] compiled from the findings of VERRIEST & ISRAEL, 1965; (14 subjects, 25 eyes).

the filter positions of the normal isopters of the Tübinger perimeter are indicated as well as the corresponding isopters of the Goldmann perimeter.

The 0.0, 1.5 and 2.0 isopters are indicated on the 90° chart and the 2.0, 2.2, 2.5 and 2.7 isopters on the 30° chart. The course of these isopters is shown in Fig. 4a and b.

TABLE III

Filter position and luminance of the normal isopters of the Tübinger perimeter and corresponding isopters of the Goldmann perimeter

filter position	asb	GP
0.0	1000	I/4
1.0	100	I/3
1.5	32	I/2
2.0	10	I/1
2.5	3.2	—

Figures for standard deviation in a large group of normal subjects are not available. These will, however, be the same as those for the kinetic results with the Goldmann perimeter. It is also true for the Tübinger perimeter that the isopters of older subjects become contracted concentrically with an average contraction of 0.5 log unit. The results of the kinetic examination with the Tübinger perimeter do not differ essentially from the results of examination with the Goldmann perimeter[7].

Static perimetry with the Tübinger perimeter.

In Fig. 5 the average normal static sensitivity curves within the 30° parallel are given.[8] The difference in the course of these sensitivity curves is slight. The maximum difference between the temporal and nasal parts of the 0–180° curve is 0.2 log unit. The difference between the results in the young age group (under 40 years) and the old age group (above 60 years) varies from 0.2 to 0.3 log unit. The two average sensitivity curves are more or less parallel, a fact which is not in agreement with the results obtained by VERRIEST & ISRAEL. The selection and

---

[7] see also Chapter VI: the topographical accuracy of the Tübinger perimeter is greater than the Goldmann perimeter in the 30° visual field.

[8] based on WEEKERS (1970), and our own results. WEEKERS examined 120 subjects in three age groups (under 40 years, 40–60 years, above 60 years); there were 40 subjects in each group but only 10 subjects per meridian. The value of M $\pm$ 2.228 sd in this case does not include 95% of the normal population.

132

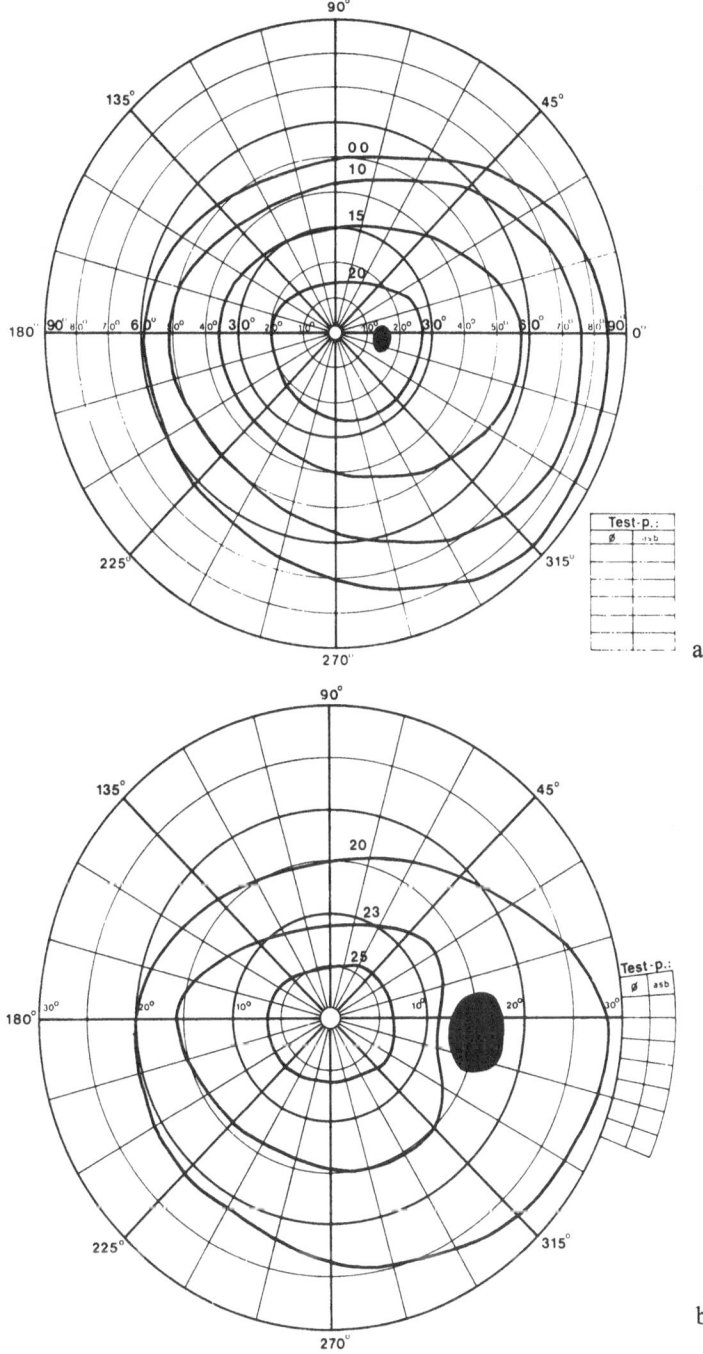

Fig. 4
Normal isopters of young subjects as measured with the Tübinger perimeter
a. 90°-field
b. 30°-field

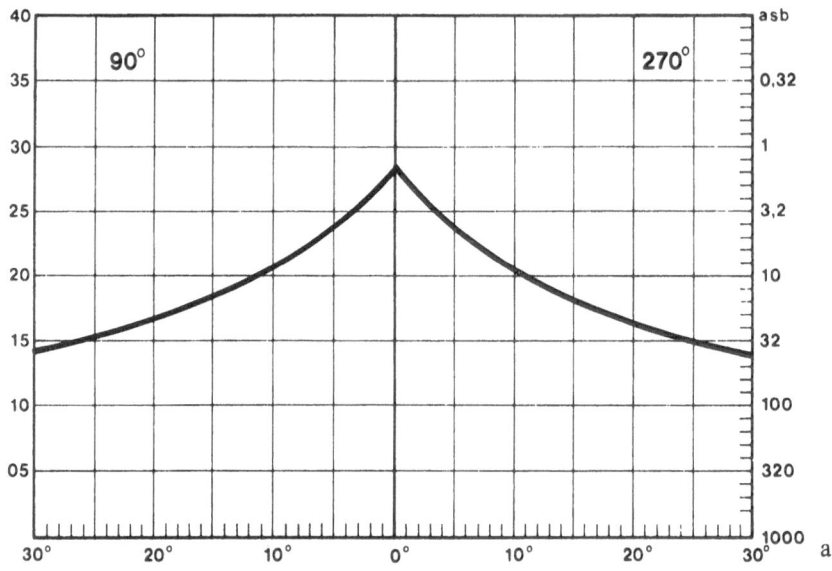

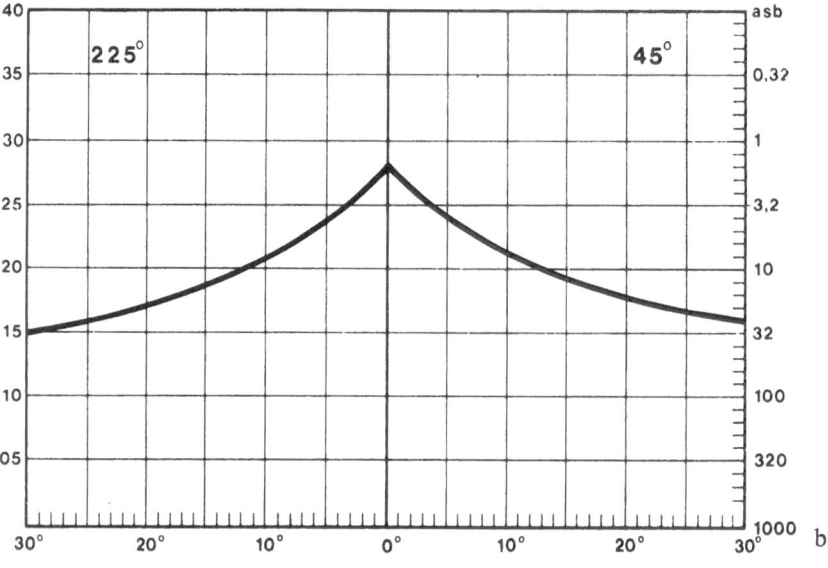

Fig. 5

Normal sensitivity curves of young subjects as measured with the Tübinger perimeter (30°-field).

134

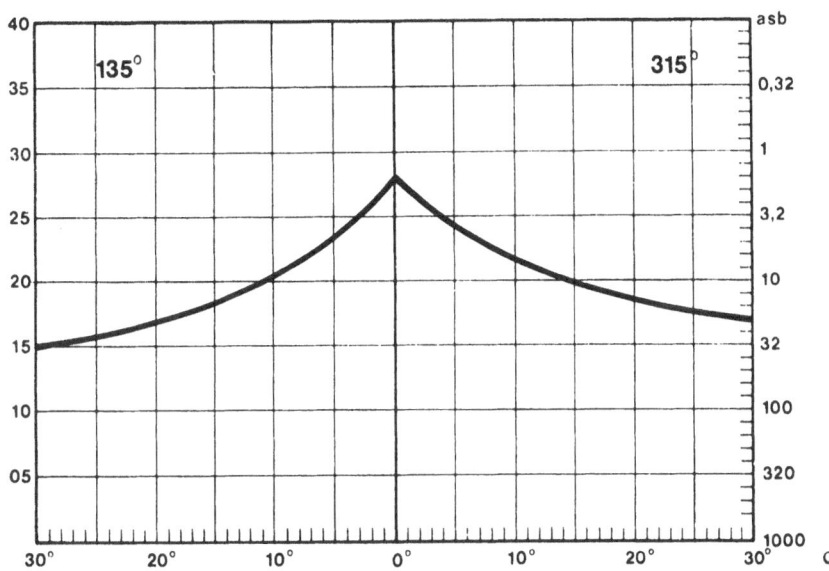

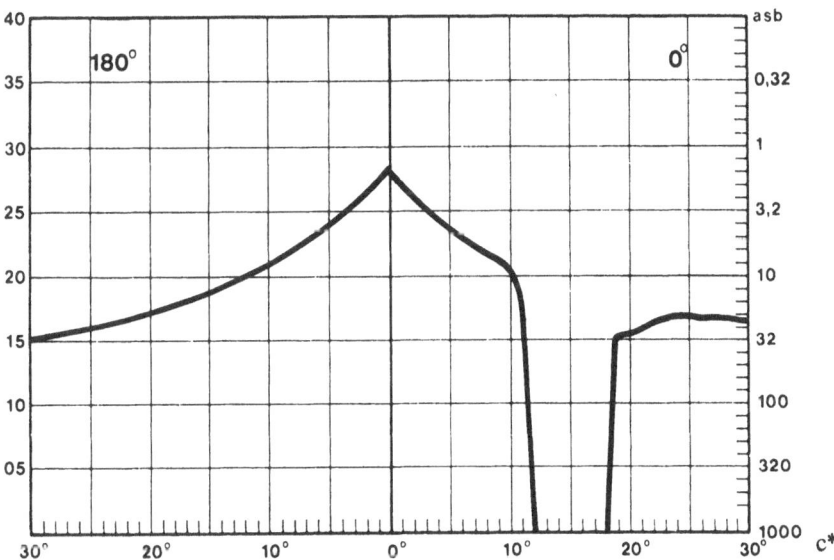

135

composition of the age groups, however, makes a precise comparison senseless. The Tübinger perimeter is the only instrument with which the peripheral visual field can be examined statically up to 90° eccentricity.

Kinetic campimetry with the Double Projection Campimeter.

The four standard isopters of the Double Projection Campimeter are obtained with luminances of 315 asb, 100 asb, 31.5 asb and 10 asb. These standard isopters are not shown here as they do not differ essentially from the isopters of the Goldmann perimeter.

Static campimetry with the Double Projection Campimeter.

The average normal sensitivity curve in the horizontal meridian with standard deviation and 95 % tolerance limit is given in Fig. 6[9].

The standard deviations for static campimetry with the Double Projection Campimeter are the smallest recorded in the literature of the visual field. Possible reasons for this were brought forward in the description of the Double Projection Campimeter[10].

In Table IV various data about the threshold measurements are given: lowest value, average value, highest value, standard deviation and 95 % tolerance limit.

From these data it is once more apparent that the standard deviation increases from the centre to the periphery. The standard deviation varies between 0.1 and 0.15 log unit.

Between the average sensitivity curve and the 95 % tolerance limit there is a difference that varies between 0.3 and 0.5 log unit. This means that the sensitivity curves of normal subjects will not lie more than 0.5 log unit below the average sensitivity curve. If the data from Table II on the older age group are combined with the Double Projection Campimeter data shown above, it follows that the sensitivity curve of a normal elderly person can lie 1.0 log unit below the average sensitivity curve for the 20–30-year-old group. The average sensitivity curve for the older group lies 0.3–0.5 log unit lower and the tolerance limit for the older group will, as for the younger group, lie not more than 0.5 log unit below this.

In addition to the inter-individual variation in the height of the sensitivity curve there is also variation in the shape of the sensitivity curve. This is among other things important for the interpretation of the results of multiple stimulus static perimetry[11]. An example of variation in the shape of the sensitivity curve

---

[9] GREVE & WIJNANS, 1973; 22 normal subjects between 19 and 22 years of age.
[10] see Chapter VI.
[11] see Chapter VIII.

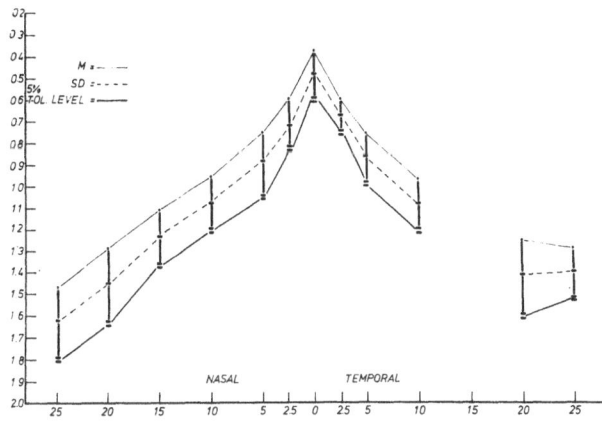

Fig. 6

Normal sensitivity curves of young subjects as measured with the Double Projection Campimeter.

m = mean sensitivity curve
SD = standard deviation
95% TOL. LEVEL = 95% tolerance level

TABLE IV

Means, highest and lowest values, standard deviations and upper 95-percent tolerance limits for the differential threshold of 22 normal subjects an 12 locations (stimulus duration: 1 s)

	Nasal					
	25°	20°	15°	10°	5°	2.5°
Lowest value	1.23	1.17	1.00	0.82	0.60	0.47
Mean value	1.47	1.30	1.12	0.96	0.76	0.60
Highest value	1.78	1.62	1.37	1.15	1.12	0.77
Standard deviation	0.145	0.149	0.110	0.107	0.128	0.097
95-percent tolerance limits	1.800	1.367	1.639	1.205	1.053	0.821

	Temporal					
	0°	2.5°	5°	10°	20°	25°
Lowest value	0.23	0.50	0.62	0.80	0.97	1.10
Mean value	0.38	0.60	0.76	0.98	1.25	1.29
Highest value	0.50	0.70	0.92	1.15	1.58	1.48
Standard deviation	0.093	0.065	0.101	0.106	0.154	0.106
95-percent tolerance limits	0.594	0.751	0.991	1.215	1.602	1.535

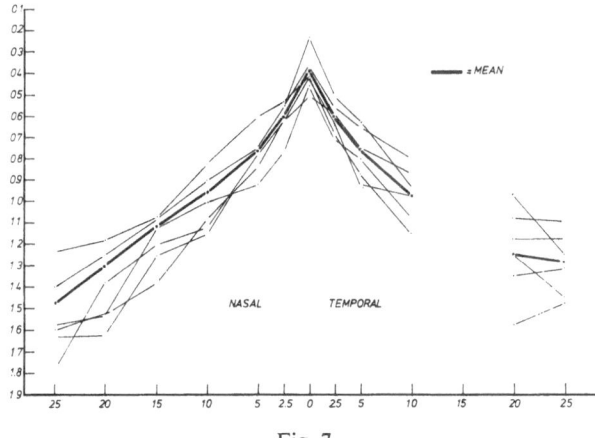

Fig. 7

Average normal sensitivity curve and 8 individual normal sensitivity curves of young subjects

is given in Fig. 7, which shows subjects with a steeper and a less steep gradient. The gradient of sensitivity from the centre to the periphery is, however, always more or less smooth.

The causes of the inter-individual variation in light sensitivity are, among others, differences in the optics of the eye, in the anatomical structure of the visual system (e.g. position of the blood vessels) and in the degree of integration within the visual system (e.g. differences in spatial and temporal interaction). Intelligence, concentration and training also play a part[12].

INTRA-INDIVIDUAL VARIATIONS.

The intra-individual variation (i.e. of one subject) is based on complex physical, physiological and psychological mechanisms. The intra-individual variation is different for each subject, although within certain limits. The intra-individual variation, as the inter-individual variation, can be examined statistically.

The significance of threshold changes, i.e. visual field defects, should be determined on the basis of average values, standard deviation and tolerance levels[13].

---

[12] see: Intra-individual variation.

[13] GREVE & WIJNANS, 1973.

138

Without dwelling on the many theories about the origin of threshold variation, we will mention a number of factors which are important in connection with visual field examination[14].

The physical factors include: an adequate fixation object, accurate positioning, the size of the steps of luminance, fluctuations in the flow of electric current

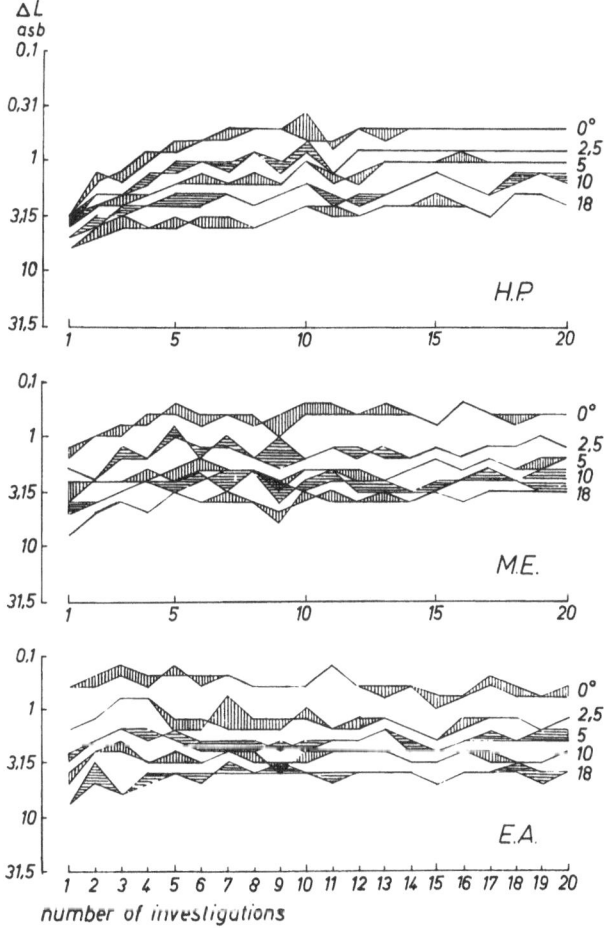

Fig. 8
Influence of training on thresholdmeasurements

[14] see: CRAWFORD & PIRENNE, 1954; BORNSCHEIN, 1961; BLACKWELL, 1952; VERPLANCK et al., 1953, 1955, 1958; BAUMGARDT, 1948; BOUMAN & VAN DEN VELDEN, 1948.

to the lamp and quantum statistics[15]. When a correction lens in a holder is used, alteration in the position of the fixation axis in relation to the lens, and in the distance between the cornea and the lens, can alter the position and size of the stimulus on the retina. The fixation nystagmus varies from person to person. Fluctuations in accommodation influence the threshold variation. The physiological factors have retinal and neural aspects. This is also known as biological variation. It is very probable that biological variation of the light sensitivity exists. The size of this under the conditions of the visual field examination is not known, as it is always a measurement of all the factors influencing variation. Among the psychological factors intelligence, concentration and training are important variables. In clinical visual field examination it is inevitable that untrained patients are examined. The threshold variation for trained patients is markedly less than for untrained patients, as is shown in Fig. 8[16] and in Fig. 9.

Every patient must first decide upon a criterion of perception for himself. This criterion can vary from the indication of the slightest change to quite definite perception. The patient's concentration can repeatedly slacken during the long visual field examination. One can try to avoid this as far as possible by inserting pauses between short periods of intensive examination and by warning the patient, verbally or otherwise, before each presentation.

Size of the intra-individual variation.

The 'frequency of seeing' curve has been mentioned already[17]. This curve is produced when the 'method of constant stimuli' is used for threshold examination. For trained subjects the range of luminance within the chance of perception varies from 1% to 99% is 0.3 log unit (Fig. 9). For untrained subjects this range is often larger, for instance 0.5 log unit. Thus the threshold value which is measured in visual field examination is not a constant value; in the vicinity of the threshold a stimulus of a certain luminance has a certain chance of being seen. The threshold measurements can vary one or more luminance steps (of 0.1 log unit) without any lesion being involved. If, in the frequency of seeing curve, the variation between 1% and 99% chance of perception covers a range of 0.3 log unit, this means that the variation is less than 0.3 log unit for visual field examination by the method of limits. In the usual static visual field examination the threshold is measured only three times in one position in

---

[15] see Chapter II.
[16] AULHORN & HARMS, 1972.
[17] see Chapter II.

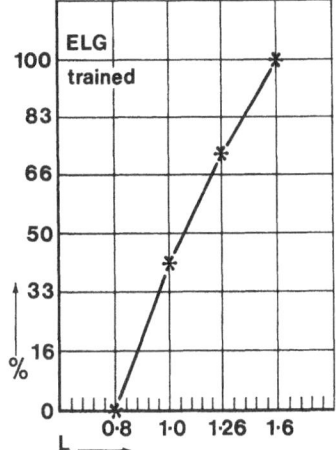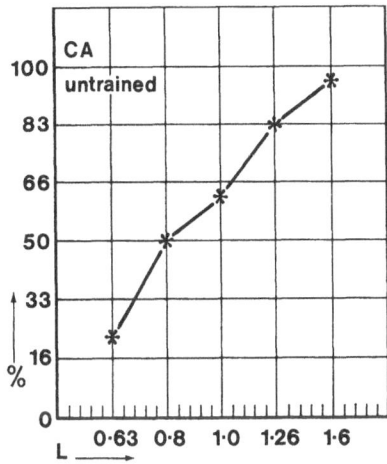

Fig. 9
Frequency-of-seeing curve of
a) trained subject and
b) untrained subject

order to get an impression of the variation. These three measurements will lie somewhere in the range between the 1% and the 99% chance of perception. It is improbable that two measurements will just fall at the extreme edges of this threshold zone. In visual field examination by the method of limits the range found in normal subjects is usually 0.2 log unit. The threshold zone thus consists of a band of width 0.2 log unit.[18]

Size of luminance steps and intra-individual variation.

The size of the luminance steps in static visual field examination is determined by the intra-individual variation. The size of the steps must be smaller than the physiological and psychological variation. The accuracy with which the intensity of a defect is recorded is also dependent on the size of the steps. As the average range is 0.2 log unit, luminance steps of 0.1 log unit have been chosen for the assessment phase of static perimetry. In trained patients the range is smaller than 0.2 log unit, so that greater accuracy can be achieved with smaller steps of luminance. In a study of the variation in threshold measurements in normal subjects we found, with luminance steps of 0.05 log unit, that a range of 0.2 log

---

[18] The relationship between variation and gradient has already been discussed in Chapter III.

141

unit was exceptional. The majority of subjects had a range of 0.1 or 0.15 log unit[19]. The most efficient approach to threshold level can naturally be achieved with steps of luminance which decrease in size as they come closer to the threshold.

The measurement of the threshold and the determination of variation become more accurate as the number of measurements in the threshold zone becomes larger. Variation cannot be assessed from one threshold measurement and without the variation it is difficult to judge the significance of the defects of slight intensity.

A distinction must be made between the size of steps in the detection phase and in the assessment phase. The above considerations apply to the assessment phase. The duration of the visual field examination is dependent on the size of the steps. In the assessment phase, the object of which is to record the intensity of a defect as accurately as possible, smaller steps are needed than in the detection phase, the object of which is to discover a defect. For the detection phase steps of 0.2 log unit are sufficient.

Significance of defects.

Reduced light sensitivity is expressed as a raised threshold. When the reduction in sensitivity is slight, the question is whether the threshold is significantly raised or still falls within the normal variation. When the range is 0.2 log unit defects of 0.2 log unit cannot be measured by means of a single measurement at one position.

When the number of measurements in the defect and in the normal zone is increased, it can be shown that the average of the threshold measurements in the defect is significantly higher than the average threshold measurements outside it. In practice, this is seldom done, so that as a general rule a reduction in sensitivity of 0.3 log unit can very probably be called pathological, at least if there are no angioscotomata in the vicinity and the size of the steps is 0.1 log unit. If the range is 0.4 log unit and a single measurement of the threshold is made, only a reduction in sensitivity of at least 0.5 log unit is significant. The greater the variation of the measurements from one patient, the more frequent the measurements will have to be.

A defect intensity of 0.3 log unit is the minimum to which a pathological significance can be attached under the conditions of the routine examination of glaucoma patients. Whether a defect of 0.3 log unit is of practical importance

---

[19] GREVE & WIJNANS, 1973.

142

for the assessment of the severity of the glaucomatous condition is a different matter.

When, as in the detection phase, steps of 0.2 log unit are chosen, the chance that defects of slight intensity will be found is still acceptable.

This is shown in Table V.

TABLE V

Chance of detection of defects of 0.3 log unit if luminance steps of 0.1 or 0.2 log unit are used and the range between 1% and 99% chance of perception is 0.3 or 0.5 log unit

range 1%–99%*	step size	number of measurements	chance %
0.3	0.1	3	99.0
0.5	0.1	3	98.0
0.3	0.2	3	98.5
0.5	0.2	3	97.5
0.3	0.1	2	95.0
0.5	0.1	2	93.0
0.3	0.2	2	92.0
0.5	0.2	2	91.0

* number of luminance steps between 1% and 99% frequency-of-seeing.

Variation between successive examinations.

Intra-individual variation includes the difference between the results obtained at different examinations. These differences, however, are of little importance for visual field examination, because they have the same influence in all positions. At most a change in the general sensitivity level can be found. The intensity of a defect as compared to the normal sensitivity level will not change[20].

In normal subjects the reproducibility of threshold measurements at different times is good, with both kinetic and static perimetry.[21] The reproducibility of visual field defects, however, is much more important. In most cases of visual field examination and certainly in glaucoma, an important question is whether progression or regression is taking place. If there is little variation in and round

---

[20] see Chapter X.
[21] DRANCE et al. 1966; BERRY et al., 1966.

a defect, any progression which has taken place can be accurately recorded in a following examination. This is only the case, however, if the investigator performs the examination on both occasions in the same way. The problems associated with kinetic perimetry in this respect have already been discussed. It is practically impossible to detect slight progression or regression by means of kinetic perimetry. Very marked variation in results can be found when different investigators, without comparable training or knowledge of visual field examination examine the same patient by means of kinetic perimetry[22]. The significance of alterations in defects decreases accordingly. When different specialized investigators with a comparable good training examine the same patient with visual field defects, in our experience the reproducibility of the results of static perimetry at different times is good.

In addition to the normal variation discussed above, pathological variation can occur, either through genuine variation in the light sensitivity or because adjacent areas of normal and defective light sensitivity alternate with each other (sieve-like defect).

INFLUENCE OF AGE

When standard values for the normal visual field are registered, these are usually taken from measurements of the light sensitivity of a group of normal subjects from 20–30 years of age. Because of the age chosen and the rigorous selection as regards other visual functions and refraction, the standard normal values are really optimum values. The majority of glaucoma patients in whom visual field defects are found are old, i.e. they have an average age of about 60 years. As has been stated above, a general reduction of sensitivity occurs between the ages of 20 and 80[23]. This reduction of sensitivity is greater for kinetic perimetry than for static perimetry[24]. According to some authors the reduction of sensitivity is greater in the periphery than in the centre, but this difference is small[25]. WOLF observed an acceleration in the reduction of light sensitivity after the age of 60[23]. With the exception of VERRIEST & ISRAEL all authors found that the variation increased with age.

The results of measurements in the older age group are largely dependent on

[22] NIESEL, 1970.

[23] see FERREE et al., 1929; WEEKERS & ROUSSEL, 1945; MANN & SHARPLEY, 1947; WOLF, 1966; DRANCE et al., 1967.

[24] Compare VERRIEST & ISRAEL, 1965 with ZEHNDER-ALBRECHT, 1950.

[25] VERRIEST & ISRAEL, 1965; ASPINALL, 1967.

144

the composition of the group (age, etc.) and on the manner of selection[26].

The reasons for the general reduction of sensitivity in older subjects are usually sought in:
1. longer reaction time;
2. a. position of the eye in the orbit;
   b. senile miosis;
   c. senile lens opacities;
   d. senile degeneration of the visual system;
   e. oxygen shortage.

Reaction time.

The longer reaction time only influences the results of kinetic perimetry[27]. This is probably one of the most important causes of the more marked general reduction of sensitivity (concentric contraction) found with kinetic perimetry than with static perimetry. The longer reaction time is clearly demonstrated by the increased difference between centrifugal and centripetal isopters in the older age group. Retinal factors may also be involved[28].

Position of the eye in the orbit.

The position of the eye in the orbit cannot influence the peripheral limitations of the visual field. The smaller extent of the visual field in the nasal periphery as compared with the temporal periphery cannot be explained either by direct obstruction by the nose or orbital rim.[28]

Senile miosis.

Senile miosis cannot explain the general reduction of sensitivity[29]. Senile lens opacities, degeneration of the visual system and oxygen shortage remain as the most important causes of the generalized reduction in sensitivity[30].

---

[26] FISHER (1968), for example, selected very rigorously on the basis of visual acuity, refraction, slit lamp appearance and the variation of the measurements obtained with kinetic perimetry. By eliminating the older subjects with a greater variation than 5° and with lens opacities he obtained an optimum group of older subjects.

[27] see Chapter III.

[28] FISHER, 1968.

[29] WEALE, 1963; ASPINALL, 1967; DRANCE, 1967; FISHER, 1968.

[30] see also WEEKERS & ROUSSEL, 1945.

Senile lens opacities.

Judging by our own experience lens opacities are by far the most important cause of general reduction of sensitivity[31]. If subjects with lens opacities are rigidly excluded, the (peripheral) reduction in light sensitivity is found to be only slight (0.25 log unit)[32]. The usual effect of lens opacities is flattening of the curve, so that the reduction of the central sensitivity is greater than the reduction of the peripheral sensitivity[33].

Senile degeneration of the visual system.

It is not clear how important senile degeneration of the visual system, with the exception of the optic part, is for the reduction of light sensitivity in the older age group. Some authors consider that the general senile reduction of sensitivity can be explained by the alterations in the lens alone[34].

Oxygen shortage.

The reduction of light sensitivity found in older subjects is the same as the reduction of sensitivity found in normal young subjects when breathing a low percentage of oxygen. Some authors consider that part of the reduction in light sensitivity in older subjects is caused by oxygen shortage[35].

The conclusion can be drawn that the generalized reduction in light sensitivity with advancing ages is only slight when preretinal anomalies are eliminated.

In kinetic perimetry the slower reaction time with advancing age plays its part in causing a general concentric contraction.

BLIND SPOT

Optic disc and blind spot.

The blind spot (Mariotte) in the visual field is caused by the optic disc. The size and position of the optic disc are variable.

---

[31] see Chapter X and WOLF, 1960.

[32] FISHER, 1968.

[33] see examples of chapter XI.

[34] MAZZANTINI, 1963; GUNKEL & GOURAS, 1963; WEALE, 1963.

[35] WOLFF, 1966; MCFARLAND, 1963.

146

The average horizontal diameter is 1.618 mm and the average vertical diameter is 1.796 mm[36].

The optic disc is usually oval, with the largest diameter in the vertical axis, but can be round or oval, with the largest diameter in the horizontal axis. The structure of the surrounding area also shows much individual variation.

If 1 mm on the retina corresponds with 4 degrees in the visual field, the average diameter of the blind spot should be 6,5°. The blind spot is in fact usually an oval scotoma in agreement with the above measurements. The values given in the literature, however, vary enormously[37]. The blind spot has a nucleus of absolute insensity surrounded by a margin of relatively reduced light sensitivity (relative intensity). The size of the relative margin varies according to the strength of the stimulus used. Furthermore the relative margin is not the same all the way round, but is larger at the top and bottom of the blind spot, almost certainly because of angioscotomata.

BJERRUM recorded the limits of the blind spot as 13° on the nasal side and 18° on the temporal side, with one third above the horizontal meridian and two thirds below it. Round these absolute limits he found a relative margin of not more than 1 degree.

Pericecal visual field.

When the blind spot is examined in eight directions by means of static perimetry, a result is obtained as shown in Fig. 10.

The absolute limits are given at the bottom of the figure by the maximum luminance. From these figures it is apparent that the size of the relative margin round the absolute nucleus depends on the strength of the stimulus. The kinetic method is the easiest way of examining the blind spot. The blind spot, like every other defect, is examined from the blind part outwards, i.e. centrifugally, and in a direction which is perpendicular to the edge. The fact must not be forgotten, however, that the gradient in the pericecal area is not the same in the various directions of investigation, and in some directions is nearly horizontal. In the section on kinetic perimetry the hazards of a flat gradient have already been pointed out. When the stimulus luminance is close to the pericecal threshold level, pseudo-enlargement of the blind spot can very easily be found with kinetic perimetry. In Fig. 10 a pseudo-blind spot is indicated. The absolute nucleus of this defect corresponds to the hole in the Tübinger perimeter through which

---

[36] ISHII, quoted by DUKE ELDER, 1961.
[37] DUBOIS-POULSEN et al., 1951.

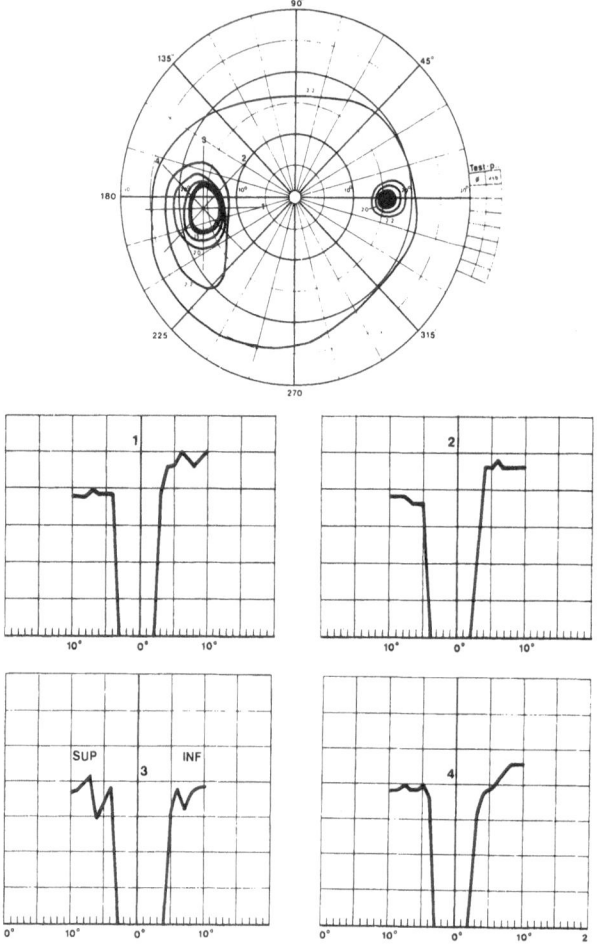

Fig 10

Sensitivity curves in the pericecal area of the visual field (see text)

fixation can be controlled. Kinetic perimetry of this hole also shows a margin of relative intensity like the normal blind spot. This is due to successive lateral spatial summation of the juxtaliminal stimuli and has clearly nothing to do with decreased sensitivity. In the case of the normal blind spot the pericecal defective area of relative intensity is much larger, so that other factors must also be involved.

If the stimulus luminance is chosen correctly, i.e. at least 0.3 log unit supraliminal, these technical artifacts do not occur. This stimulus luminance corre-

148

sponds with the luminance of a stimulus, the isopter of which lies at least 20°
outside the temporal edge of the blind spot. If this rule is adhered to the influence
of changes in the strength of the stimulus due to preretinal factors is also avoided
(Fig. 11).

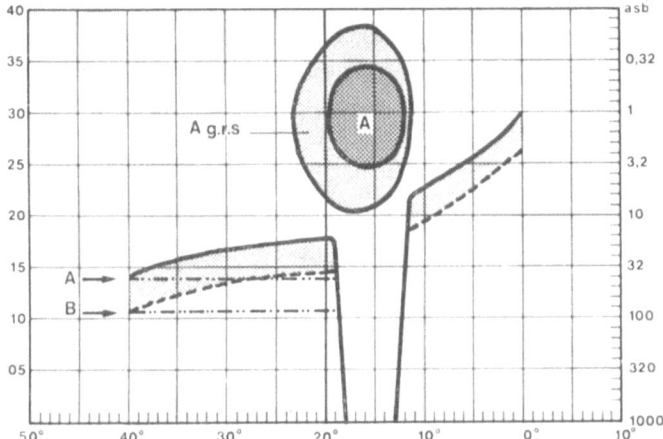

Fig. 11

A stimulus which is 20° outside the temporal rim of the blind spot is 0.3 log unit above
threshold level. If a general reduction of sensitivity occurs one has to choose a stronger
stimulus to achieve the same result

TABLE VI

*Limits of the blind spot as measured with the I/2 and I/4 stimulus of the Goldmann
perimeter*

	I/2		I/4	
	mean	sd	mean	sd
1. nasal limit	10.0	0.94		
2. temporal limit	20.3	0.91		
3. portion above horizontal meridian	6.7	1.04	see text	
4. portion below horizontal meridian	7.7	0.96	see text	
5. height (i.e. 3 + 4)	13.7	0.20	8.0	0.10
6. width (i.e. 2 − 1)	9.6	0.11	6.1	0.09

Size and position of the blind spot.

The size of the normal blind spot has recently been noted for kinetic perimetry with the I/4 and the I/2 stimulus of the Goldmann perimeter; these results are given in Table VI[38].

It appears that the average relative horizontal limits of the blind spot for the I/2 isopter are at 10° and 20° eccentricity, with a standard deviation of a little less than one degree. About 45% of the relative blind spot lies above the horizontal meridian. For the absolute blind spot (I/4), however, it appears that BJERRUM's old rule is correct: on the average one third above and two thirds below the horizontal meridian.

The relative margin of the blind spot is mainly found at the poles, and more

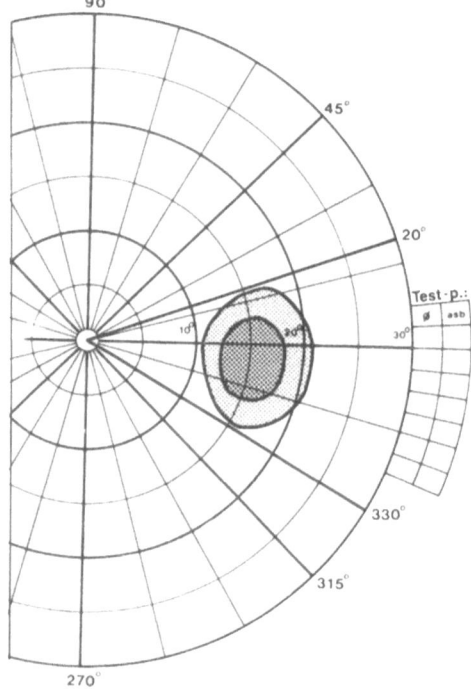

Fig. 12
The normal blind spot

---

[38] ARMALY, 1969, size given in degrees; the difference in the values 5 as compared to 3 and 4 and 6 as compared to 1 and 2 is due to different composition of the groups.

particularly at the superior pole, as appears from the differences in height and width between the relative and absolute blind spots. This polar extension is almost certainly due to angioscotomata. The relative extension of the blind spot is larger than the zone of one degree already mentioned. As the absolute limits of the blind spot measured with the Goldmann or Tübinger perimeter, we take a height of 8° and a width of 6° (Fig. 12). The absolute nasal limit of the widest part of the blind spot lies at 12°, the absolute temporal limit at 18°. We allow one degree variation on both sides in height and width of the absolute blind spot. The width of the relative blind spot must be less than 10° and the height less than 14°. This means that the relative blind spot of the right eye is bounded at the bottom by the 330° meridian and at the top by the 20° meridian.

Enlargement of the blind spot outside these limits must always be investigated by means of meridional static perimetry. On the grounds of these results (and the fundus picture – peripapillary area) a conclusion can be drawn as to whether an enlargement of the blind spot is pathological or not.

The blind spot can be displaced upwards or downwards as a whole without alteration of the normal limits; in this case the meridional boundaries naturally do not apply.

The size of the blind spot does not alter significantly with age[39]; there is no significant difference between the blind spots of normal subjects and glaucoma-patients.

Slight or moderate ametropia, if corrected, does not affect the size and position of the blind spot. If strongly positive lenses are used the blind spot becomes smaller and is displaced towards the centre; if strongly negative lenses are used the blind spot becomes larger and more peripheral (prisma effect)[40]. In the pericecal visual field reduced inhibition has been demonstrated in normal subjects[41].

ANGIOSCOTOMATA

Entoptic observation shows clearly how a large number of blood vessels of different diameters bend around the fovea on their pathway from the disc (PURKINJE's images).

The largest vessels run in the inner layer of the retina under the internal limiting membrane. The blood vessel wall is almost transparent. The column of blood in the blood vessels forms a filter for the perimetric stimulus. Only the largest

---

[39] BECK, 1955; ARMALY, 1969.

[40] see Chapter X.

[41] ENOCH et al., 1970.

of these blood vessels are of significance for visual field examination (Fig. 13[42]). The blood vessels have their largest diameter on and near the disc (± 0.1 mm). These produce a filter with a diameter of a little less than half a degree (± 24′). At the level of the receptors the 'shadow' of the vessels will be a little larger, depending on the distance between the blood vessel and the receptors. This distance is greatest round the disc. As they leave the disc the blood vessels often run very close together and can thus form one large filter with a diameter of 1°.

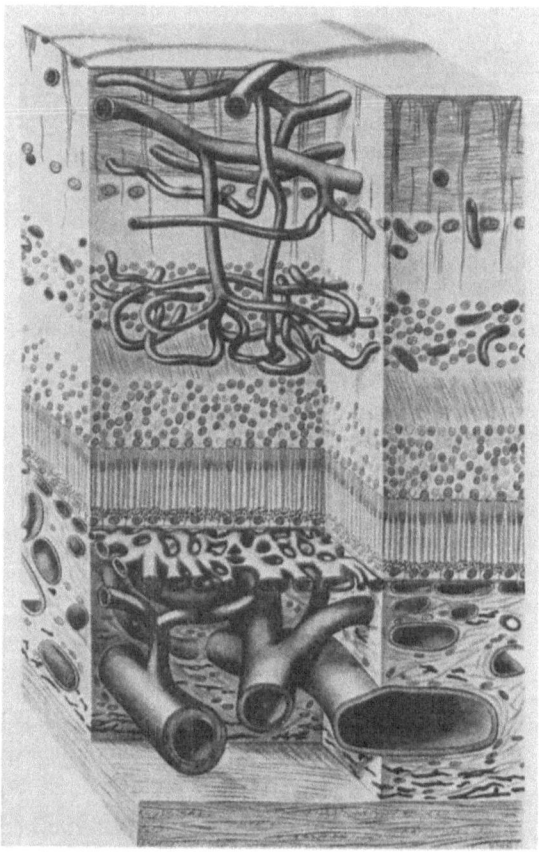

Fig. 13
Section through the retina showing the position of the blood vessels in the inner part of the retina

---

[42] after BARGMANN, 1967.

Normal angioscotomata.

The visual field defects produced by normal blood vessels, the angioscotomata, are important for visual field examination for many reasons. The position, size, intensity and variability of the physiological angioscotomata must be known in order to be able to delimit pathological defects. In our experience, in single stimulus and multiple stimulus static visual field examination the presence of physiological angioscotomata must be taken into account all the time. Angioscotomata are particularly apparent with short presentation times (such as with Xenon flash lamps).

From the literature it appears that the angioscotomata are seldom larger than 1°[43].

Because the diameter of the angioscotomata is so small, their chance of detection with kinetic perimetry is limited by the speed with which the stimulus is moved.

The determination of the size of the angioscotomata by means of kinetic perimetry is, as with the blind spot and every other scotoma, dependent on the strength of stimulus used. The closer the stimulus is to threshold level, the larger the angioscotomata. For the examination of angioscotomata stimuli are recommended the corresponding isopters of which run just outside the blind spot, i.e. juxtaliminal stimuli. The objections to such stimuli have been discussed under the heading of the blind spot.

The positions in the visual field in which angioscotomata can be found are limited to the positions in which there are large retinal blood vessels. At the poles of the blind spot angioscotomata play a large part in causing pseudo-enlargement of the blind spot. An important area for glaucoma is the intermediate visual field, the Bjerrum area. The large blood vessels run in this area and the majority of angioscotomata are found here. In the central visual field the diameter of the blood vessels is too small to give rise to angioscotomata of any significance. Angioscotomata are generally regarded as relative defects; only Goldmann feels that they can be absolute close to the blind spot. In the older literature no particulars are given about the detailed intensity of angioscotomata, expressed in log units; recently an intensity of 0.3–0.5 log unit has been recorded[44].

We have investigated the size and intensity of angioscotomata by means of static campimetry (DPC). Photographs of the fundus oculi of 15 normal subjects

---

[43] EVANS, 1948; GOLDMANN, 1947; WEEKERS & HUMBLET, 1945; DUBOIS-POULSEN, 1952.
[44] WEEKERS, 1969; static perimetry with Tübinger perimeter.

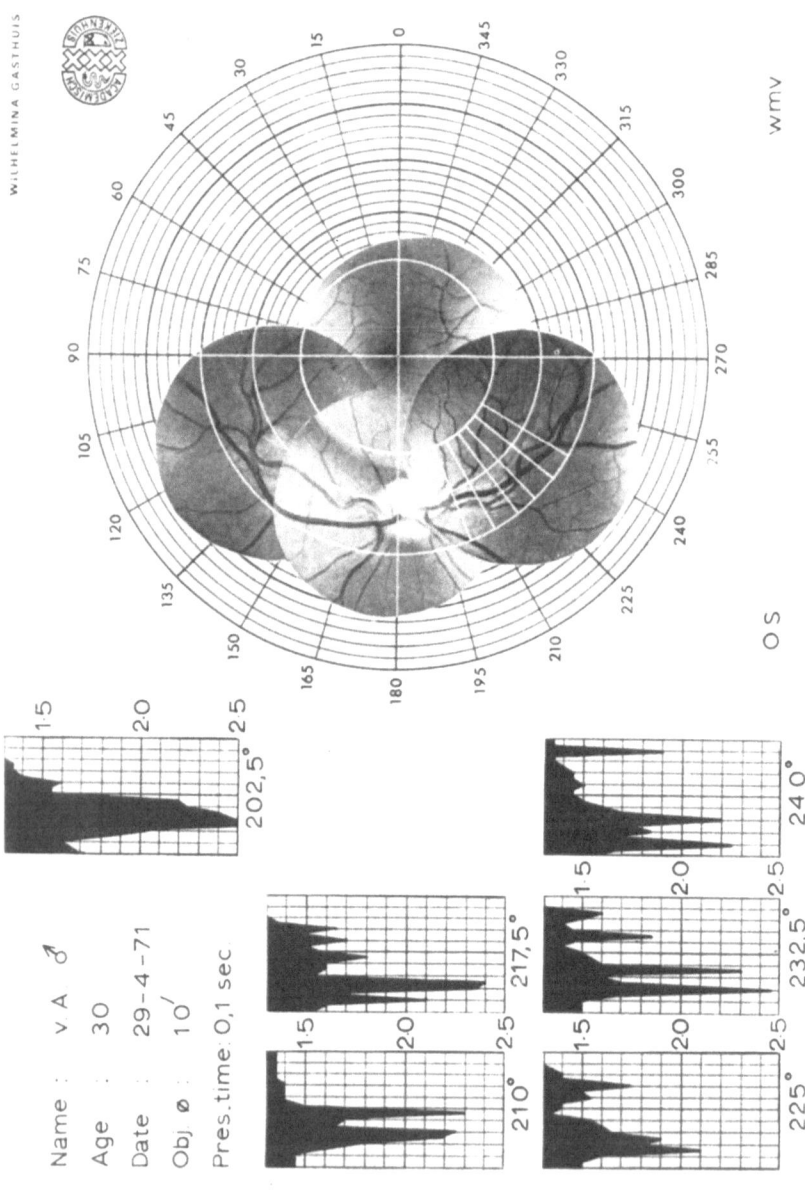

Fig. 14

Photograph of a fundus showing blood vessels and relation to the visual field chart. Partial meridional static campimetry (DPC) was performed across the location of the blood vessels as indicated

were made. These photographs were enlarged in such a manner that they corresponded with the visual field chart of the Double Projection Campimeter. On the photographs a number of areas were selected in which large blood vessels were present and in these areas meridional static campimetry was performed. In Fig. 14 the results obtained from a subject of 20 years of age are given. The maximum intensity in every case was less than 1 log unit. The deepest part of the angioscotomata only had a diameter of 30'[45]. When the diameter was measured at the level at which the intensity of the scotomata was 0.5 log unit, this was usually found to be 1° or less; occasionally 2°, especially when two blood vessels ran close together. In older subjects the angioscotomata were usually a little wider than in younger subjects but the intensity was not greater. The diameter of the margins of the angioscotomata varies between 1° and 6°. Angioscotomata are usually funnel-shaped, i.e. as the intensity increases the diameter decreases. The reason for the relative margin has been sought in the perivascular sheath. It seems to us to be more probable that the size of the local areas of spatial summation and the physiological fixation nystagmus determine the shape of the angioscotomata.

Variation in the size of the angioscotomata

According to some authors the size of the angioscotomata varies under the influence of numerous conditions: time of day, temperature, time since the last meal, menstruation, pregnancy, fatigue, fear, infections of the nose or sinuses and various medicines[46]. We mention in particular pressure on the jugular vein, artifically raised intra-ocular pressure and shortage of oxygen. These three last factors cause enlargement of the angioscotomata.

GOLDMANN considered that this enlargement was the result of retinal or neural processes[47]. It is not the blood vessels or their sheaths which alter in size, but the light sensitivity of the retinal perceptive units which changes under the influence of a decreased supply of oxygen, whether this is produced by raised intra-ocular pressure, pressure on the jugular vein or shortage of oxygen in the air breathed[48]. Opinions are divided about the existence of enlarged angioscotomata as an early symptom of visual field damage in glaucoma.

---

[45] presentation time 0.5 s.

[46] EVANS, 1948; DUBOIS-POULSEN, 1952; WELT, 1945.

[47] GOLDMANN, 1947.

[48] EVANS (1948); suggested that the synapses function less efficiently when there is shortage of oxygen.

Conclusion

Normal angioscotomata are in general limited to the intermediate visual field and usually have a diameter of 1° (maximum 2°). The intensity is less than 1 log unit.

The deepest point of the funnel-shaped angioscotomata is seldom larger than 30′. This diameter is in agreement with the diameter of the large blood vessels. Round the deepest part there is a margin of decreasing intensity.

The fact that lesions in the fundus of a spherical eye must be represented on a flat surface leads to cartographic deformation of defects[49]. This deformation increases from the centre to the periphery. Polar azimuthal equidistant projection is generally used. An approximation of this projection method making use of La Hire's centre of projection (distance to centre of chart is 2.71 R) is shown in Fig. 15. The relative distances in the meridional direction remain the same,

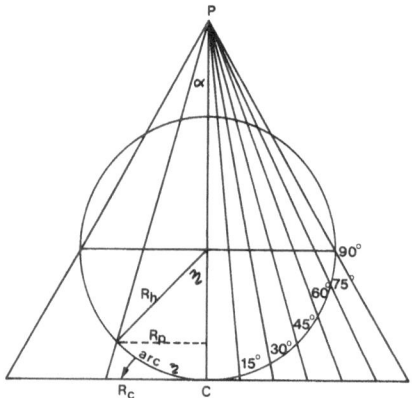

Fig. 15

Polar azimuthal equidistant projection.

R_h = radius of hemisphere
R_p = radius of parallel at eccentricity η in hemisphere
η = eccentricity
c   = centre of chart
R_c = radius of parallel at eccentricity η on chart
$R_c \approx$ arc η
P   = La Hire's centre on projection; PR $\approx$ 2.71 R

---

[49] see also GROENOW, 1895; TEN DOESSCHATE, 1947; DUBOIS-POULSEN, 1952; MAGIS, 1957; FRISEN, 1970.

but in the direction at right angles to this, i.e. along the parallels, the size of the defect appears to increase.

The deformation of defects along the parallel is proportional to the ratio arc η/R sin η (arc $\eta \approx R_c$). With the aid of Fig. 15 this can be explained as follows:

$$\frac{R_c}{R_p} = \frac{\text{arc } \eta}{R_h \sin \eta} = \frac{\frac{\eta}{360} \cdot 2\pi R_h}{R_h \sin \eta} = \frac{\eta \cdot \pi}{\sin \eta \; 180}$$

As η increases from 0° to 90°, sin η increases from 0 to 1.

The numerator thus increases more rapidly than the denominator, i.e. as the eccentricity increases the deformation becomes steadily greater. For example:
at 15°: 1.02
at 30°: 1.05
at 60°: 1.2
at 90°: 1.5

Within the 30° visual field the deformation is negligible. In the outer periphery a defect is represented as 1.5 times too large in the circular direction by the cartographic distortion.

CHAPTER VIII

MULTIPLE STATIC STIMULI IN THE DETECTION PHASE

In previous chapters it has been shown that the static method is to be preferred for the detection of visual field defects, particularly those in the central and intermediate visual field. The capacity of a method to detect defects depends upon the number of positions examined and whether or not the examination is performed at threshold level. In Chapter V a number of 150 positions has been chosen.

It is possible to examine this number of positions by means of static perimetry. The larger the number of positions, the longer the duration of the examination will be. Probably on account of the time factor some authors have compromised on the principle that visual field examination should be an investigation of thresholds and they use supraliminal stimuli. A stimulus at a supraliminal luminance level, only has to be presented once. The duration of the examination can thus be reduced to a half or a third of the time needed for threshold measurements.

In the detection phase, however, the duration of the examination can also be reduced by simultaneous presentation of a number of stimuli (2, 3 or 4), while the principle of threshold measurements is maintained. This method of static visual field examination with multiple stimuli will be described in this chapter. The multiple stimulus method means nothing more than the simultaneous presentation of stimuli in order to shorten the duration of the investigation[1].

Our own study of multiple stimulus presentation consists of four parts: the maximum number of stimuli which a normal subject can indicate correctly, an accurate comparative study (frequency-of-seeing method) of the difference threshold on single and on multiple stimulus presentation, the value of the multiple stimulus method for mass visual field investigation and the value of the multiple stimulus method for the clinical visual field examination of glaucoma patients[2].

SPECIFIC PROBLEMS OF MULTIPLE STIMULI

Some specific problems arising when the multiple stimulus method is used, will be listed first:
1. simultaneous threshold approach;
2. supraliminal stimuli;

---

[1] see page 195.
[2] We are deeply indebted to Prof. AULHORN and Prof. HARMS who provided research facilities for the first two parts of this study and assisted us with their advice.

3. neural interaction;
4. 'Gestalt'psychological phenomena;
5. counting and indicating;
6. localized attention;
7. maximum number of stimuli;
8. threshold level and variation;
9. pseudo-variation;
10. multiple stimuli and visual field defects.

1. Simultaneous threshold approach.

Simultaneous presentation of stimuli does not necessarily imply simultaneous perception. If simultaneous perception of simultaneously presented stimuli is achieved the maximum amount of time is won by the multiple stimulus method. Simultaneous perception means perception after an equal number of luminance steps. As is the case in the single stimulus method, the examination with multiple stimuli starts at an infraliminal level. In the ideal case the luminance of all the stimuli in a simultaneously presented group should be the same number of steps under the expected individual threshold level at the commencement of the measurement. The individual threshold level, however, is unknown, so that the calculations must be based on the average threshold level. In order to achieve the highest possible degree of simultaneous perception the luminance of all the stimuli in a group must be equally infraliminal with respect to the average

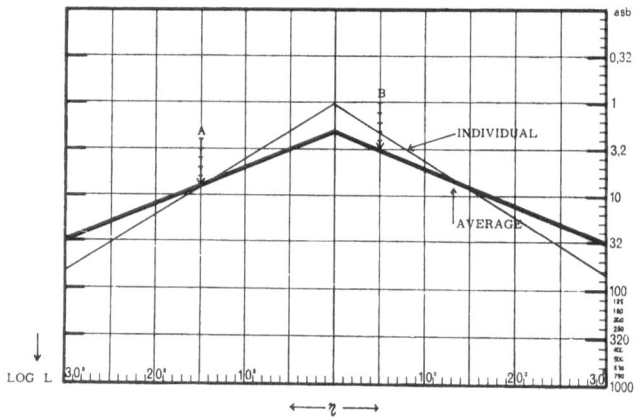

Fig. 1

Stimuli A and B are equidistant to the average sensitivity curve but not to an individual sensitivity curve

160

threshold level. For this situation we have chosen the term 'equidistant stimuli'; it is represented in Fig. 1.

When the individual sensitivity curve equals the average sensitivity curve the equidistant stimuli A and B will be seen simultaneously. In this case the time saved is proportional to the number of stimuli. Many individual sensitivity curves, however, differ not only in level but also in shape from the average sensitivity curve on account of the individual variations in light sensitivity between normal subjects[3].

An example of a normal individual curve which differs in shape from the average sensitivity curve is shown in Fig. 1. The equidistant stimuli A and B will not be seen simultaneously. As soon as stimulus B has been seen and the threshold level of stimulus A still has to be found, the multiple stimulus presentation ceases to save time, since the simultaneous presentation of stimulus B with stimulus A does not provide any new information. The time saved by the multiple stimulus method is the time before the perception at threshold level of stimulus B.

As the difference in threshold luminance between stimulus A and stimulus B increases the time saved by simultaneous approach to the threshold decreases. In normal cases the differences in threshold luminance between two positions in the visual field are limited. If visual field defects are present, however, the differences in threshold luminance between simultaneously examined positions can be very large, so that much of the time saved by the multiple stimulus method as compared with the single stimulus method is lost (Fig. 2).

As the saving of time is practically the only reason for using the multiple stimulus method, its application will be limited to the detection phase, the object of which is to differentiate between normal and pathological visual fields.

A second reason why the perception of equidistant stimuli will not always be simultaneous may be found in the physiological intra-individual variations. Usually the triplo-range of threshold measurements covers 0.2 lu.

It is not known whether the normal threshold fluctuations occur simultaneously at different points, so that all positions reach a maximum or minimum light sensitivity at the same time. If one position in a simultaneously examined group has optimum light sensitivity while another position at the same time has suboptimum sensitivity, this might result in the perception of equidistant stimuli not being simultaneous.

If perception is not simultaneous it will be necessary to ask the patient where he saw the stimuli, and these questions and answers take time.

---

[3] see Chapter VII.

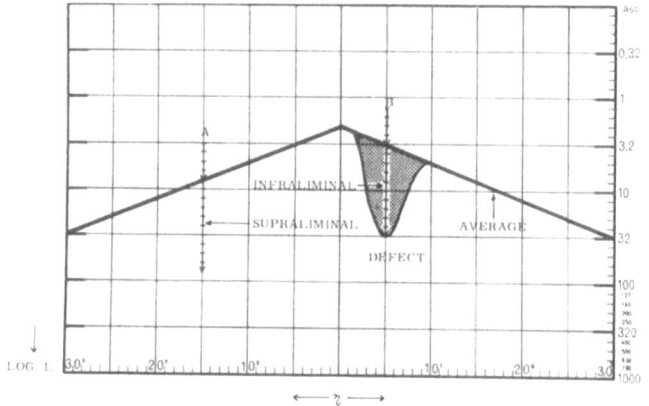

Fig. 2

Equidistant stimuli and a visual field defect

2. Supraliminal stimuli.

The time saved by the simultaneous perception of stimuli is maximum when supraliminal stimuli are presented. This is done in all the methods which have been recommended up to now. The advantage of the time saved by the use of supraliminal stimuli is coupled with the disadvantage that the capacity to detect relative defects is reduced. This is true both for single stimulus and multiple stimulus presentation. The use of supraliminal stimuli means inevitably that relative defects will be overlooked. In our opinion, if false negative results are to be avoided, the multiple stimulus examination should start at an infraliminal level[4]. From this level the threshold is measured by increasing the luminance step by step.

A second equally important reason for the use of infraliminal stimuli is that defects can better be distinguished from false positive results. The reason, which will be dealt with extensively in Chapter X, is that the intensity of a defect must not be expressed as compared with the average normal sensitivity, but as compared with the patient's reconstructed normal level of sensitivity, i.e. the intensity of a defect is expressed in its relationship to the patient's individual sensitivity curve. In order to do this, not only the threshold value in the defect should be known, but also a number of normal threshold values, from which the patient's sensitivity curve can be reconstructed.

Only when these values are known is it possible to reach a decision about the

---

[4] GREVE, 1971; GREVE & WIJNANS, 1973.

162

degree of decrease of sensitivity and to determine whether the result is a normal variation (the so-called false positive result) or a real defect[5].

In the multiple stimulus method threshold measurements are to be preferred to the presentation of supraliminal stimuli.

3. Neural interaction.

Various authors have suggested that some sort of interaction might take place between the stimuli in a simultaneously presented group, and that this interaction might influence the threshold perception[6]. Direct neural interaction is improbable. Anatomical connections between receptive fields can only be demonstrated over a maximum area of 4°[7], and the greatest distance over which spatial interaction has been demonstrated in psychophysical experiments is also 4°[8]. Interaction over larger areas, as demonstrated in electrophysiological experiments[9], could not be confirmed in psychophysical experiments.[10]

The distance between simultaneously presented stimuli will have to be at least 4°. Stimuli which are not presented simultaneously are naturally not subject to any spatial restrictions. The perception of a stimulus can, however, be influenced at a higher perceptual level by the simultaneous presentation of other stimuli. The extent to which this affects the visual field examination with multiple stimulus presentation will be discussed below.

4. 'Gestalt' psychological phenomena.

'Gestalt' psychological phenomena undoubtedly occur when multiple stimuli are presented[11]. From every combination of stimuli presented a pattern is involuntarily formed. If a familiar pattern of 8 stimuli is presented, the presence of the 8 stimuli can be recognized by the completeness of the pattern, and the presence of 7 stimuli by the absence of one stimulus from the complete pattern. When the stimuli are repeatedly presented in a regular pattern, e.g. the corners of a square, the danger arises that the pattern will be completed even when a stimulus at one of the corners of the square is not seen.

In practice this hardly ever happens, partly because the same group is never

---

[5] see Chapters VII and X.

[6] BEDWELL, 1967; FANKHAUSER & GIGER, 1968; GOLDMANN, 1969.

[7] POLYAK, 1941; DOWLING & BOYCOTT, 1967.

[8] V. D. BRINK, 1965; V. D. BRINK & REYNTJES, 1966.

[9] MCILLWAIN, 1964; LEVICK et al., 1965.

[10] SPILLMAN & GAMBONE, 1971.

[11] see FANKHAUSER & GIGER, 1968.

presented twice. It is certainly advisable when using the multiple stimulus method to keep on altering the number and pattern of the stimuli all the time. However, when a varying number of stimuli are presented continually in the same familiar pattern, the influence of 'Gestalt' psychological phenomena is only slight, as has appeared from our experiments[12]. When lines or circles are used instead of small round stimuli, as in HARRINGTON & FLOCKS' method[13], the danger is greater that a line or circle will be seen completely while actually part of it falls in a defect. The pattern is filled in, completed, at the site of the defect. The example of the normal blind spot as negative scotoma is well-known. The 'completion phenomenon' has only been described for more complex figures that the simple stimuli which are used for visual field investigation[14]. When the multiple stimulus method is used, it is advisable to confine oneself to the classical small round perimetric stimuli.

5. Counting and indicating.

Although counting the number of stimuli and indicating their positions asks more of the patient than the simple 'yes' or 'no' answer in the single stimulus method, in practice we have encountered no difficulties. It appears that nearly every patient who can stand a lengthy visual field examination is capable of indicating the number and position of the stimuli correctly.

6. Localized attention.

Since the time of HELMHOLTZ it has been known that a subject can direct his attention towards a certain part of the visual field even during steady fixation. This process depends upon external and internal factors. The former are determined by the stimulation and are involuntary, the latter depend upon the subject himself and are voluntary. The external stimulation factors determine the conspicuousness of the stimulus[15]. If the stimulation pattern is somewhat complex, knowledge of where the stimulus is going to appear (localized attention) does influence the perception of the stimulus[16]. If, however, the stimulus is isolated and thus very conspicuous, localized attention does not affect the perception of the stimulus[17]. In other words, if the stimulus is presented against a neutral

---

[12] GREVE, 1972.

[13] see page 171.

[14] see e.g. GERRITS & TIMMERMAN, 1969.

[15] ENGEL, 1971.

[16] GRINDLEY & TOWNSEND, 1968, 1970; LIE, 1969; ENGEL, 1971.

[17] MERTENS, 1956; GRINDLEY & TOWNSEND, 1968, 1970.

background in visual field examination, localized attention does not influence the level of the difference threshold.

The results of our own experiments are in agreement with this. A subject who knows nothing of the position of the multiple stimuli can still count and localize them correctly; the threshold does not change. This means that even if a subject purposely directs his attention towards another part of the visual field, under normal fixation, the perception of multiple stimuli in the visual field is not affected.

7. Maximum number of stimuli.

This is a subject which has been studied by psychologists. Generally in psychological experiments an attempt was made to determine the maximum number of letters which could be reproduced correctly after a short presentation. Some investigators used round stimuli which are comparable to those used in perimetry. These experiments are usually limited to the central visual field and therefore not directly applicable to visual field examination, but it appears from these experiments that the maximum number of letters which can be repeated correctly is 4 or 5, and the number of round stimuli is 7 or 8.[18]

We performed experiments, under conditions similar to those in clinical perimetry, to determine the largest reproducible number of stimuli in the area within the 30° parallel. The apparatus used for these experiments has been described elsewhere[19].

[19] GREVE, 1972; the most important points are: In a hemisphere of radius 1 metre, painted white inside, 8 projectors could project stimuli. Diameter of stimuli 10′; luminance variable in steps of 0.1 log unit by means of neutral density filters (SCHOTT); stimuli could be presented by means of synchronized electromagnetic shutters during 0.5 s. The subject's head was in the middle of the hemisphere; fixation target was a red circular fixation light, diameter 30′. The 8 stimuli could be presented in any desired position and combination.

From these experiments it appeared that, in the 30° field, 2, 3, 4 and usually 5 simultaneously presented supraliminal stimuli could be recognized correctly at one glance, by which we mean that the stimuli did not have to be consciously counted[20]. In a few cases, where a difficult pattern was involved, the 5 stimuli had to be counted consciously, so that the correct number was not seen at

---

[18] GLANVILLE & DALLENBACH, 1929; HUNTER & SIEGLER, 1940; MILLER, 1956; SPERLING, 1960; AVERBACH & CORIELL, 1961; MACWORTH, 1963; KLEMMER, 1963; KAUFMAN et al., 1963.

[20] All stimuli were equally supraliminal; in most cases 0.5 log unit above the threshold.

one glance. When 5 stimuli were presented the correct number was always recognized, either at one glance or after being counted.

Six stimuli are either seen as two groups of 3 stimuli or are consciously counted. Seven and 8 stimuli always have to be counted unless they form a complete pattern or a complete pattern less one, in which case the number can be recognized without counting. With 6, 7 and 8 stimuli the result was dependent upon the pattern in which the stimuli were presented and upon the eccentricity. If 7 or 8 stimuli were presented in a semicircle at 20° eccentricity even a trained subject made a few mistakes. At 30° eccentricity counting was impossible. Counting 7 or 8 stimuli in an irregular pattern, however, presented no difficulty. We recommend these irregular patterns for the multiple stimulus method[21]. Although 8 stimuli can be recognized correctly, it is clear that 5 stimuli is the limit in practice for visual field examination. Five stimuli can usually be recognized correctly at one glance. Counting 6, 7 or 8 stimuli takes time. In addition, it becomes increasingly difficult to localize large numbers of stimuli. Training and concentration play too great a role, when larger numbers of stimuli are used, to be of practical value. The presentation of 2, 3 or 4 stimuli to a normal subject is a procedure which presents no problems. This is not only apparent from these experiments but also from observations made during mass investigations with the Visual Field Analyser[22].

There is still a large margin between the number of stimuli used and the largest possible number: 8 or more.

From the psychological literature it is known that short visual impressions like these are stored in a 'short-time memory'[23]. The amount of information available for recognition, i.e. the information which reaches the cortex, is much greater than the amount which can be reproduced from the short-time memory.

8. Threshold level and variation.

Normal subjects.

There is no information in the literature about the level and variation of the difference threshold in multiple stimulus presentation. When measuring the threshold with single and with multiple stimulus presentation, using the method of constant stimuli, it became apparent that the level and variation of the threshold is the same in both cases.

---

[21] see page 199.

[22] GREVE & VERDUIN, 1972.

[23] see also BROADBENT, 1958 and BROWN, 1958.

166

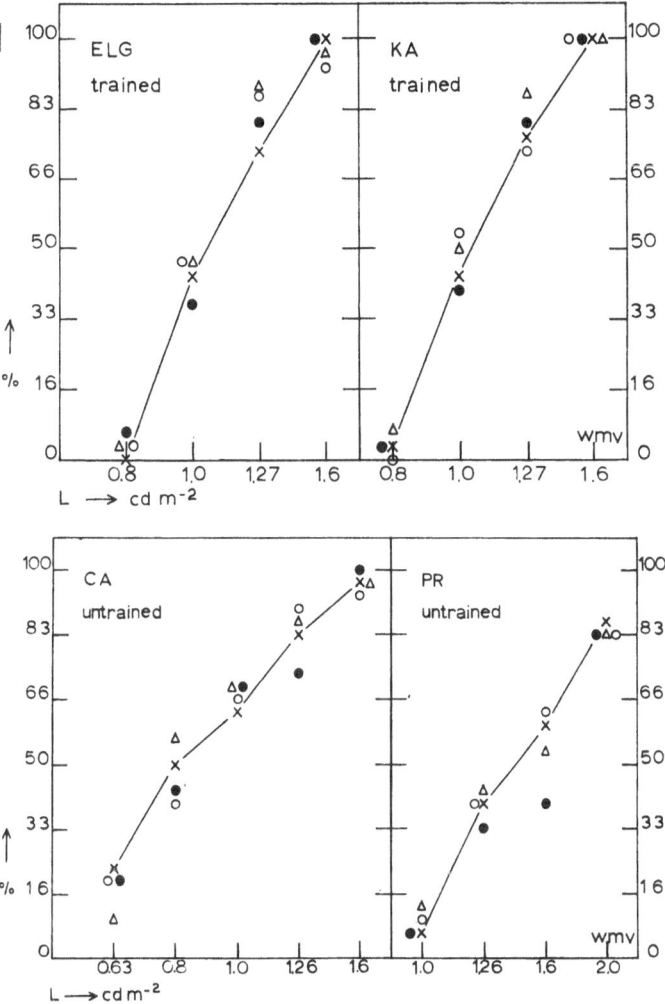

Fig. 3

Frequency-of-seeing curves of four normal subjects. Two of the subjects were trained in visual experiments; the two other subjects had no previous experience. Right eye; regular spatial arrangement; basis of triangle temporal; 5° eccentricity; curves shown for stimulus in 171° meridian.

Δ = stimulus presented with two more stimuli
O = stimulus presented with one more stimulus (45° meridian)
● = stimulus presented with one more stimulus (325° meridian)
+ = single stimulus
abscissa: luminance of stimulus in cd/m²
ordinate: frequency-of-seeing

The results for 10 normal subjects and using 4 stimuli have been published elsewhere[24]. When we increased the number of stimuli to 8, we found that when 8 stimuli are presented simultaneously the threshold is the same as on single stimulus presentation, at least when the stimuli can be counted correctly.

Figure 3 shows some results in the form of frequency-of-seeing curves. From these experiments it appears that in normal subjects the level and variation of the difference threshold are not affected by multiple stimulus presentation.

Whatever the theoretical chances of interaction and the role of the higher perceptual functions may be, the threshold is not altered by them. The multiple stimulus method therefore does not differ fundamentally from the classical single stimulus method. The difference thresholds of a number of positions are measured more or less simultaneously, but this procedure does not alter the threshold.

It is therefore possible to obtain more information in a given period of time about the condition of the visual system with the multiple stimulus method than with the single stimulus method without reducing the reliability of the visual field examination.

9. Pseudo-variation.

One argument brought against the multiple stimulus method is that the variation in the threshold measurements is greater than when single stimulus presentation is used. It appears from our experiments that this is not the case. The multiple stimulus method does, however, give an impression of greater variation. This pseudo-variation occurs because the stimulation is repeated more frequently in the multiple stimulus method. If 4 stimuli are presented several times at threshold

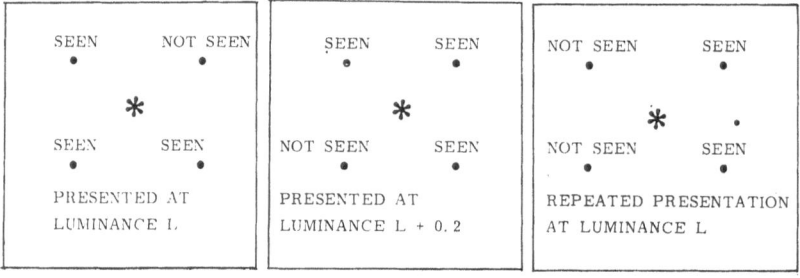

Fig. 4

Pseudo-variation of the multiple stimulus method on repeated presentation; groups of 4 simultaneously presented stimuli.

---

[24] GREVE, 1972.

level, it is not always the same stimuli in the pattern of four which are seen. The situation represented in Figure 4 can be a normal result of multiple stimulus presentation at threshold level and is produced by the normal threshold variation. If all 4 stimuli separately were repeatedly tested, the same result would be obtained.

In the multiple stimulus method the presentation of a group of stimuli is repeated regularly at the same level of luminance, if one or more stimuli from the group has not been seen. As explained above, this will usually occur at threshold level. There is a good chance that, on repetition, stimuli which were seen the first time will be missed and vice versa. This can even occur when the repetition takes place at a higher level of luminance, as long as both levels lie within the normal range (0.2 log unit).

A second cause of variation is formed by the angioscotomata. These physiological pseudoscotomata are so small ($< 1°$ diameter) that a stimulus may partially fall in the defect on the first presentation and fall outside it when the presentation is repeated, or vice versa. This is an established fact which can be explained by the physiological fixation nystagmus[25]. This type of variation arises in exactly the same way when a single stimulus is presented repeatedly in or near to an angioscotoma. It is only the more frequently repeated stimulation of one position in the multiple stimulus method which gives rise to this pseudo-variation.

A similar type of variation occurs with visual field defects with steep margins, when the stimulus falls on the margin of the defect.

10. Multiple stimuli and visual field defects.

If the simultaneous presentation of stimuli does not affect the level and variation of the difference threshold of normal subjects, this does not automatically hold true for patients. It is conceivable that in patients with cerebral lesions, in whom the higher perceptual functions are disturbed[26], the multiple stimulus method might produce incorrect results. This does not apply to glaucoma patients. If a disturbance of the higher perceptual functions (counting, indicating, completion) is present in neurological patients, this is only of importance for the investigation if this disorder leads to false negative results. Since this study does not deal with patients with defects like these, it is sufficient to say that we have seldom encountered false negative results of this origin. In addition, it should be remem-

---

[25] see Chapter VII.
[26] see e.g. BATTERSBY et al., 1953; WARRINGTON, 1967.

bered in these cases that the detection phase, does not only consist of the multiple stimulus method but that the periphery is also examined by the kinetic method.

Phenomenon of extinction.

When stimuli are presented simultaneously in the nasal and temporal hemifields the phenomenon of extinction may occur[27]. This is the phenomenon that a hemianopsia can be more easily demonstrated when a stimulus is presented simultaneously in both halves of the visual field than when a single stimulus is presented.

Knowledge of this phenomenon dates from many years back. We do not know of any recent information confirmed by static perimetry. The extinction phenomenon only occurs in hemianopsia. The lesion of the visual system causing this phenomenon is localized behind the lateral geniculate body and usually in the parietal lobe. For the study of glaucomatous visual field defects this phenomenon is of little importance.

INSTRUMENTS FOR MULTIPLE STIMULUS VISUAL FIELD EXAMINATION;
VISUAL FIELD ANALYSER

Although SALZER in 1927 had introduced a form of multiple stimulus visual field examination, the instrument of HARRINGTON & FLOCKS[28] was the first important application of the multiple stimulus principle. HARRINGTON & FLOCKS' instrument has been the precursor of, and model for, the other multiple stimulus instruments, such as the Fincham-Sutcliffe Screening scotometer[29] and the Visual Field Analyser[30]. We shall describe the Harrington-Flocks instrument and the Visual Field Analyser in detail. When considering these instruments we have to find out to what extent they meet the three chief requirements for visual field examination in the detection phase, i.e. static perimetry, 150 positions and threshold investigation. As all the methods considered here follow the principle of static presentation, this point needs not be discussed further. The other requirements for good visual field examination have been summed up on page 15. A very important requirement, which some multiple stimulus instruments cannot meet, is that of standardization.

---

[27] BENDER & FURLOW, 1945; BENDER & TEUBER, 1946; THIEBAULT et al., 1947.

[28] HARRINGTON & FLOCKS, 1954.

[29] SUTCLIFFE & BINSTEAD, 1961. We have no personal experience with the Feedback D.C.B. Screening Scotometer.

[30] FRIEDMANN, 1966; BEDWELL, 1967.

170

Method of Harrington and Flocks.

The 'Harrington-Flocks Multiple Pattern Method of Visual Field Examination' was presented to the American Ophthalmological Society in 1953 (Fig. 5).

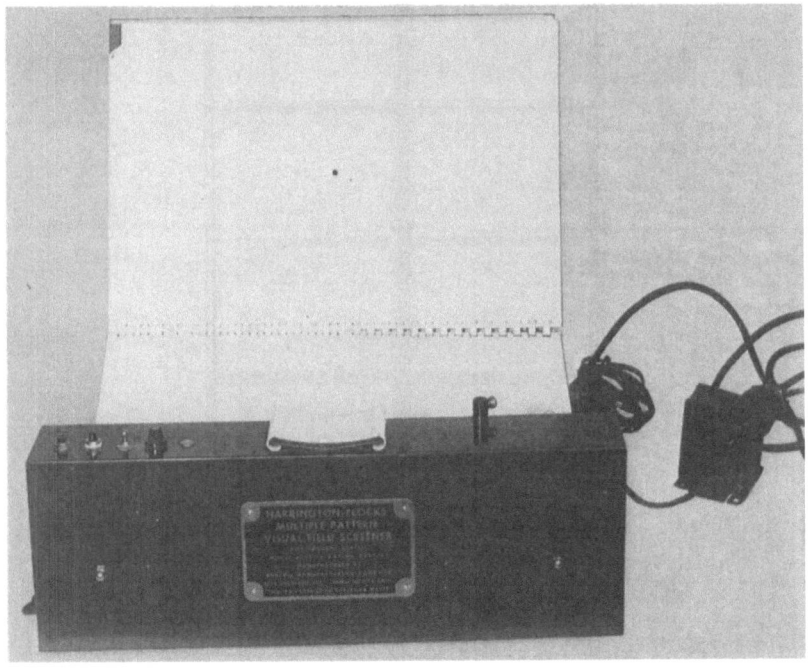

Fig. 5
Harrington-Flocks Multiple Pattern method of visual field examination

The principle of the instrument is that near ultra-violet light, provided by a fluorescent tube surrounded by a Corning 5874 filter, causes stimuli of fluorescent ink on a background of white paper to light up for 0.25 s.

The data of this instrument are given in Table I. The position of the stimuli in the 25° visual field and the groups of simultaneously presented stimuli are shown in Fig. 6a and b[31].

The instrument has no background illumination. The authors recommend a background illumination of 5 ft-cd.

If we assume that the reflection coefficient of the greyish paper is ± 0.6, the

---

[31] HARRINGTON, 1964.

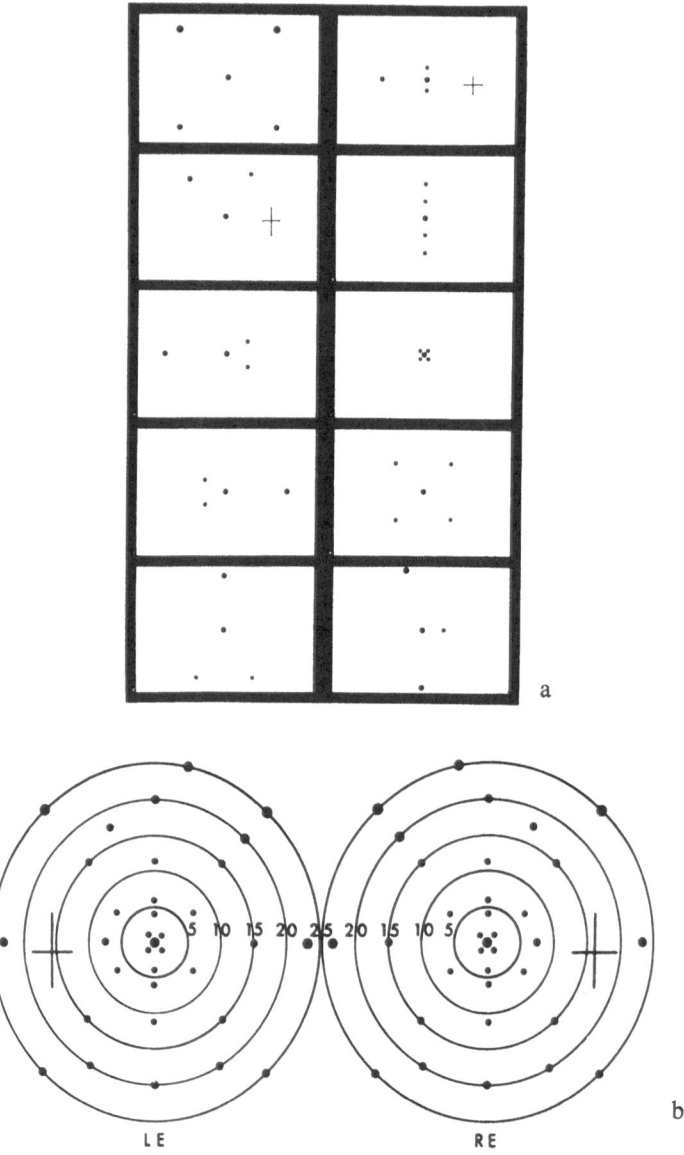

Fig. 6a, b
Positions of the stimuli of the Harrington-Flocks instrument

background luminance obtained with the recommended illumination is ± 30 asb (9.7 cd/m²). The fact that the Harrington-Flocks instrument has not got its own background illumination is one of its disadvantages. In practice many

TABLE I

Particulars of Harrington-Flocks Instrument

Distance between eye and background :	33 cm
Background luminance	: $\pm$ 30 asb (9.7 cd/m²) (recommended)
Number and position of stimuli	: 33 stimuli as in Fig. 6. With 2 crosses in the position of the blind spot; 10 patterns (Type III)
Examination of central light sensitivity:	not possible
Stimulus luminance	: equivalent to luminance of white paper illuminated by 7 ft.cd $= \pm$ 56 asb (14.7 cd/m²). One source of light; alteration of luminance not possible
Standardization	: not possible
Stimulus size	: 11' at 2° eccentricity (1 mm); 1°28' at 25° eccentricity (8 mm); more or less following the sensitivity gradient
Presentation time	: 0.25 s
Fixation control	: good

examiners do not possess a suitable room with a constant source of light which can be regulated and measured. A practical disadvantage associated with the background illumination of the HF instrument is that the examiner may cast a shadow on the background.

The stimulus luminance is, according to the authors, equal to the luminance of white paper illuminated with 7 ft-cd. This will be approximately a luminance of 56 asb (14.7 cd/m²; reflection coefficient 0.75).

An advantage of the HF instrument is that one source of light is used for all the stimuli. The short-wave light which is reflected from the objects is distracting when aphakics are being examined[32]. The maximum emission of the lamp-filter combination is at 364 nm.

An important disadvantage of the HF instrument is that the luminance is not variable. This means, in the first place, that every patient, regardless of age, is examined with the same stimulus luminance and in the second place, that the stimulus luminance is supraliminal. The luminance is also difficult to measure and to standardize.

---

[32] SLOAN, 1956.

An approximate calculation can be made of the degree to which the stimuli of the HF instrument are supraliminal. The background luminance is comparable to that of the Goldmann perimeter. Against this a stimulus of 11'diameter with a luminance of $\pm$ 56 asb is shown at 2° eccentricity.

By comparison with the normal sensitivity curve of the Goldmann perimeter we see that this luminance at 2° is 0.9 log unit supraliminal. As the size of the stimulus in the Goldmann perimeter is only 7' the stimulus of the HARRINGTON-FLOCKS instrument will be a few tenths of a log unit more supraliminal (0.2 log unit with a summation exponent of 0.5). The stimulation of the HF instrument is thus more than 1 log unit supraliminal. As the decrease in light sensitivity towards the periphery of the visual field is compensated by an increase in stimulus size, the stimulus will be about equally supraliminal at every degree of eccentricity. However, the authors never intended to construct a sensitive instrument for visual field examination; the HARRINGTON-FLOCKS instrument was intentionally constructed as a 'screener'. The authors' chief consideration was time: the examination had to be performed in 5 min. This aim is responsible for serious disadvantages. The stimuli are too strongly supraliminal. From the fact that one does not know how far above the threshold the examination is being carried out, it follows that one does not know the intensity of defects which are being missed. This is a fundamental objection to every screening method which works at a supraliminal luminance level. Absence of constant background luminance and standardizing methods for the various luminances means that the standardization of many important factors is insufficient.

The number of stimuli (33) is too small. The choice of the positions of the objects is disputable as far as the localization of stimuli (4) on the horizontal meridian is concerned. The positions are not well chosen for glaucomatous defects. When a fibre-bundle scotoma is sharply limited by the horizontal meridian, the stimuli on this meridian will be seen because the light sensitivity in the other half of the visual field is still good. A further disadvantage is that the central light sensitivity cannot be examined. This sums up the most important points concerning the Harrington-Flocks instrument. This method of examination does not fulfil fundamental criteria for rapid visual field examination.

The correctness of these theoretical objections was demonstrated in practice by comparing one year's results of examination with the Harrington-Flocks instrument with the results obtained with the Visual Field Analyser and the Goldmann perimeter. Relative defects (0.5–1.0 log unit), dependent on the age of the patient and the condition of the media, were missed with the Harrington-Flocks method. If only absolute defects or defects of large intensity are being looked for the Harrington-Flocks instrument can produce useful information.

174

Because the number of positions is so small, however, small absolute defects can also be missed. In the first part of this chapter it has already been pointed out that lines, crosses and circles as stimuli are not to be recommended[33].

The real importance of HARRINGTON & FLOCKS' work is that they showed that the principle of multiple stimulus presentation is useful for the practice of visual field examination.

Results obtained with the Harrington-Flocks instrument have been recorded in the literature[34].

In most publications the instrument was used as a 'screener', i.e., the patients were examined with the Harrington-Flocks instrument and additional examination was only carried out if defects were found with this instrument. An investigation like this can only provide information about false positive results and not about false negative results. Only HARRINGTON himself reports that he performed comparative studies with his method and the Tangent Screen. The author gives no figures and states that there is good correlation between the two methods but that some small glaucoma defects can be missed. HARRINGTON also considers that the sensitivity of the method might be increased by increasing the number of stimuli and decreasing the size of the stimuli, but he does not wish to make these alterations for fear of false positive results and too long examination time. It is emphasized again that false positive results are no problem if the examination is not performed with the all-or-nothing supraliminal method but by means of a threshold examination starting from an infraliminal luminance level. Unfortunately such an examination is not possible with the Harrington-Flocks instrument as the luminance of the stimuli is not variable. Moreover it does not seem justified to make such an all-important point of the examination time when constructing an instrument for the rapid detection of visual field defects.

A good result with the Harrington-Flocks instrument, i.e. all stimuli seen, gives an unjustified feeling of safety; the visual field has only been partially examined and the absence of defects has not been definitely proved.

Fincham and Sutcliffe's instrument.

The 'Fincham-Sutcliffe Screening Scotometer' was introduced in 1961 (Fig. 7). The aim was the construction of a 'screening' instrument which could also function as campimeter background for the Juler-Stimulus-Projector. Data of this

---

[33] see stimuli of the original Harrington-Flocks instrument, 1954.
[34] HARRINGTON & FLOCKS, 1959; ROBERTS, 1957; HILTON, 1958; CASSIDY & HAVENER, 1959; KUHN, 1957; ROBERTSON, 1956; HARRINGTON, 1971, 3rd edition book.

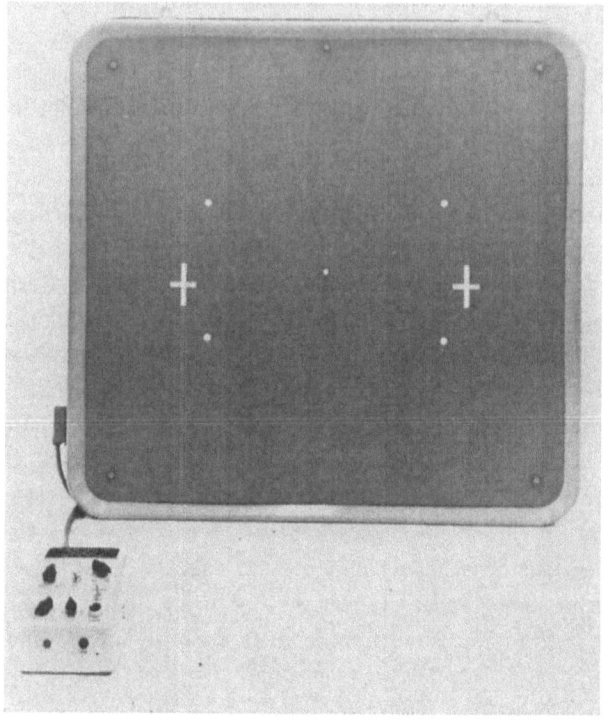

Fig. 7
Fincham-Sutcliffe screening scotometer

instrument are given in Table II. The instrument consists of a grey screen covering the 25° visual field at a distance of 1 m from the eye.

In the screen there are 58 holes with translucent plugs, behind which are low-voltage lamps. The use of 58 different lamps introduces a large variation in luminance and presentation time. It is very difficult, if not impossible, to standardize 58 lamps. 58 lamps also undergo changes at different rates. We measured the luminance of the lamps in the FS instrument we were using and found differences of factor 2 between individual lamps (0.3 log unit). Problems concerning the use of lamps have also been noted by Gloster[35] using the Globuck screen. The use of a number of lamps, which are difficult to standardize, is not to be recommended for multiple stimulus instruments.

The objections to the absence of standardized background luminance as part of the instrument have already been given.

---

[35] GLOSTER, 1971.

TABLE II
Particulars of Fincham-Sutcliffe Instrument

Distance between eye and background :	100 cm
Background luminance :	not part of instrument. Recommended: 30–40 lux on background with reflection coefficient of 0.3–0.35 = ± 10 asb (3.14 cd/m²)
Number and position of stimuli :	58 stimuli in 18 patterns (Fig. 8)
Examination of central light sensitivity:	not possible
Stimulus luminance :	unknown. Source of light: 58 different low-voltage tungsten filament lamps behind plastic translucent plugs. Luminance adjustable by means of rheostat
Standardization :	none
Stimulus size :	only 2 stimulus diameters: 2.0 and 3.0 mm (± 7′). Not following the sensitivity gradient
Presentation time :	variable between 0.1 and 0.9 s, 0.25 s recommended
Fixation control :	good

The number of stimuli in the Fincham-Sutcliffe instrument is larger than in the Harrington-Flocks instrument, and thus the chance of detecting a defect is greater (Fig. 8). The stimulus size, in which there is only a choice of two, does not compensate the decreasing sensitivity towards the periphery.

The poor standardization of this instrument made us decide not to continue

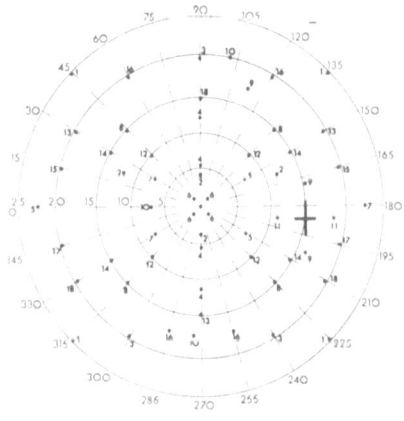

R.E.

Fig. 8
Positions of the stimuli of the Fincham-Sutcliffe instrument

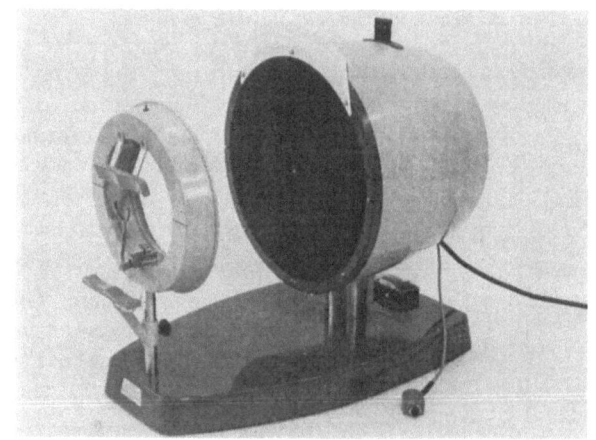

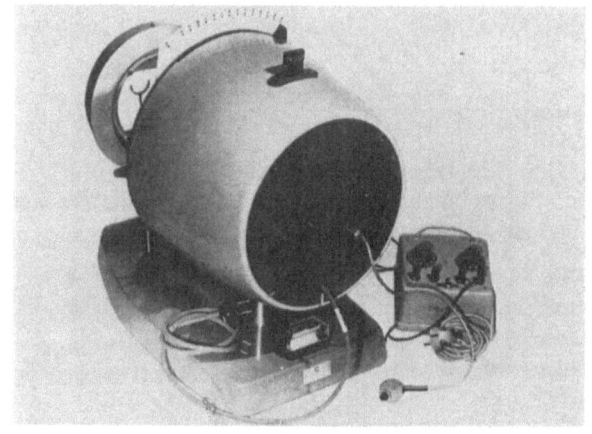

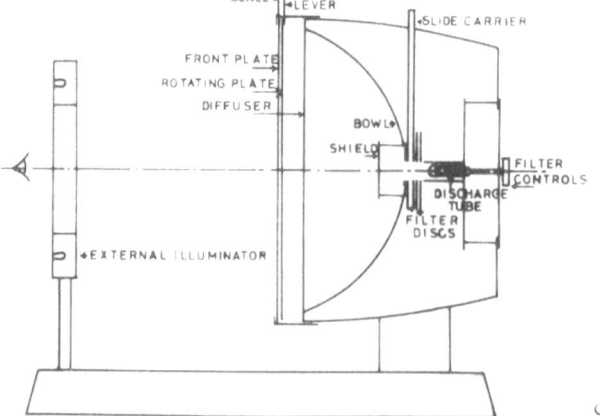

Fig. 9a, b, c
Visual Field Analyser

using it in our investigation after a trial period of six months. On the other hand the attempt to combine the detection phase and the assessment phase in one instrument is to be welcomed.

The Friedmann Visual Field Analyser.

The Friedmann Visual Field Analyser was described by FRIEDMANN (1966) and BEDWELL (1967). We chose this instrument for multiple stimulus examination in the detection phase because it is the best available instrument at the moment.

A technical description and discussion of the Visual Field Analyser will be given first. A number of data are summarized in Table III. The instrument is illustrated (with section) in Fig. 9a and b, and in Fig. 10a and b the positions of the stimuli in the 25° visual field and the groups of stimuli which are presented simultaneously are shown. The Visual Field Analyser is a compact instrument, with which groups of 2, 3 or 4 stimuli are presented by means of a fixed plate and a rotating plate, in which a number of openings have been made. In each of the 15 positions of the rotating plate a number of openings in the two plates correspond. Through the openings the subject sees the diffuser of opal plastic, which lies just behind the plates. The diffuser is illuminated for a short time by means of a system consisting of a Xenon flash tube and an integrating hemisphere.

TABLE III

Particulars of Visual Field Analyser

Distance between eye and background :	33 cm
Background luminance	: built-in background illumination of 10 lux on dull black background with reflection $\pm$ 0.05; 0.5 asb (0.16 cd$\pm$m²)
Number and position of stimuli	: 46 stimuli presented in 15 groups (Fig. 10)
Examination of central light sensitivity:	possible
Stimulus luminance	: with presentation time of 380 µs $\pm$ 6 $\times$ 10⁴ cd/m² (see text); one source of light: Xenon flash tube
Alteration of luminance	: with neutral filters in steps of 0.2 log unit
Standardizing apparatus	: not built in (see text)
Stimulus size	: smallest stimulus at 2° is 15′30″ (1.5 mm); approximately in agreement with course of sensitivity gradient (see text)
Presentation time	: 130 µs at top of flash; 380 µs at one third from the top (see text)
Fixation control	: very difficult

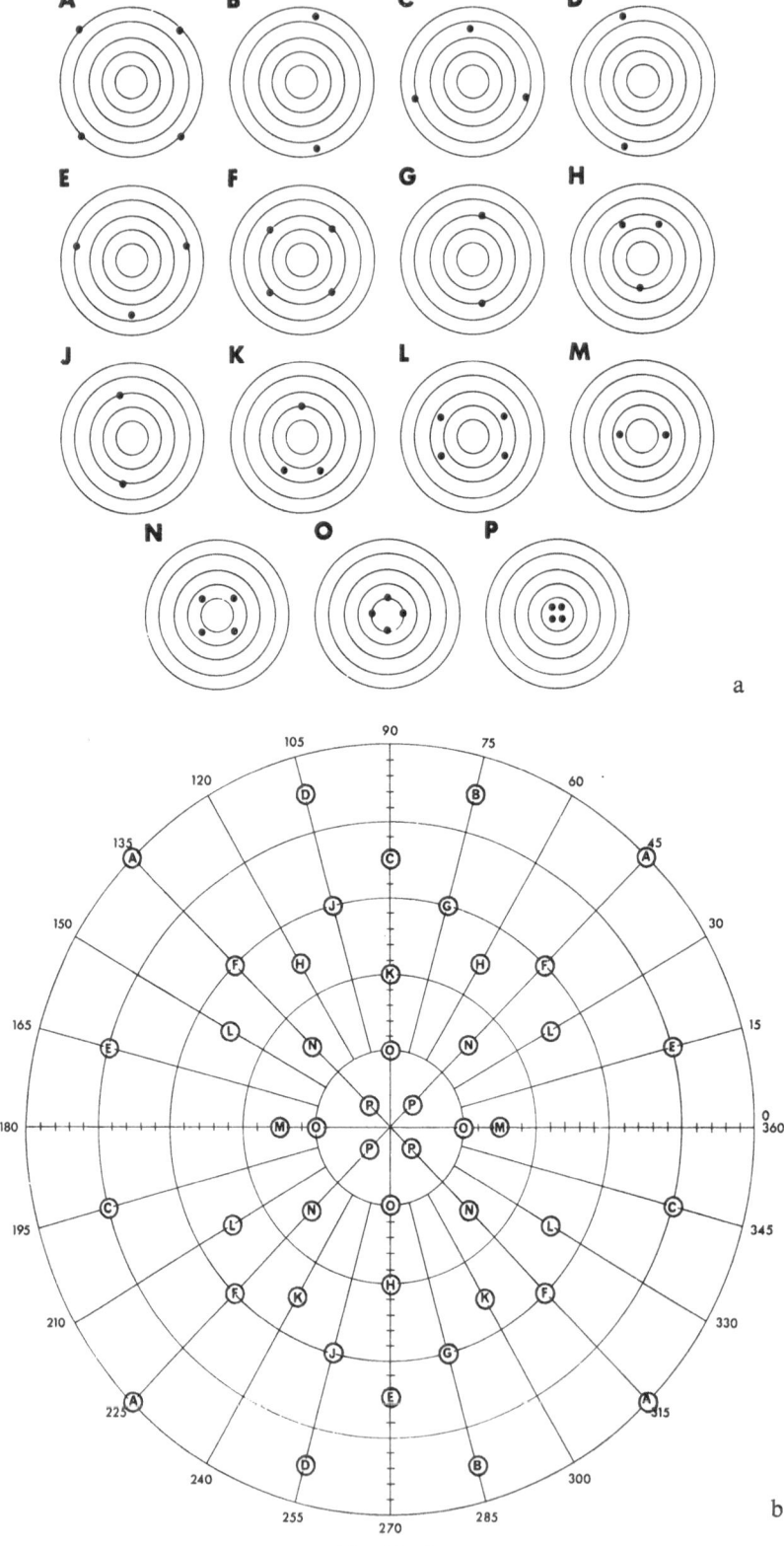

Fig. 10a, b

Positions of the stimuli of the Visual Field Analyser and groups of simultaneously
presented stimuli

In addition to the peripheral stimuli there is a stimulus for the examination of the central light sensitivity. The construction of the Visual Field Analyser is simple and efficient for multiple stimulus presentation; the designers have found an ingenious way of using one source of light for all the stimuli.

Unfortunately the construction is not very stable, so that the instrument sways when it is touched by the examiner or the subject. This is not a fundamental objection but it is disagreeable in practice. A second objection to the construction is that it is difficult to check the subject's fixation. This has become apparent during the examination of thousands of patients with this instrument.

The advantages and disadvantages of the Visual Field Analyser are as follows:

Advantages.

1. ingenious presentation system for multiple stimuli;
2. one source of light for all stimuli;
3. variable stimulus luminance;
4. large range of stimulus luminance;
5. short presentation time;
6. built-in background illumination;
7. central light sensitivity can be examined;
8. easy to use.

Disadvantages

A. Fundamental

1. poor fixation control;
2. too few stimuli; choice of positions in some cases not suitable for glaucomatous defects;
3. choice of stimulus size does not completely compensate the sensitivity gradient; compensation by altering luminance is preferable;
4. the same strength of stimulus for nasal and temporal intermediate visual fields;
5. low background luminance (with reservations, see text);
6. no built-in standardizing method.

B. Minor disadvantages

7. openings in the front plates are visible;
8. unstable construction;
9. no holder for a correcting lens;
10. no headband;
11. Xenon flashtubes and electrical system change with time (see 6);

A few important points will now be considered.

Luminance

The great advantage of the Visual Field Analyser is that the *luminance is variable.*

The Visual Field Analyser is the only multiple stimulus instrument with variable luminance. Together with the built-in background illumination and the use of one source of light for all the stimuli, the fact that the luminance is variable made us decide to use the Visual Field Analyser for our investigation. It has already been emphasized that the measurement of the difference threshold is essential for the detection ('screening') of defects as well as for their assessment. Without variable luminance this is impossible. The luminance steps of 0.2 log unit are obtained by means of Kodak Wratten neutral density filters. The range of luminance is $\pm$ 2.4 log unit for all stimuli for a normal subject. This range is easily sufficient compared, for instance, with the Goldmann perimeter which only has this range at the centre, whereas at 25° eccentricity the range is reduced to 1.2 log unit[36]. A Xenon flashtube has the disadvantage that it is difficult to standardize. The advantage of such lamps is the very short presentation time[37]. The presentation time of the Visual Field Analyser is far under the critical time. A second advantage of Xenon flashtubes is the large light output. The stimulus luminance of a Xenon flashtube cannot be measured in the usual way with a luminance- or lux-meter, like lamps which burn constantly. We measured the light coming from the diffuser (without the front plate) in 3 different Visual Field Analysers: a new instrument (no. 1), an instrument which had been used for a short time (no. 2), and an instrument which had been intensively used for 2 years (no. 3).

Our measurements concern the complete illumination system of the Visual Field Analyser, i.e. the flashtube, the feedingsystem, the hemisphere and the diffuser. A few measurements were also made with neutral density filters. The measuring apparatus consisted of a vacuum photo-electric cell[38] and a storage oscilloscope[39].

---

[36] see Chapter VII. If one stimulus size is used.

[37] see Chapter IV.

[38] type 150 AV Philips with Kodak Wratten filter 106.

[39] These measurements were made possible thanks to Ir. K. VAN DEN BERGE of the 'Laboratorium voor Medische Fysica' in Amsterdam. We are very grateful to him for his valuable advice. Data concerning these measurements can be found in the Technical Note of BRUNETTE & MOLOTCHINNIKOFF, 1970.

TABLE IV

Results of measurements of the light source of 3 Visual Field Analysers; see text

instrument	V_0	$T(V_0)$	$T(1/3V_0)$*[40]	light flux in lumen	luminance[41] in cd/m²
no. 1 max.	3.55	0.13	0.38	2.6	6×10^4
no. 2 max.	2.65	0.12	0.38	1.9	4.45×10^4
no. 3 max.	1.85	0.14	0.43	1.3	3×10^3

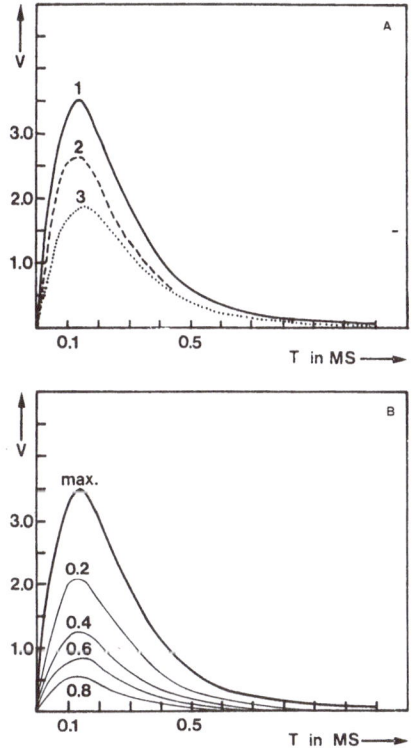

Fig. 11

A Registration of the flashes of the light sources of 3 different Visual Field Analysers
B Registration of a flash with and without neutral density filters

---

[40] time in microseconds.
[41] for a presentation time of $T(1/3V_0)$.

The results of the measurements are given in Table IV and Fig. 11.

In Fig. 11a the curves of the 3 different instruments are represented graphically and in Fig. 11b the maximum curve (without filters) and the curves with respectively 0.2, 0.4, 0.6 and 0.8 log unit filters are given. The light flux increases very rapidly for a short time up to a maximum (V_0) and then decreases exponentially. The energy content of a flash like this can be roughly compared to a rectangular flash with V_0 as indicator for the light flux and a presentation time of $T(1/3V_0)$. The flash from Xenon tube no. 1 can thus be compared with a rectangular flash of 6×10^4 cd/m² with a presentation time of 0.38 ms. The effect of this flash is the same as that of a flash of 0.038 s with a luminance of 600 cd/m² (total temporal summation). Roughly speaking (partial temporal summation) this flash can be compared with a flash of 1.0 s. with a luminance of $\pm$ 300 cd/m² (with stimulus size 15′ and background luminance 0.16 cd/m² $= 0.5$ asb)[42].

The neutral density filters are Kodak Wratten gelatine filters, the properties of which are known. From the measurements shown in Fig. 11 it appears that the steps of luminance correspond fairly well with the given 0.2 log unit (deviation 10%).[43]

[42] The luminance of the Visual Field Analyser at 2° eccentricity is 2.6 log unit above threshold level; the threshold level would be $\pm$ 300/400 $= 0.75$ cd/m²; for instrument no. 3 the threshold luminance would be $\pm$ 0.37 cd/m²; stimulus II (14′) of the Goldmann perimeter has a threshold luminance of 0.16 cd/m² at 2° eccentricity with a background luminance of 0.5 asb. These luminances are all of the same order of magnitude.
[43] This table indicates the measured luminance values in percentage of the maximum luminance.

filter	expected value	measured value
0.2	63%	60%
0.4	40%	36%
0.6	25%	23%
0.8	16%	16%

From these measurements the following conclusions may be drawn about the light source of the Visual Field Analyser:

1. the light flux from the flash of the Xenon tube only varies slightly on repeated presentations ($\pm$ 5%). This variation is negligible for clinical visual field examination.

2. if the interval between flashes is too short for recharge of the flashtube the light flux decreases. This decrease was perceptible with instrument no. 3 as soon as the recharging time was less than 2 s. When the recharging time is too short the light flux decreases; with a recharging time of 1 s the light

flux is about 0.1 log unit lower. When the recharging time is 3 s the decrease in light flux is negligible.

3. the whole system of flash tube, feeding system, hemisphere and diffuser changes considerably with use, at least if we may assume that the original light flux of each instrument was the same. Instrument no. 3 only produced 50 % of the light flux of instrument no. 1[44].

There are considerable differences in the level of luminance in Visual Field Analysers which have been used for longer or shorter periods of time.

These differences emphasize the necessity of a good method of standiardization for the Visual Field Analyser. The light flux of the instrument should be standardized regularly and the lamp renewed if necessary.

4. The time needed to reach the V_o value is $\pm$ 0.13 ms (130 μs); the time for the light flux to decrease to one third of the V_o value is between 380 and 400μs. After 1 ms the V_o value is practically 0.

A Xenon flashtube is a good source of light for multiple stimulus static visual field examination. A relatively simple and cheap standardization method still has to be found[45].

Background.

The Visual Field Analyser has a built-in system for the illumination of the dull black front plate. This is a definite advantage as compared with the other instruments described here. This source of light produces an even illumination of 10 lux[46].

Behind the ring-shaped dull white diffuser are 8 lamps, burning on low voltage, in order to secure a longer life and reduce the effects of fluctuations in the electric current.

The lamps are easy to change. The background illumination can be measured with a luxmeter (which is unfortunately not supplied with the instrument). The reflection coefficient of the background, according to our measurements, is $\pm$ 0.05. The resulting luminance is 0.5 asb (0.16 cd/m²), which brings the adaptation level into the low photopic area[47]. A disadvantage of every dull black background is that scratches and shiny areas can be disturbing, but this is an inconvenience of minor importance.

---

[44] see Table IV.

[45] FRIEDMANN himself uses a Patterson CDS Endarging Computer (personal communication).

[46] Our measurements showed that this illumination is uniform within acceptable limits.

[47] AEG Lux meter, Mc Beth illuminometer.

The background luminance of 0.5 asb (0.16 cd/m²) was partly chosen because the authors thought that visual field examination was more sensitive at the mesopic adaptation level than at the photopic level (on account of JAYLE's work). By our definition background luminance of 0.5 asb is not mesopic but low photopic. This is apparent from Fig. 12, in which the sensitivity curve of a stimulus

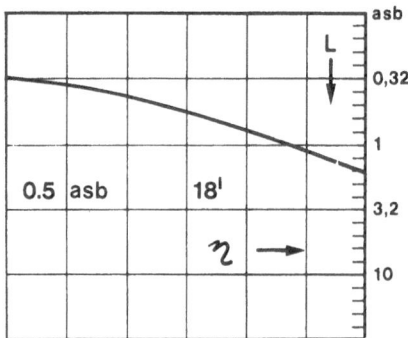

Fig. 12

Sensitivity curve of a stimulus of 18′ on a background luminance of 0.5 asb (Tübinger perimeter)

of 18′ angular subtense with background luminance of 0.5 asb is given. The matter of the supposed mesopic sensitivity has been extensively dealt with[48]. As long as it has not been convincingly proved that it is advantageous to examine glaucomatous visual fields under mesopic conditions, the photopic adaptation level is to be preferred. The most important arguments in favour of this are the adaptation time and the adaptation sensitivity (for light from outside). Experience with the Visual Field Analyser has shown that one must wait several minutes before the patient is adapted, and that changes in the surrounding illumination have a disturbing effect.

Central sensitivity.

A point in favour of the Visual Field Analyser is that it is possible to examine the central light sensitivity. To this end the white fixation object is removed and, in the central opening which now appears, the central stimulus is presented in the same way as the peripheral stimuli. The central stimulus is single. Examination of the central light sensitivity is an essential part of every visual field examination. Central and peri-, para- or ceco-central scotomata can only be

---

[48] see Chapter IV.

assessed correctly if the central light sensitivity is known. The comparison of the visual acuity with the central light sensitivity is an important check on the results of the examination and in some cases it is of diagnostic importance (amblyopia, cataract).

In the instruments used by us, the diameter of the central stimulus is larger than that of the stimuli at 2°, so that the central threshold level is usually 0.4 log unit lower (i.e. higher filter density) than the peripheral threshold levels.

Number and position of stimuli.

The Visual Field Analyser has 46 stimuli, divided into 15 groups. The number of stimuli is insufficient. Small defects, or in some positions even large defects, can be missed with the Visual Field Analyser because the distance between the stimuli is too large (Fig. 13). For technical reasons the number of stimuli in the Visual Field Analyser cannot be increased. The limited number of stimuli is an important disadvantage of this instrument, which is ingenious in so many ways. This disadvantage can, however, be overcome, by using a second front plate, for instance, by means of which the number of stimuli can be doubled.

The stimuli on the horizontal meridian are badly placed for the visual field

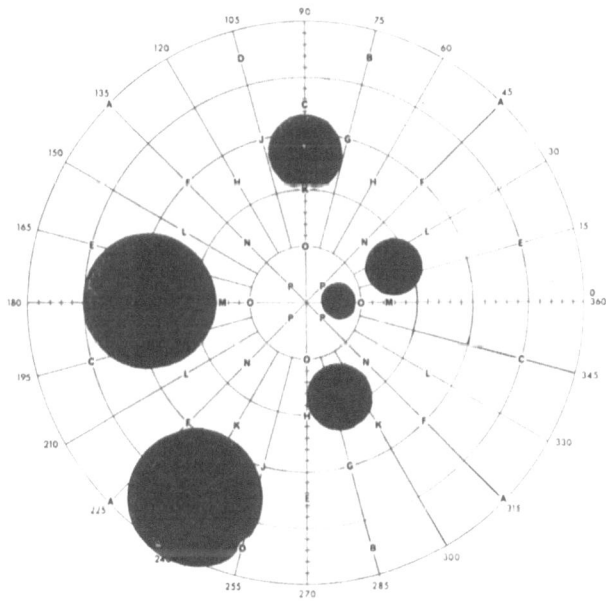

Fig. 13
Some defects that can theoretically be missed by the Visual Field Analyser

187

examination of glaucoma patients. When a defect has a sharp horizontal boundary stimuli 0 and M often just fall in the intact half of the visual field.

The important nasal area on both sides of the horizontal meridian is only covered by 2 stimuli: P at 2° and E or C at 20°. The number of stimuli in the central visual field is insufficient. The right and left eyes are examined with stimuli in the same position and of the same strength. In the central visual field there is no difference in the topography of the light sensitivity between the two eyes, but at 20° eccentricity the temporal visual field is 0.1–0.2 log unit more sensitive than the nasal visual field. This means that the stimuli A (25°) and C (20°) cannot be equidistant with regard to the average sensitivity curve for both the nasal and the temporal visual field. The difference of 0.1–0.2 log unit may give rise to a difference in perception of one step of luminance, which means that the nasal stimulus of group C will be seen one filter-step later than the temporal stimulus.

Stimulus size.

The size of the stimuli in the Visual Field Analyser increases from 2° to 25° eccentricity in order to compensate the decrease of light sensitivity towards the periphery. For several reasons it is preferable to keep the size of stimulus unchanged and to compensate the sensitivity gradient by means of neutral filters[49]. Bedwell[50] has listed the angular subtense of the stimuli in the Visual

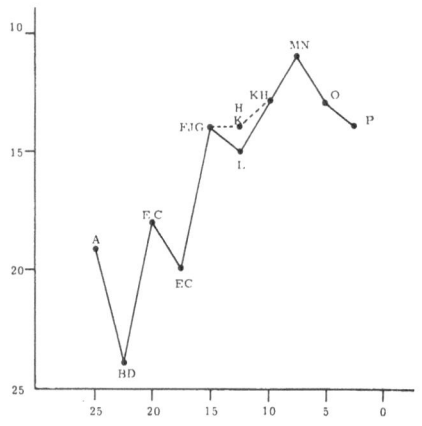

Fig. 14

Angular subtense of the stimuli of the Visual Field Analyser; abscissa: eccentricity; ordinate: angular subtense in degrees

---

[49] see Chapter IV.
[50] BEDWELL, 1967.

188

Field Analyser. If a sort of sensitivity curve is drawn from these data the result is the curve shown in Fig. 14. It appears that the stimuli at 2° (P) and 5° (0) are larger than the stimuli at 7.5° (MN) and the same size as the stimuli at 10° (KH). Furthermore the curve does not follow the smooth, nearly linear course of the normal sensitivity gradient.

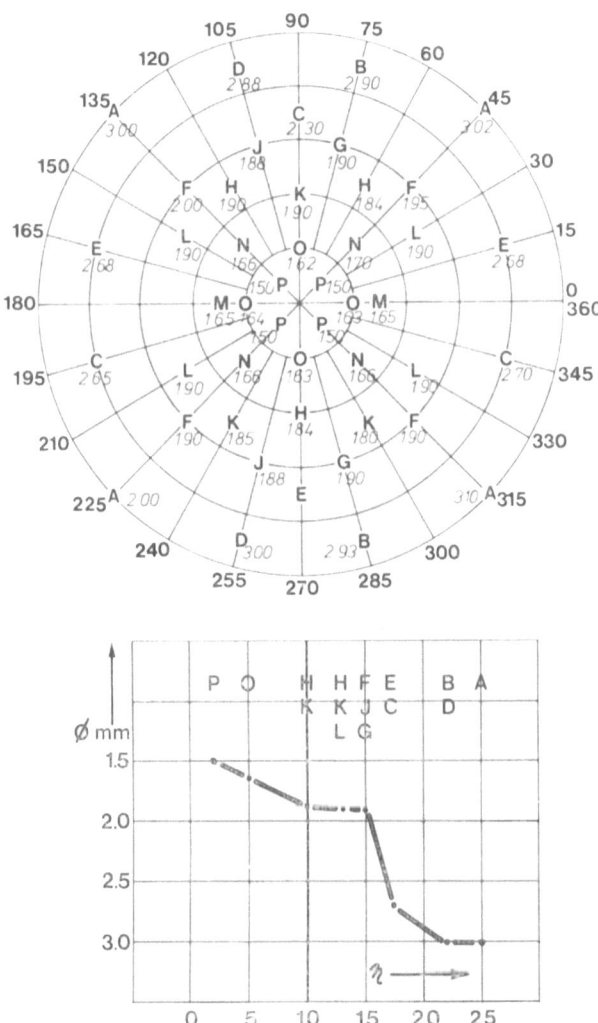

Fig. 15

Measurements of the sizes of the holes of the Visual Field Analyser frontplate (in mm.).

We measured the diameter of the openings in the front plate (i.e. not the same as the angular subtense) and found the results shown in Fig. 15a and b. It is again apparent that the choice (or the technical realization) of the stimulus size is not completely infallible. The most striking facts are:
1. the pericentral stimuli (0 and P) are too big;
2. the stimuli at 15° (FJG) are too small.

If the effect of these size anomalies is calculated in log units of difference in luminance, taking into account the spatial summation coefficient, differences of 0.1–0.15 log unit are obtained. These discrepancies may give rise to a difference of one step (0.2 log unit) in the thresholds of simultaneously presented stimuli.

Imperfections like these can be avoided by working with neutral filters instead of stimuli of different sizes.

The sizes of the stimuli were chosen after experimental examination of normal subjects[51]. The subjects were examined without correction for near vision. This is probably the reason why the pericentral stimuli are too big. The average stimulus size as given by Bedwell is 14′; in our measurements the smallest stimulus at 2° has a diameter of 15′30″.

Conclusion.

For multiple stimulus presentation the Visual Field Analyser is at present the instrument of choice. In a number of details it is susceptible of improvement. The ultimate aim should be the construction of an optimum multiple stimulus instrument as described on page 199.

Examination with the Visual Field Analyser.

In the instructions provided with the instrument, one is advised to examine the patient with a certain stimulus luminance according to his age. This luminance is chosen so that all normal subjects in the age group are able to see the stimuli. It follows that this luminance must at least be equal to the tolerance limit in the age group[52]. From our own experiments it appears that the tolerance limit lies about 0.3 log unit above the average sensitivity curve; in subjects with high sensitivity the tolerance level can be 0.6 log unit supraliminal. In such cases defects of 0.5 log unit may be missed. The fundamental objections to this method of examination have been brought forward. We therefore performed all our examinations with the Visual Field Analyser starting from the infraliminal level.

---

[51] FRIEDMANN, personal communication.

[52] see first part of this chapter and Chapter VII.

For every position a threshold luminance is determined. The examination is performed as follows: a group of stimuli is presented infraliminally. The patient does not see anything. The luminance is increased by 0.2 log unit and the stimuli are presented again; when the patient's threshold level is reached he will see one or more stimuli of the group. When not all the stimuli are seen the patient is asked to indicate which he saw. Of these positions the threshold is now known. To determine the threshold luminance of the stimuli in the group which were not seen, the luminance is again raised by 0.2 log unit. In a number of cases the patient will now see all the stimuli. The threshold luminance at the positions examined is noted. When one or more stimuli from a group are missed we repeat the examination of these positions twice at the same level of luminance, in order to be sure that the threshold is not raised as the result of blinking, diminished attention or inaccurate fixation. The repeat examination does not take place straight away, so that the same group is never presented twice consecutively. When the stimuli are seen with two of the three presentations with a given luminance we record this luminance as the threshold luminance. When the threshold luminance of one or more stimuli lies 0.4 log unit lower than that of other stimuli, this is theoretically a significant loss of sensitivity.

In practice, however, this need not be the case.[53] The reason for this is, on the one hand, the imperfections in the choice of stimulus size in the Visual Field Analyser and, on the other hand, the interindividual variations in the shape of the sensitivity curve. If the latter is the reason this can be recognized. When a subject's sensitivity curve is clearly steeper or flatter than the average, the difference in threshold luminance between the central and peripheral stimuli will be larger than expected from interindividual variation. Generally speaking the divergence from the average gradient of sensitivity will appear in all meridians. This is expressed, on examination with the Visual Field Analyser, as a gradually increasing (steeper gradient) or decreasing (flatter gradient) threshold luminance from the centre to the periphery in all meridians. In Fig. 16 an example of normal variation in the results of examination with the Visual Field Analyser is given. When an isolated reduction in sensitivity of 0.4 log unit is found (which is thus not part of an inter-individual gradient variation) the cause can be an angioscotoma, a pathological defect, or one of the above mentioned imperfections in the Visual Field Analyser. The differentiation between these takes place in the assessment phase.

When evaluating the results of examination with the Visual Field Analyser

---

[53] see also Chapter XI.

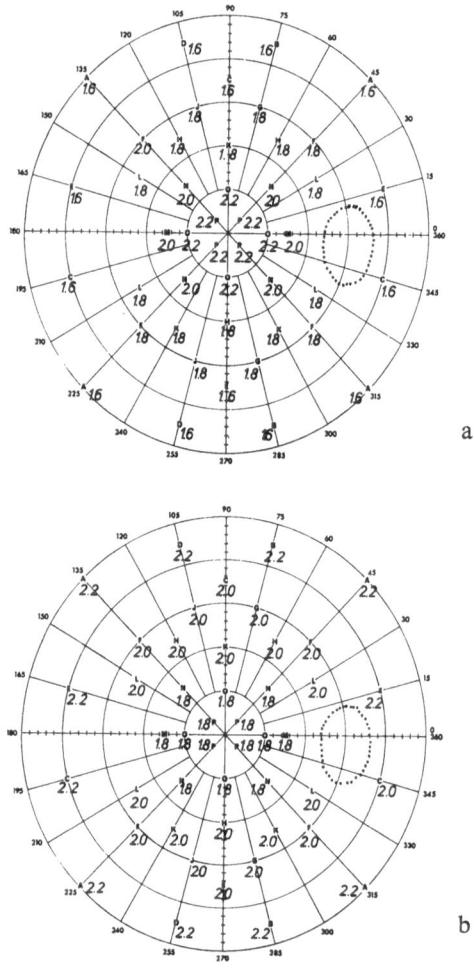

Fig. 16
Example of the effect of a steep gradient (a) and a flat gradient (b) on the result of the examination with the Visual Field Analyser

it should be taken into account that the central openings (P,O) in the front plate are rather too large and that therefore a lower threshold luminance (higher filter density) will often be found in the centre[54].

Although strictly speaking it is not necessary in the detection phase to do more than detect significant loss of sensitivity (i.e. reduction of 0.4–0.6 log unit)

[54] A detailed description of our method is given elsewhere, GREVE & VERRIEST, 1971 (Dutch text).

192

we always complete the examination with the Visual Field Analyser, i.e. we determine the exact level of every reduction in sensitivity. To understand the reason for this, one should be familiar with the organization of a department for visual field examination[55].

The examination, which is performed by specialized technical assistants, is supervised by the perimetrologist. For the perimetrologist the comparison of the results of a complete investigation with the Visual Field Analyser (intensity of defects accurate to 0.2 log unit) with the results of the assessment phase is an important check on the quality of the examination. The fact that the measurements are partially repeated increases the reliability of the examination.

Normal visual field with the Visual Field Analyser.

As has been explained, differences between the threshold luminances of the 46 positions examined with the Visual Field Analyser are often found. In our experience it seldom happens that the thresholds of all 46 stimuli lie at the same luminance level. In a study of 21 normal subjects differences of 0.2 log unit were found in 11 cases, of 0.4 log unit in 6 cases and of 0.6 log unit in 3 cases (see Table V)[56]. The reason has already been discussed.

TABLE V

Differences in threshold level of stimuli of the Visual Field Analyser; 21 normal subjects

Greatest difference	No. of subjects
0.6	3
0.4	6
0.2	11
Total	20

A quite different cause of raised threshold luminance is the existence of physiological angioscotomata. The angioscotomata are limited in position, size and intensity[57]. When examined with the Visual Field Analyser the angioscotomata can have a maximum intensity of 0.8 log unit.

---

[55] see also Chapter XI.

[56] after GREVE, 1972.

[57] see Chapter VII.

TABLE VI

*Highest filter dial positions at which one or more
stimuli were seen by 21 normal young subjects*

Higher filter dial position	No. of subjects
2.6	3
2.4	14
2.2	4
Total	21

Many normal subjects of 20–35 years of age can see the stimuli of the Visual Field Analyser with a filter density of 2.4 or even 2.6.

The inter-individual variation is $\pm$ 0.6 log unit in this age group. In the older age groups ($>$ 60 years) the variation in level and form of the sensitivity curve increases on account of opacities in the media (chiefly lens opacities), which show marked individual differences. Some 70-year-old subjects see the majority of the stimuli with a filter density of 2.0, while other 70-year-old subjects only begin to see stimuli with a filter density of 1.0. There is no point in giving normal values for this age group.

THE VISUAL FIELD ANALYSER IN THE DETECTION PHASE

Literature and introduction.

Only a few publications have appeared in the literature, on comparative studies with the Visual Field Analyser. We have not been able to find an account of a comparative study between single stimulus static visual field examination and multiple stimulus static visual field examination, as described in this study.

Favourable results have been obtained by FECHNER & HEAFNER and by WENC-KER[58]. FECHNER & HAEFNER followed the instructions for use of the Visual Field Analyser and compared the results with kinetic projection campimetry[59] and kinetic perimetry with the Maggiore perimeter. These authors recommend the Visual Field Analyser for the detection of visual field defects. From their data it appears that only defects of fairly large size and intensity were compared. We

---

[58] FECHNER & HAEFNER, 1971; WENCKER, 1970.
[59] Projector held in the examiner's hand.

have only been able to obtain information about WENCKER'S work from publications by DEMAILLY[60].

WENCKER compared the results obtained with the Visual Field Analyser with results obtained with the II/1-object of the Goldmann perimeter and, as was to be expected, found a number of defects with the Visual Field Analyser which were not found with the Goldmann perimeter.

Some of our own experiences have already been reported in preliminary publications[61]. In this work these studies have been extended and further elaborated, with a number of alterations.

As has already been emphasized at the beginning of this chapter the saving of time is the only reason for using multiple stimulus presentation.

If the 46 stimulus positions of the Visual Field Analyser are examined by means of kinetic perimetry – which means examination of 7 isopters (Fig. 17) –

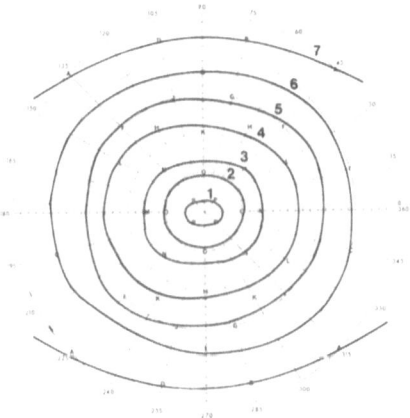

Fig. 17

Seven isopters necessary to examine the 46 stimulus positions of the Visual Field Analyser with kinetic perimetry.

it is found that the examination of a normal subject takes about 9 minutes. If the same examination is performed by means of single stimulus static perimetry (steps of 0.2 log unit), it takes about 12 minutes. If the same normal subject is examined with the Visual Field Analyser this takes about 4 minutes. The ratio examination time Visual Field Analyser: examination time kinetic perimetry:

---

[60] DEMAILLY, 1971; DEMAILLY et al, 1973.

[61] GREVE, 1970; GREVE & KINDS, 1970.

195

examination time single stimulus static perimetry is 4:9:12. A considerable amount of time is thus saved by using multiple stimulus presentation.

In a comparative study between the Visual Field Analyser on the one hand and the Goldmann and Tübinger perimeters or Double Projection Campimeter on the other hand, the differences between these methods must be taken into consideration. A number of characteristics in which the Visual Field Analyser differs from the classical methods are given in Table III of Chapter VI. The most important points are:

1. 46 fixed positions in the 52° field;
2. cartographic accuracy;
3. background luminance of 0.5 asb;
4. luminance steps of 0.2 log unit;
5. presentation time of 380 µs;
6. multiple stimuli.

When the results of the Visual Field Analyser are compared with the results of *kinetic visual field examination*, in the first place the fundamental differences between static and kinetic visual field examination must be taken into account[62]. In the second place the outcome of the comparison depends on the number of positions examined with kinetic perimetry.

In most cases this is, with the usual kinetic procedures, about 32 positions within the 30° parallel and the examination of the blind spot. This means that less positions are examined than with the Visual Field Analyser, so that the detection chance is reduced proportionally. The blind spot, on the other hand, is usually more closely examined with the kinetic method than with the Visual Field Analyser. The Visual Field Analyser has 4 stimuli round the blind spot while, in the kinetic method, the limits of the blind spot are determined in at least 8 positions working from the blind spot outwards. Finally, in kinetic perimetry larger steps of luminance are generally used (0.5 log unit for the Goldmann perimeter instead of 0.2 log unit for the Visual Field Analyser).

When the results of the examination with the Visual Field Analyser are compared with those of *static perimetry*, the first consideration is again the number and localization of the positions examined. In the detection phase the examination of two oblique meridians has its limitations as, although great spatial accuracy is achieved in these meridians, outside them large areas of the visual field remain unexamined. The same applies to circular static perimetry along one parallel. Distribution of the positions to be examined as in the Visual Field

---

[62] see Chapter III.

Analyser is better for the detection phase, although the number of stimuli is too small.

In the assessment phase, as has been explained, degree-by-degree meridional or circular perimetry is the method of choice. When a defect has once been discovered, it will be more accurately registered by means of classical static perimetry. Comparison of the results obtained with the Visual Field Analyser and with classical perimetry is only worthwhile as far as the detection phase is concerned.

The cartographic accuracy of the Visual Field Analyser is optimum as there is no transmission system, and localization of the stimulus is not necessary because the stimuli have fixed positions.

The question of the background luminance has already come up several times. It cannot be said with certainty whether defects have the same intensity at the low photopic adaptation level of the Visual Field Analyser (0.5 asb) as at the higher adaptation levels of the Goldmann perimeter (31.6 asb,) the Tübinger perimeter (10 asb) and the Double Projection Campimeter (31.5 asb).

It is possible that the intensity of visual field defects is not the same when the examination is performed with different presentation times. We have no adequate data on this point.

If the value of the multiple stimulus method for the detection of visual field defects is to be investigated, a distinction must be made between false-negative and false-positive results.

False-negative results are obtained when, on performing detection with the multiple stimulus method, defects are missed which are found with another method. If the multiple stimulus method were to give a high percentage of false-negative results it would be useless.

False-positive results are obtained when, on performing detection with the multiple stimulus method, defects are found which cannot be reproduced with another method, and the existence of which cannot be made plausible in any other way. False-positive results in the detection phase reduce the efficiency of the examination, but they do not make the method completely useless, as the results are in any case examined more closely in the assessment phase.

False-negative results.

The only way to show that the multiple stimulus method offers the same detection chance as the classical single stimulus method is to examine the visual fields of the same patients with both methods. The results of an investigation like this are discussed in Chapter XI.

False-positive results.

To show the data obtained with the multiple stimulus method are correct, the data from the examination of patients can be used (see Chapter XI). Valuable information can also be obtained from the examination of a large number of supposedly normal subjects. We performed a study like this on 1834 subjects[63]. This mass investigation also furnished data on the average duration of the examination with the Visual Field Analyser (special method) and the percentage of visual field defects found in a group of supposedly normal subjects. We shall deal shortly with this large-scale visual field investigation. In this investigation one concession was made to the examination time: a standard luminance was used, which was chosen so that a normal subject could see all the stimuli. This luminance lies about 0.2 log unit above threshold level and differs from the luminance used in Friedmann's original supraliminal method. With this examination method, which is only justified for investigations in which a large number of visual fields must be screened in a relatively short time, we obtained the following results:

1. large-scale visual field screening is quite possible with the multiple stimulus method;
2. an examination of this sort takes an average of 6 minutes for 2 eye s;
3. in nearly 2% of the 1834 supposedly normal subjects visual field defects were found; half of these defects had an intensity of more than 0.4 log unit;
4. in this large number of subjects only 2 false-positive results were found (about $1^0/_{00}$).

Screening.

In addition to the information about false-positive results, the mass investigation was set up in order to see how far relatively accurate screening of the visual field (up to 25°) can be realized. A screening method can be made more or less precise, depending upon the data which one expects to obtain from the screening. In the case of visual field examination, the number of positions examined can be made larger or smaller and the stimulus luminance chosen can be liminal or supraliminal. As the number of positions becomes fewer and the examination becomes more supraliminal, the number of defects found will decrease and the duration of the examination will become shorter. If the purpose of the screening of the visual field is selection and prevention, the detection phase of the visual field examination is best performed as described in detail on page 199. The kinetic

---

[63] GREVE & VERDUIN, 1972.

examination can then be omitted. The optimum screening method for the visual field is then the same as the optimum multiple stimulus method, which will be considered below. Numerous modifications are possible, depending on what one requires from the screening.

A description is given below of the requirements for an optimum multiple stimulus method. These requirements follow from the considerations given above on the visual field examination in general. Optimum multiple stimulus examination is considered to be the most important part of the detection phase. Our initial considerations are that the stimuli are presented according to the principles of static perimetry and that the differential light sensitivity is investigated, i.e. a threshold determination.

The best solution would be to build the multiple stimulus method into one of the good perimeters. This would have the advantage that the detection and the assessment phase could be carried out with one instrument under the same standardized conditions. Furthermore the useful properties of the perimeter could be utilised: even background, isolation from the surroundings, control of fixation and possibilities of standardization.

The most important consideration apart from those given above is the number and distribution of the stimuli. It is sensible to limit the multiple stimulus method to the 30° visual field. The number and distribution of the stimuli in the 30° field has been dealt with in detail. As a compromise between an acceptable duration of the examination and the greatest detection chance 150 positions were chosen, the distribution of which is given in Fig. 3 of Chapter V.

A maximum of 4 stimuli can be presented simultaneously. 2, 3 or 4 simultaneous stimuli are presented at random. The changing of the groups should be carried out rapidly and easily.

The stimuli presented simultaneously should have varying, preferably irregular, configurations. In other words, the stimuli must not repeatedly be presented as the corners of regular quadrilaterals or triangles. To facilitate the indication of the position of the stimuli they should be distributed over different quadrants.

The decrease in photopic light sensitivity from the centre to the periphery is best compensated by neutral density filters. The compensation is such that the stimuli are equidistant from the average sensitivity curve. At the photopic level, with a stimulus of 7' diameter, the average light sensitivity decreases nasally with about 0.1 log unit per 2 degrees eccentricity (temporally the decrease is

199

less rapid). The differences in the average sensitivity curves between the right and the left eyes will have to be compensated for separately.

The stimuli should have a sufficient range of luminance, preferably 3 log units above the average sensitivity curve. A Xenon flash tube is a suitable source of light. A standardizing instrument for this lamp must be built in. A short presentation time is one of the properties of a Xenon flash tube.

Steps of luminance of 0.2 log unit are sufficient. The stimulus size will have to be adapted to the size of the standard stimulus in the perimeters into which the multiple stimulus method is built. Only one size of stimulus is necessary as the gradient of sensitivity can be compensated for with neutral density filters.

TWO OTHER DETECTION METHODS

Two other methods for the detection of glaucomatous defects have been described by ARMALY[64] and GLOSTER[65].

ARMALY'S *method.*

ARMALY'S 'selective perimetry' consists of a combined kinetic and static exam-

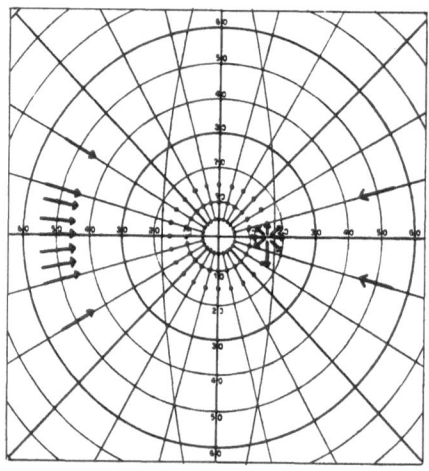

Fig. 18
Selective perimetry of Armaly.

---

[64] ARMALY, 1969.
[65] GLOSTER, 1970.

ination with the Goldmann perimeter, as shown in Fig. 18. In this method supraliminal stimuli are used. By means of kinetic perimetry the threshold is examined in 9 positions in the nasal periphery and 2 positions in the temporal periphery. The blind spot is also examined kinetically in 8 directions. With a stimulus, the isopter of which runs outside the blind spot, usually I/2/e, sometimes I/3/e, 72 positions are examined supraliminally using static perimetry. These positions lie on the 5°, 10° and 15° parallels.

This method has the advantage that a large number of positions are examined in the paracentral area, although the area outside 15° receives little attention. The distribution of the 72 stimuli could be chosen much more efficiently. The method is actually a form of supraliminal circular static perimetry. The disadvantage of this method is that, as the position examined comes nearer to the centre, the stimulus becomes increasingly supraliminal (Fig. 19).

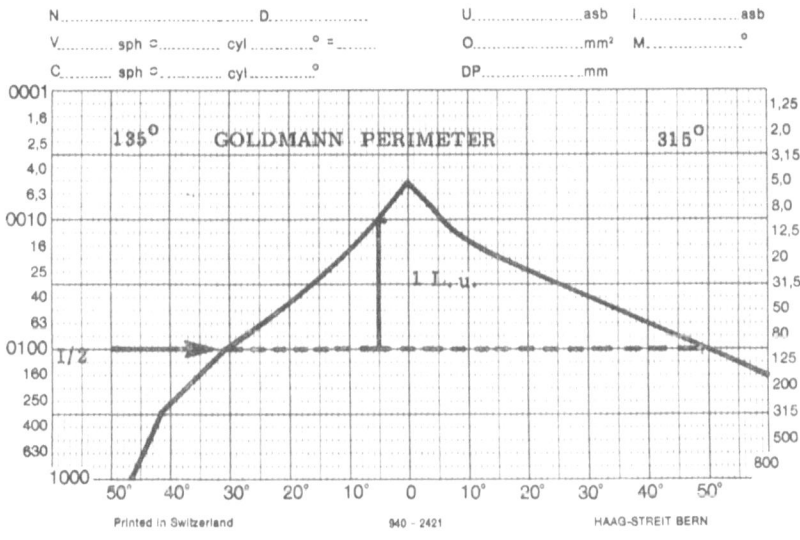

Fig. 19

Stimulus I/2 of the Goldmann perimeter and its relation to the normal sensitivity curve.

In the area inside the position of a normal I/2 isopter the I/2 stimulus at 5° is one log unit above threshold level. Defects of 0.9 log unit and less will be missed. This makes it particularly difficult to find the relative margin around small absolute defects. We prefer the multiple stimulus static threshold examination to ARMALY's 'selective perimetry'.

201

Essentially GLOSTER's method is comparable to ARMALY's method. Both tests are supraliminal and consist of the examination of a number of selected positions in the central and intermediate visual field with the help of the Goldmann perimeter. GLOSTER invented a means of presenting stimuli semi-automatically in random order. He used the I/3 or I/4 stimulus of the Goldmann perimeter, sometimes the I/2. This gives rise to the same objections we have mentioned with regard to ARMALY's method. The number and distribution of the stimuli in GLOSTER's method, however, is better (Fig. 20). He presents the stimuli at

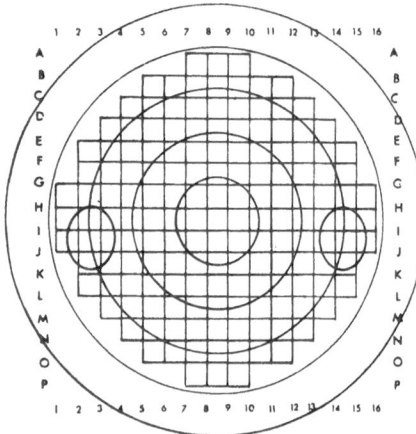

Fig. 20
Stimulus positions of Gloster's detection method

the intersections and angles of a rectangular network with meshes of $\pm$ 2.5° diameter. This method results in good spatial accuracy (because 188 positions are examined in the 20° visual field). Although a number of relative defects can be missed, nearly all defects of great intensity will be found. For the examination of the peripheral visual field GLOSTER used stimulus positions according to ESTERMAN's method[66].

The essential difference between ARMALY's and GLOSTER's methods on the one hand, and the multiple stimulus method on the other, is that ARMALY and GLOSTER gain time by presenting supraliminal stimuli, whereas in the multiple stimulus method time is saved by the simultaneous presentation of stimuli while the principle of threshold examination is maintained.

---

[66] ESTERMAN, 1967, 1968.

PRERETINAL FACTORS

Before a stimulus reaches the retina it must pass through the optical system of the eye. This consists consecutively of the cornea, anterior chamber, pupil, lens and vitreous body. In the optical system refraction, reflection, absorption, diffusion and diffraction occur[1]. On the retina a diminished and inverted image is formed[2].

---

[1] see e.g. WEALE, 1956. The equivalent strength of the optical system is $\pm$ 60 dioptres. The cornea accounts for the largest part of this ($\pm$ 40 dioptres) and the lens for the rest ($\pm$ 20 dioptres).

[2] The size of the retinal image can be calculated approximately from the formula below

(DAWSON, Vol. 4): $h' = \dfrac{-\tan \omega}{F^e}$

in which h' is diameter of retinal image in metres, ω = angle at which object is seen and F^e = equivalent power in D.

The most important factors in the optical system – as far as visual field examination is concerned – are the diameter of the pupil, the condition of the lens, accommodation and ametropia.

PUPIL

The illumination of the retina is partially determined by the surface area of the pupil. This is expressed in the formula:

$D = 0.36\ \tau_\lambda$. S.L, where D is the retinal illumination, S the surface area of the pupil and L the luminance of the stimulus (or background). The transmission factor τ varies according to the wavelength of the stimulus between 0.1 and 0.7[3]. The retinal illumination is approximately proportional to the square of the pupil diameter.

TABLE I

Decrease in effective diameter of pupil with distance from axis of fixation: Correction factors for each location to compensate for reduction in amount of light reaching the retina

Distance from Axis of Fixation	Ratio of Horizontal to Vertical Diameter of Pupil	Correction Factor (log units*)
10° N	0.98	—0.01
0°	1.00	0.00
10° T	0.998	—0.01
20° T	0.946	—0.02
30° T	0.905	—0.04
40° T	0.851	—0.07
50° T	0.756	—0.12
60° T	0.629	—0.19
70° T	0.505	—0.28
75° T	0.488	—
80° T	0.414	—0.41
90° T	0.242	—0.62
92° T	0.210	—
96° T	0.175	—0.76

* Computed from data read from smoothed curve.

---

[3] DAWSON, Vol. 2. This formula is an approximation; because of the STILES-CRAWFORD effect the retinal illumination with larger pupil diameters is less than would be expected on the basis of the formula (see next page).

The effective surface area of the pupil becomes steadily smaller as the angle at which the pupil is seen increases[4]. The influence of the decrease in effective pupillary surface area is negligible up to 50° eccentricity, i.e. less than 0.1 log unit, as appears from Table I[5]. Only in the extreme temporal periphery need a correction factor be applied.

Changes in the pupil diameter between 2 and 6 mm generally have a negligible influence on the visual field[6]. We found in our experiments that in a normal 20-year-old subject a change of the pupil diameter from 6 to 2 mm, produced by illuminating the eye which is not being examined, has no noticeable influence on the level of the sensitivity curve (Fig. 1). A pupil diameter of less than 2 mm could not be obtained by this method.

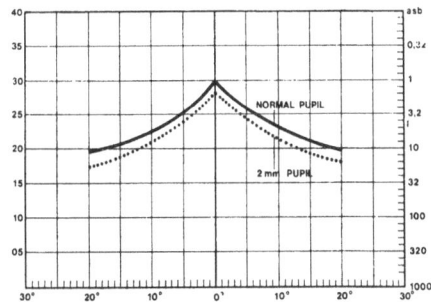

Fig. 1
Sensitivity curve of a normal subject with different pupil diameters.
a) 6 mm
b) 2 mm

The effect of the increase in retinal illumination when the pupil diameter is large is reduced by the increase in spherical and chromatic aberration and the resulting less sharp image of the stimulus.

At the retinal level the effect of a larger pupil diameter is reduced by the STILES-CRAWFORD effect[7]: rays of light which enter the eye through the centre of the pupil give a greater sensation of brightness than rays of light which pass through the pupil eccentrically. The greater amount of light which passes

[4] SPRING & STILES, 1948; SLOAN, 1950; JAY, 1961.
[5] SLOAN, 1950.
[6] FERREE, RAND & SLOAN, 1934; ENGEL, 1942; DUBOIS-POULSEN, 1952; ASPINALL, 1967. A positive relationship between pupil diameter and size of visual field was found by MAZZANTINI & WIRTH, 1962.
[7] STILES & CRAWFORD, 1933; CRAWFORD, 1972.

through the pupil when the diameter is larger does not contribute proportionally to the subjective brightness.

When the pupil diameter is less than 2 mm a generalized reduction in sensitivity can occur. The chief cause of this is probably the reduced retinal illumination, although diffraction may also be concerned when the pupil diameter is less than 1.5 mm[8].

When the pupil diameter is 1 mm the light reaching the retina is reduced 16 × (1.2 log unit) as compared with a pupil diameter of 4 mm. In a young subject this makes little difference, but in older subjects, where the lens also absorbs a portion of the light, the retinal illumination can be so far reduced that the examination takes place more or less at the mesopic adaptation level. This can be recognized by the fact that the sensitivity curve is not only lower but also less steep.

Senile miosis.

It is well known that the pupil diameter decreases with age[9]. Although the light sensitivity decreases with age, a correlation between this and senile miosis can hardly be found[10].

The importance of the pupil diameter is relative, as narrowing of the pupil can only affect the general sensitivity. Variations in the diameter of the pupil do not influence the intensity of defects[11]. Mesopization of the sensitivity curve can be recognized directly.

LENS.

In addition to the refraction of light, absorption and diffusion of light occur in the lens. This absorption is selective in so far that light of short wavelength is more strongly absorbed than light of long wavelength (Fig. 2)[12].

When the pupil diameter is large, spherical and chromatic aberration occur. These effects influence the position of the normal isopters and the level of the sensitivity curve. With advancing age the density of the lens increases and thus also the absorption and diffusion. The absorption has the effect of a filter and the diffusion the effect of ground glass.

---

[8] RIGGS, 1965.

[9] BIRREN et al., 1950.

[10] DRANCE, 1967; ASPINALL, 1967.

[11] as opposed to FORBES, 1966; at least when this intensity is determined as described in Chapter X.

[12] DAWSON, Vol. 2; SAID & WEALE, 1959; RUDDOCH, 1965; MELLERIO, 1971.

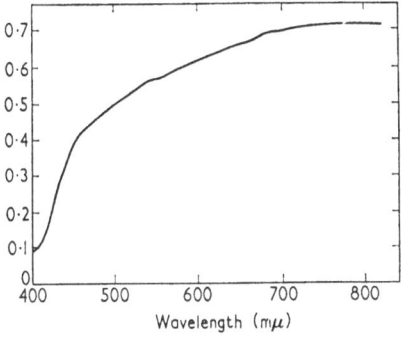

Fig. 2

Selective absorption in the lens. The transmission factor $\tau\lambda$ for young human eyes is indicated along the ordinate; wavelength in mμ along the abscissa (reproduced from The Eye vol. 2: after Ludvigh and McCarthy, 1938).

When diffuse senile lens opacity is present, the effect on the visual field will not be more than a generalized decrease in sensitivity. As has already been noted this does not disturb the interpretation of the results of visual field examination unless the opacity is so dense that visual field examination is impossible. When the lens opacity is not diffuse but localized and irregular, localized reduction in sensitivity can occur. This effect of such a localized lens opacity has been described[13]. When the opacity is more posterior in the lens, the effect will be more localized. In our experience sharply defined defects do not occur, so that the differentiation between defects due to cataract and glaucomatous defects is usually no problem. Cataractogenous defects usually have sloping edges; irregular, more or less localized peripheral cataractogenous defects have been described[14]. In the literature data about the effect of localized cataract on the visual field are very scarce. A more detailed investigation, using red and blue stimuli for instance, would be worthwhile. A study of the visual field before and after cataract extraction would also provide interesting information[15].

---

[13] BOYNTON & CLARKE, 1964.

[14] DUBOIS-POULSEN, 1952; LYNE & PHILLIPS, 1969.

[15] Recently a study concerning cataract extraction has been carried out (BIGGER & BECKER, 1971) on 90 eyes from 64 patients, some of which had glaucomatous defects and some non-specific defects. All the eyes had glaucoma simplex and cataract. Generalized reduction in sensitivity, enlargement of the blind spot and baring of the blind spot were regarded as non-specific. In all 49 eyes with non-specific defects the general light sensitivity improved after cataract extraction. 23 of the 41 visual fields with specific defects remained unchanged, showing that the defects were not caused by the cataract. In 17 cases scotomata disappeared or decreased in intensity. These authors

207

The denser the cataract becomes, the more difficult it is to assess the visual field. When a cataract causes a reduction in sensitivity of more than 2 log units, accurate quantitative perimetry as described here can no longer be carried out. In the discussion of the pupil diameter it has already been noted that the combination of a narrow pupil and lens opacity can cause such a reduction in the retinal illumination that the examination takes place at mesopic adaptation levels. As has been pointed out the fraction $\dfrac{\Delta L}{L}$ increases when the adaptation shifts from the photopic to the mesopic level. The threshold is thus relatively higher; the sensitivity curve is lower, especially in the centre (Fig. 3). This effect

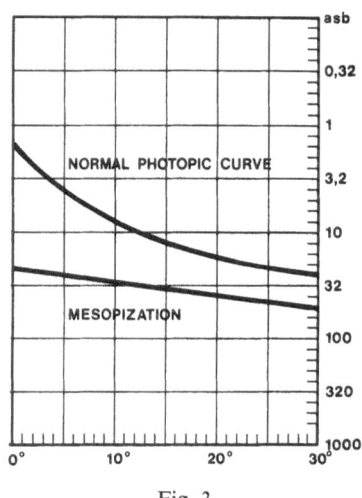

Fig. 3

Mesopization of the sensitivity curve due to decrease of retinal illumination.

on the sensitivity curve is called mesopization. A progressive general reduction of sensitivity (or mesopization) and increasing myopia generally indicate cataract formation[16].

---

consider that some of the reversible defects must have been due to lens opacity and senile miosis, but that a number of the defects were reversed as the result of the reduction in intra-ocular pressure. The fact that most of the reversible defects were found to have been of short duration is an argument in favour of the author's last suggestion. This study had, however, not really proved that local lens opacities cannot simulate glaucomatous defects.

[16] DAY & SCHEIE, 1953.

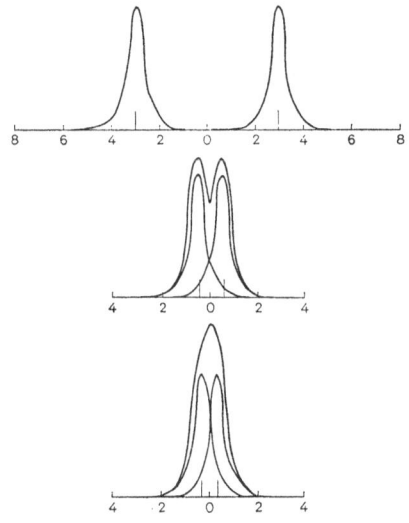

Fig. 4

Light spread in the images of two stars and summed intensity distribution as the two stars approach each other; alsscissa: minutes of arc.

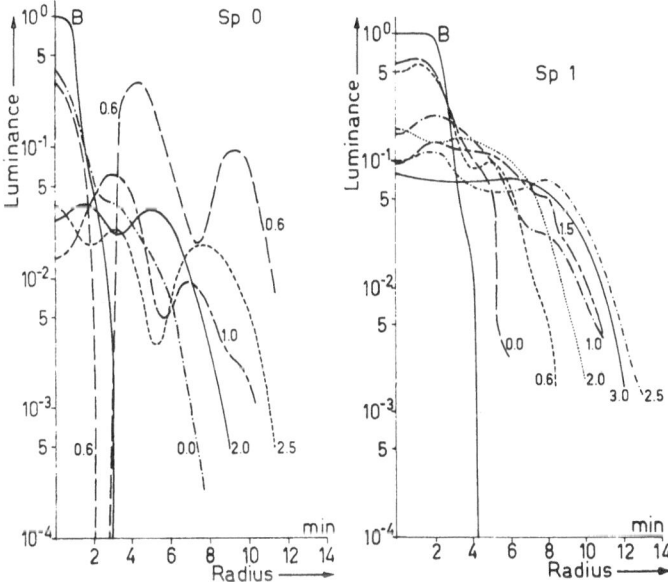

Fig. 5

Retinal light distribution of stimulus 0 and stimulus I of the Goldmann perimeter under conditions of emmetropia and several degrees of ametropia.
B indicates the light distribution in object space.

Image formation in the emmetropic eye.

The optical apparatus of the eye transforms each luminous point in object space into a retinal light distribution called point-spread function (Fig. 4)[17]. The image of a perimetric object formed on the retina is dependent on the properties of the optical apparatus of the eye. Every object is composed of a large number of punctate objects, the point-spread function of which determines the image on the retina. When the object is large a proportionally smaller part of the object is spread over the retina than when the object is small; in other words, the deviation of the retinal light distribution with respect to the light distribution in the object space is less for a large object than for a small object.

In Fig. 5, as illustration, the retinal light distribution of stimulus 0 and stimulus I of the Goldmann perimeter are shown[18].

Image formation in the ametropic eye.

In the ametropic eye the image is not formed at the level of the retina but in front of or behind it. The result is that every point of the emmetropic retinal image is now represented as a diffusion circle. The greater the ametropia, the larger the diffusion circle will be (see Fig. 5)[19]. The effect of the ametropia, however, is not only enlargement, but also alteration of the light distribution and particularly of the marginal contrast gradient. As shown in Fig. 5 the gradient contrast becomes less steep. Since the perception of stimuli depends on this contrast gradient, the threshold in ametropia will be higher. A poor retinal image has little or no effect on the perception of large stimuli; with small stimuli, on the other hand, the treshold level is raised considerably. With a stimulus diameter of 0.6' the foveal threshold level is 1 log unit higher when the subject is made 1 dioptre ametropic[20]. With stimulus III of the Goldmann perimeter (27'10'') a poorly defined image has hardly any effect on the foveal threshold[21].

---

[17] FLAMANT, 1955; WESTHEIMER & CAMPBELL, 1962; KRAUSKOPF, 1962; RÖHLER, 1962; figure after WESTHEIMER, 1972.

[18] FANKHAUSER & RÖHLER, 1967.

[19] The diffusion circle can be calculated from the formula (DAWSON, Vol. 4):
$b = \dfrac{p.k.}{K + Fe}$, where b = diameter of diffusion circle in mm, p = pupil diameter in mm, K = ametropia in D, F_e = equivalent power in D.

[20] OGLE, 1960, 1961, 1962.

[21] SLOAN, 1962.

With increasing eccentricity the effect of the poorly defined image on the threshold decreases, partly because of the greater spatial interaction in the periphery and because physiological ametropia in the periphery is normally present[22]. On adaptation to background luminances lower than the usual photopic level, the effect of the poor image decreases because of the increase in spatial interaction[23].

Central ametropia scotoma.

In visual field examination the result of a poor retinal image due to ametropia is a relative central scotoma, which decreases in intensity from the centre to the periphery (Fig. 6). Outside 30° the ametropia has no more effect[24]. The blind

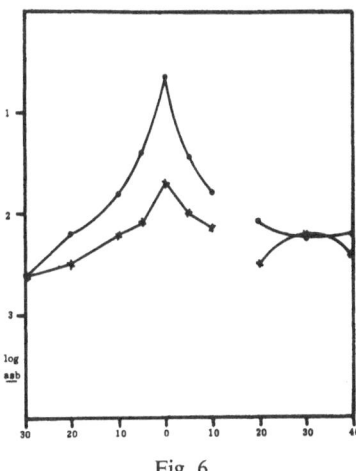

Fig. 6

The effect of a presbyopia of 3.0 diopters on the sensitivity curve; stimulus size 0 of Goldmann perimeter (after SLOAN, 1961).

spot is enlarged in uncorrected ametropia[25]. If there are defects in the visual field, these will appear enlarged in cases of ametropia, because the strength of the stimulus is reduced by the ametropia.

Correcting lenses.

In order to avoid central ametropia scotoma the patient's eye must be corrected for the distance at which the perimetric examination is carried out. Naturally

---

[22] see next page.

[23] BAIR, 1940.

[24] MONJE & OFFERMANN, 1954; FANKHAUSER & ENOCH, 1962; SLOAN, 1961; ARMALY, 1967.

[25] JACQUES, 1946.

only lenses with a thin frame are suitable. These lenses are placed in a correcting lens holder supplied with the instrument.

When correcting lenses are used the following factors should be considered:

1. the transmission depends on the strength of the lens;
2. the visual field is limited by the edge (and frame) of the correcting lens;
3. the position of the stimulus on the retina is altered by the prismatic effect of strong lenses.

The transmission of lenses depends on the colour, thickness and strength of the lens. Positive lenses converge most of the light rays onto the area of the pupil. Hence more light should enter the eye with a positive lens than with a negative lens[26]. When colourless lenses are used the consequences of the above mentioned effect for the visual field are small (less than 0.3 log unit).

The limitation of the visual field by the edge of the lens lies at about the 40° parallel.

The displacement of the position of the stimulus by the prismatic effect can be calculated from the formula $\Delta\eta \sim 0.8 \, (\tan \eta) \, F$, in which the eccentricity is expressed in degrees and the strength of the lens in dioptres[27]. As the lens becomes stronger the displacement is greater. The disturbing effects of correcting lenses are most marked in aphakics. At 12° eccentricity an S + 15.00 lens causes an alteration in position of 2.5°. This means, for example, that the edge of the blind spot is displaced from 12° to 9.5°. It is therefore better to examine aphakics with contact lenses[28].

Strong positive lenses give rise to an absolute ring scotoma directly outside the boundary drawn by the edge of the lens. This ring scotoma arises because the rays of light within the edge of the lens are bent towards the centre by the prismatic effect, whereas outside the edge of the lens the rays follow the normal straight course.

Similarly strong negative lenses cause a double image of the stimulus directly outside the edge of the lens.

Peripheral ametropia; refraction scotoma.

When speaking of ametropia, the refraction anomaly of central vision is generally referred to. For visual field examination the peripheral refraction is also im-

---

[26] MILLODOT, 1970.

[27] FANKHAUSER & ENOCH, 1962.

[28] JAYLE & OURGAUD, 1953; MASSIN & PIOT, 1963; BEASLY, 1965.

212

portant. It is well known that high degrees of astigmatism can occur outside the fixation axis.[29]

Large inter-individual differences in peripheral refraction have been found, even in subjects with the same central refraction.

In all cases the severity of the ametropia increases with the eccentricity. This means that the retinal image of a peripheral stimulus will be very bad in many cases. The peripheral ametropia is found in most cases to be the same for the left and the right eyes of the same subject and for the nasal and temporal parts of the same eye. In 3.2% [30] of cases, however, there is a marked difference in peripheral ametropia between the nasal and temporal parts of the eye. In most cases marked astigmatism of the nasal side (temporal half of visual field) was found and seldom marked astigmatism of the temporal side (nasal half of visual field). In one case there was homonymous asymmetry in the form of marked astigmatism on the right side.

These forms of peripheral refraction asymmetry may be caused by an asymmetrical form of the eyeball and can give rise to a refraction scotoma (peripheral ametropia scotoma). In most cases these will be bi-temporal refraction scotomata[31], which can be readily differentiated from glaucomatous defects by their typical shape (but may cause difficulties in the differential diagnosis of chiasmal bi-temporal defects). The rare bi-nasal defects might be mistaken for glaucomatous defects[32], but have no 'nasal step'.

ACCOMMODATION

Presbyopia and fatigue of accommodation.

With advancing age the range of accommodation decreases; this results in:
1. ametropia, i.e. presbyopia;
2. accommodation fatigue.

Uncorrected presbyopia gives rise to a central ametropia scotoma. The influence of presbyopia is naturally less with the Bjerrum screen at a distance of 2 metres than with perimeters with a radius of 30 cm.

Accommodation fatigue can give rise to progressively decreasing light sensitivity (spiral visual field, great variation of measurements). It is well known that the total range of accommodation cannot be used for long without trouble.

Accommodation fatigue can also occur in uncorrected hypermetropia.

---

[29] FERREE et al., 1931, 1932, 1935; REMPT et al., 1971.

[30] 14 cases out of 442, REMPT et al., 1971.

[31] SCHMIDT, 1955; GREVE & VERDUIN, 1972; AULHORN & HARMS, 1972.

[32] KOMMERELL, 1969.

Miotics can have a disturbing effect on visual field examination for other reasons than miosis alone. The myopia-producing accommodation spasm, which can be caused by miotics especially in young people, varies in strength according to the time. Maximum myopia is present after about 30 minutes (Fig. 7)[33]. The average myopia, according to various authors, is 2.17 dioptres, depending upon the miotic used. After about 2 hours the myopia has practically disappeared.

Both the degree of myopia and the variation with time reduce the reliability

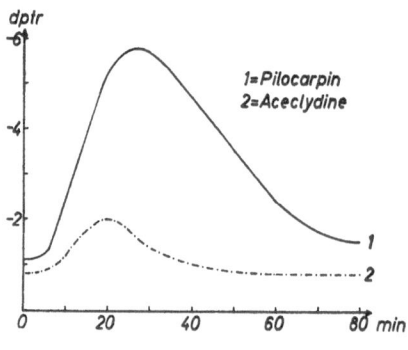

Fig. 7

Myopization by pilocarpine; abscissa: time after pilocarpine; ordinate: myopia in diopters.

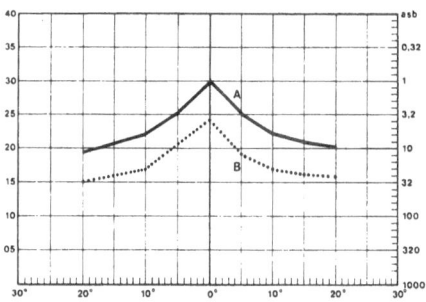

Fig. 8

Effect of myopization due to pilocarpine on the sensitivity curve of a normal young (20 years) subject.

A: normal pupil

B: 30 minutes after administration of pilocarpine without correction

---

[33] DAY & SCHEIE, 1953; MEYTHALER & RUPPERT, 1971; FECHNER, 1971; AUST & MORLANG, 1970 (figure).

of visual field examination in the first two hours after administering a miotic. In Fig. 8 the effect of pilocarpine 2% on the sensitivity curve of a normal subject (20 years old) is shown. After 30 minutes the diameter of the pupil is 2 mm and the myopia 4.5 dioptres; the result is a reduction of sensitivity of 0.6 log unit in the centre and 0.4–0.5 log unit in the periphery.

Some investigators use mydriatics for the routine examination of glaucoma patients. As the effect of miosis is easy to recognize and has no influence on the intensity of defects we do not use mydriatics for routine examinations. In some cases with a dense cataract the use of mydriatics can be advantageous.

CHAPTER X

DESCRIPTION OF VISUAL FIELD DEFECTS

Topography
Definitions
Numerical topographical classification
Intensity
Absolute and relative defects
Quantitative determination of relative defects in static perimetry
Intensity of defects in kinetic perimetry
Distribution of intensity in defects

The evaluation of visual field defects should be based on:

1. topography   a. size
                    b. shape
                    c. localization.
2. intensity   a. *degree* of reduction of light sensitivity
                    b. *distribution* of light sensitivity, i.e. homogeneous or not; sloping or steep edges.

TOPOGRAPHY

Definitions.

The description of the size of a defect is usually limited to large or small. The shape of glaucomatous defects is expressed in terms like; arcuate scotoma, 'baring of the blind spot', step, enlargement of the blind spot, etc.

The position of defects is usually described in terms as: central or peripheral; inferior or superior; temporal or nasal.

In the case of glaucoma the Bjerrum area between the 10° and 20° parallels has always played an important part. By a Bjerrum scotoma is usually meant a complete arcuate bundle scotoma, extending between the blind spot and the nasal part of the horizontal meridian. Further indications of position are central, paracentral, pericentral, juxtacecal and pericecal.

A number of these terms do not indicate an accurately defined area; we shall therefore give a more detailed description:

1. central scotoma: a scotoma the greatest intensity of which is in the centre of the visual field;
2. paracentral scotoma: a scotoma the greatest intensity of which is close to the centre of the visual field and within the 10° parallel;
3. pericentral scotoma: a scotoma largely surrounding the centre but still within the 10° parallel;
4. centrocecal scotoma: a scotoma mainly localized in the area between the centre and the blind spot, usually associated with reduced sensitivity at the centre;
5. juxtacecal scotoma: a small scotoma localized on the temporal or nasal side of the blind spot and connected with it;
6. pericecal scotoma: enlarged blind spot in all directions.

Polar enlargement of the blind spot indicates that the blind spot is only enlarged at the inferior or superior pole. An isolated scotoma is a scotoma which is well defined on all sides and does not form part of a larger scotoma, unless that scotoma is of slight intensity (see below). The length of an isolated scotoma, measured in circular direction (i.e. the direction of the fibre bundles) will not be more than 45° (Fig. 1). Larger scotomata will be called partial fibre bundle defects. When describing glaucomatous defects we shall use the above definitions.

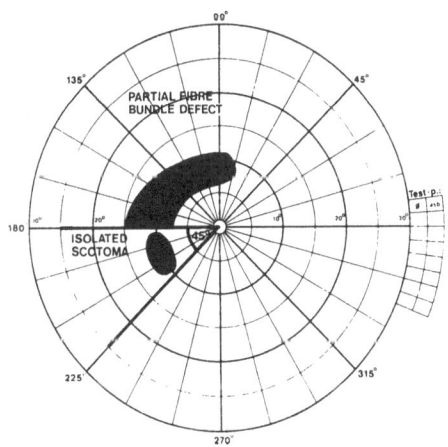

Fig 1

Demonstration of an isolated scotoma and a partial fibre bundle defect.

217

The position of a defect can be more precisely recorded by indicating the meridian(s) and parallel which are involved.

Numerical topographical classification.

It was felt that the descriptions used in general are insufficient, particularly to indicate the size of a defect, nor can they be used for mechanical codification. In an attempt to make better description and mechanical classification possible we have introduced the concept of topographical units. The visual field is divided into 180 topographical units, 45 in each quadrant (Fig. 2a and 2b).[1] The choice of the number and size of the topographical units was based on the following considerations:

1. the paracentral visual field and the Bjerrum area are relatively more important than the peripheral visual field;
2. the paracentral visual field is important for good visual function;
3. the size of the summation areas under photopic conditions increases towards the periphery;
4. defects smaller than 3 degrees are difficult to detect except in the central visual field;
5. the subdivision into topographical units should as far as possible make use of the parallels and meridians;
6. the subdivisions should be the same in the four quadrants of the visual field.

As is the case with every subdivision into groups it has been impossible to avoid arbitrary limits. In this topographical classification there are 30 units per quadrant in the 30° field, 12 units between the 30° parallel and the 55° parallel and only 3 units outside the 55° parallel (uniocular temporal crescent).

In each quadrant the topographical units are numbered from 1 to 45; numbers 1 and 2 are close to the centre. The higher the number of the topographical unit, the further it will be from the centre. The size of the topographical units increases towards the periphery in inverse proportion to the importance of the various parts of the visual field[2].

---

[1] A classification of this sort was proposed by ESTERMAN (1967); his units are different from ours.

[2] This subdivision into topographical units is very simular to the number and position of the stimuli in the detection phase. This simularity has been chosen intentionally. Theoretically in the detection phase there is one stimulus per topographical unit. Exceptions to this rule are: firstly, the area within the 5° parallel – there are 4 extra stimuli here in the detection phase which do not correspond with topographical units; and secondly the topographical units 25–30, where 2 stimuli per unit are chosen – one of these 2 stimuli lies on the 30° parallel.

218

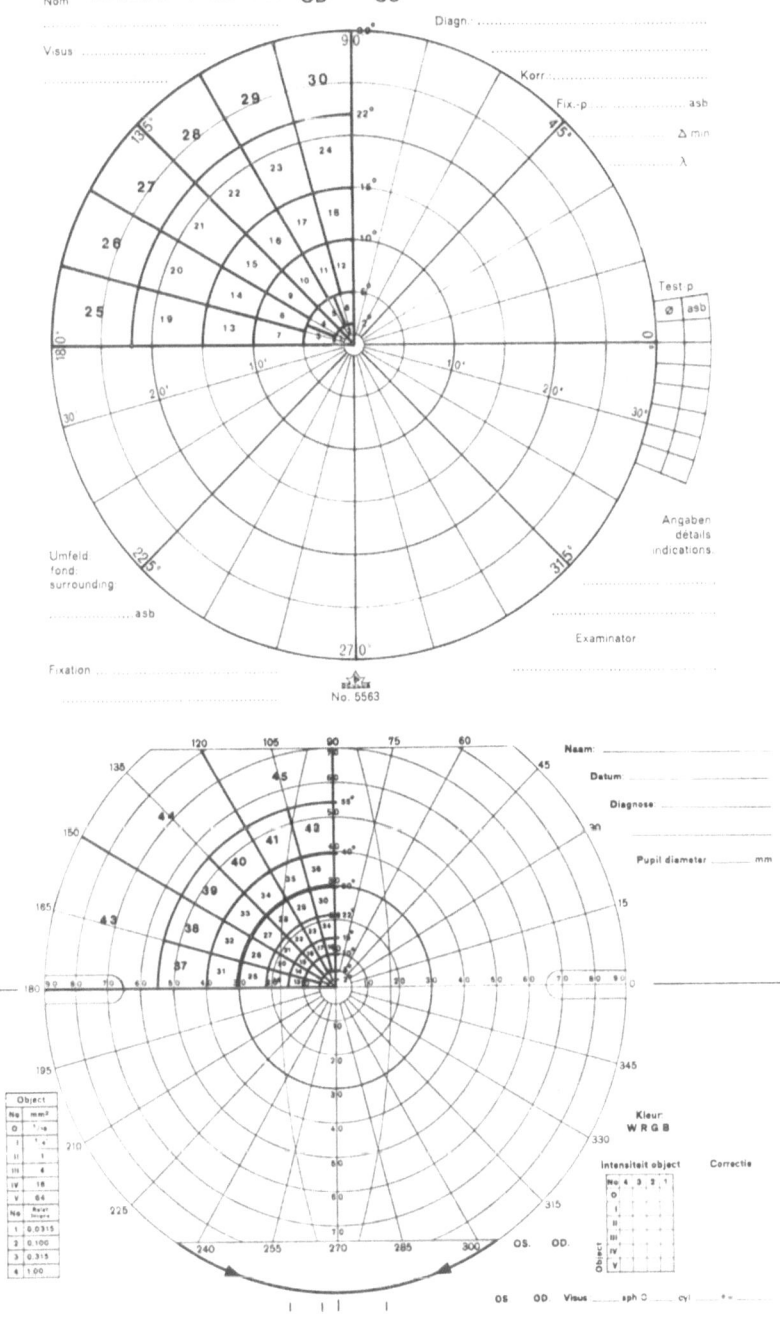

Fig. 2
Topographical units.

With the help of these topographical units the localization and size of a defect can easily be described. The localization is defined by giving the quadrant in which the defect is found – superonasal, superotemporal, inferonasal or inferotemporal – and the numbers of the topographical units which the defect occupies. The size of the defect can be recorded by noting the number of topographical units involved; the numbers can be read off from a transparent plastic diagram on which the units are shown. We have diagrams of this sort suitable for the charts of all instruments.

INTENSITY

Absolute and relative defects.

The topography of visual field defects has always been important in the description of visual field defects. The intensity of defects, on the other hand, has only received scant attention. By intensity we mean the degree of reduction in sensitivity in a visual field defect.

The intensity of a defect can be absolute or relative. This distinction is arbitrary. By an absolute defect we mean a defect in which the largest object of the perimeter (e.g. object size V of the Goldmann perimeter) with maximum luminance is not seen.

Every other defect is relative. Thus we also include under relative defects, defects in which the standard objects of the usual perimeters (7' or 10') with maximum luminance are not seen. We call this a defect for maximum luminance and not an absolute defect. Actually an intensity 'for maximum luminance' is not an exact definition; it merely indicates that the luminance of the perimeter is insufficient to allow further measurement of the exact intensity of the defect. In all cases in which the intensity is less than 'for maximum luminance' the exact intensity can be recorded. Generally, however, the description of the intensity of the defect is limited to the distinction between absolute and relative. In the results of kinetic perimetry the strength of stimulus with which a given defect was detected, is sometimes recorded. This only provides information about the intensity of a defect, however, when all possible stimulus luminances were used to examine the defect, and the course of the isopters involved is known.

The quantitative evaluation of the intensity of visual field defects has many advantages; the greatest advantage is that insight into perimetry increases when the intensity of defects is consistently evaluated. Significant defects can be differentiated from insignificant ones.

220

Quantitative determination of relative defects in static perimetry.

The accuracy with which the intensity is defined depends upon the accuracy with which the measurements are made. In static perimetry steps of 0.1 log unit are used. We therefore express the intensity of defects in tenths of a log unit, i.e. the number of luminance steps which the threshold lies above the normal level.

In the older literature suggestions have been made for the more accurate definition of the intensity of defects, but these were not based on the refinements of static perimetry.

BAIR[3] expressed the intensity of a defect as the logarithm of the ratio between the normal light sensivity and the measured light sensitivity. If the light sensitivity is expressed as $\dfrac{L}{\Delta L}$, the logarithm of the ratio;

$$\frac{\text{normal light sensitivity}}{\text{measured sensitivity (defect)}} = \log \frac{\dfrac{L}{\Delta\,Ln}}{\dfrac{L}{\Delta\,Ld}} = \log \Delta\,Ld - \log \Delta\,Ln.$$

If both sensitivities are the same the ratio becomes 1 and the logarithm of the ratio. The intensity of the defect is thus 0.

GOLDMANN[4] has drawn up a diagram for the determination of the sensitivity of a given position from the results of kinetic perimetry (Fig. 3). The position is found

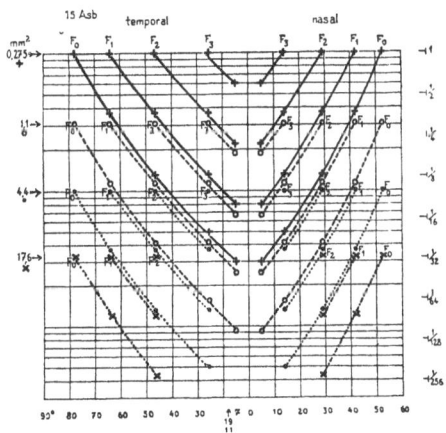

Fig. 3

Diagram of Goldmann for the determination of intensity.

---

[3] BAIR, 1940.

[4] GOLDMANN, 1946. If one wishes to express the intensity in ordinary fractions these can be read off directly from the table on the next page:

where a given stimulus size-luminance combination is seen and the sensitivity of this position can then be read off from the diagram. GOLDMANN expressed the sensitivity in fractions, which is essentially the same as expressing it in logarithmic units of loss of sensitivity.

GOLDMANN's diagram can only be used for object I (0.25 mm²) because it assumes a spatial summation coefficient of 0.85 for the larger objects over a large part of the visual field. As has already been explained this figure of 0.85 is susceptible to large variations.

We have given the preference to the expression of the intensity of a defect in log units, because this can be read off simply and directly from the sensitivity curve of static perimetry.

TABLE

Intensity of a visual field defect expressed in log units with the corresponding value in fractions

intensity of defect	remaining sensitivity		
log units	fraction	log units	fraction
0.1	$\dfrac{1}{1.25} = \dfrac{4}{6}$	1.1	$\dfrac{1}{12.5} = \dfrac{2}{25}$
0.2	$\dfrac{1}{1.6}$	1.2	$\dfrac{1}{16}$
0.3	$\dfrac{1}{2}$	1.3	$\dfrac{1}{20}$
0.4	$\dfrac{1}{2.5}$	1.4	$\dfrac{1}{25}$
0.5	$\dfrac{1}{3}$	1.5	$\dfrac{1}{30}$
0.6	$\dfrac{1}{4}$	1.6	$\dfrac{1}{40}$
0.7	$\dfrac{1}{5}$	1.7	$\dfrac{1}{50}$
0.8	$\dfrac{1}{6.3}$	1.8	$\dfrac{1}{63}$
0.9	$\dfrac{1}{8}$	1.9	$\dfrac{1}{80}$
1.0	$\dfrac{1}{10}$	2.0	$\dfrac{1}{100}$ etc.

The intensity of a defect is measured as compared with the reconstructed individual 'normal' sensitivity. The normal sensitivity curves have been described in Chapter VII. The individual sensitivity curves can differ in height and shape from the average normal sensitivity. An individual sensitivity curve can be lower than the average sensitivity curve and still be normal. Because of preretinal factors an individual sensitivity curve can even be much lower than the average sensitivity curve without abnormal light sensitivity of the perceptional part of the visual system being involved.

An essential point in our determination of sensitivity is that we differentiate between general reduction of sensitivity (g.r.s.) and localized reduction of sensitivity, i.e. a local defect. Generalized reduction of sensitivity implies that the whole curve is lowered in a direction parallel to the ordinate without essential change of shape: g.r.s. $= \Delta Lg - \Delta Ln$ (Fig. 4). This shifted sensitivity curve (ΔLg) is the patient's individual curve. The intensity of a defect is determined with respect to this curve. When the sensitivity curve is not too much deformed by defects it can be reconstructed adequately from the parts of the visual field which are still intact.

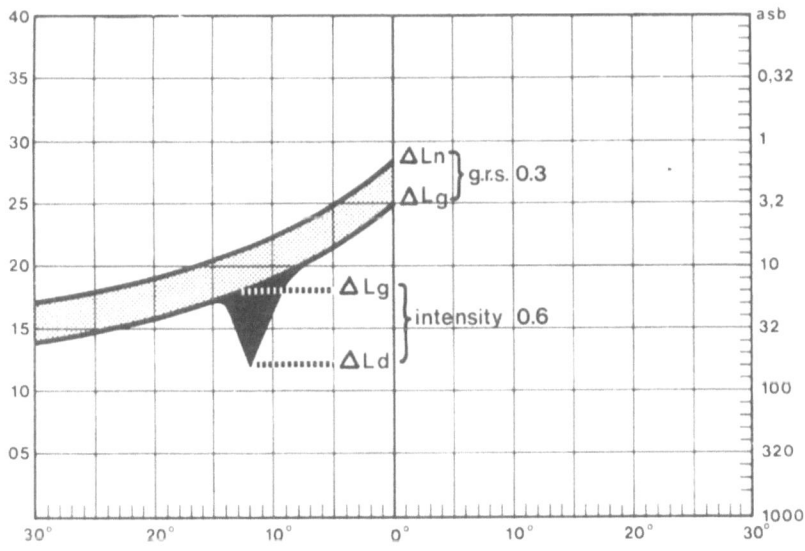

Fig. 4
Demonstration of general reduction of sensitivity and localized defect.
$\Delta L n =$ normal threshold
$\Delta L g =$ individual 'normal' threshold after general reduction of sensitivity
$\Delta L d =$ threshold in the defect

223

The intensity of a defect is thus the difference between the threshold in the defect (ΔLd) and the average normal threshold (ΔLn), with the general reduction of sensitivity (ΔLg — ΔLn) subtracted from the difference:

intensity (ΔLd — ΔLn) — (ΔLg — ΔLn)
$\quad$ = ΔLd — ΔLg (see Fig. 4).

When the results of static perimetry are available, the general reduction of sensitivity of a defect can easily be expressed in this way.

Intensity of defects in kinetic perimetry.

The intensity of defects found with kinetic perimetry can also be expressed in log units. The interpretation is more difficult and the intensity is usually determined with steps of 0.5 log unit. Also the accuracy of kinetic perimetry is limited.

In kinetic perimetry we make use of the average normal kinetic sensitivity curve. In the first place the general reduction of sensitivity is determined. In kinetic terminology this is a concentric contraction of all isopters. It must be shown whether the distance between the isopters is correct. This distance is determined by the difference in luminance between the stimuli with which these isopters were measured and the gradient in the part of the visual field in which the isopters lie. By comparison with the normal sensitivity curve one can see whether the distance between two isopters in one meridian is correct. We shall demonstrate this with the example in Fig. 5. When the isopter measured with stimulus A crosses the horizontal meridian at 22°, the isopter measured with stimulus B should cross that meridian at 9°. With the help of the normal sensitivity curve in a given meridian, starting from a position A, a position B is looked for with a threshold 0.5 log unit lower. With adequate experience one can judge very rapidly whether the relationship between the isopters is normal. An abnormal relationship, i.e. when the distances between isopters are either too long or too short, indicates an alteration in the sensitivity gradient: too short indicates a steep gradient; too long indicates a flat gradient.

When the relationship between the isopters is normal – and in the large majority of cases this is so – the degree of concentric contraction can be determined, expressed in log units. Theoretically any isopter can be used for this determination, but we generally use an isopter in the intermediate visual field, and naturally in a position where there are no local defects. The starting point is the position where an isopter should normally be. When, for instance, the isopter measured with stimulus A crosses the horizontal meridian at 12°, this means that the 12° position has a light sensitivity of 0.4 log units under the

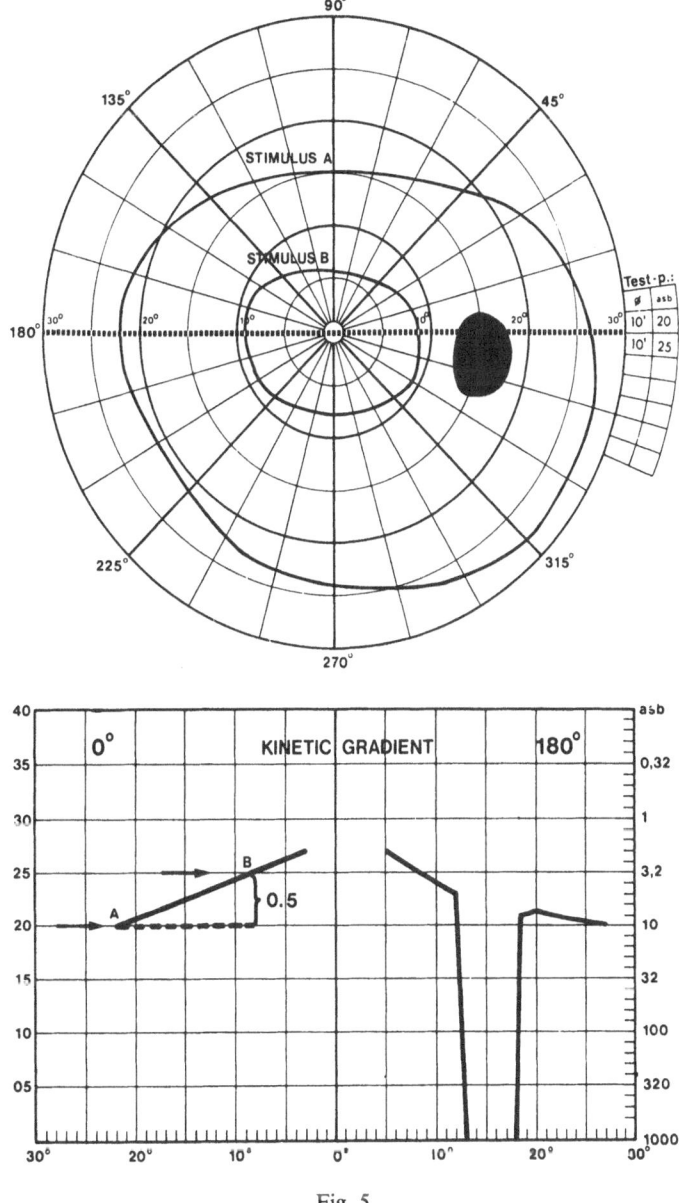

Fig. 5

Determination of the normal or abnormal distance between isopters.

225

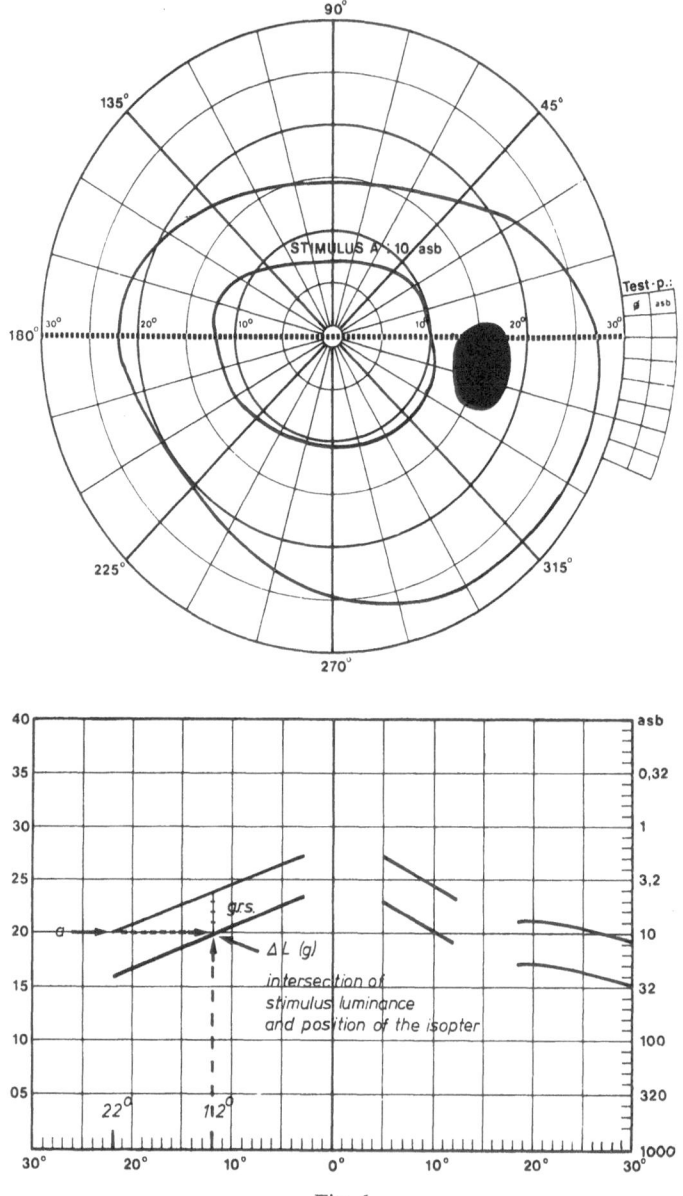

Fig. 6
Determination of concentric contraction.

normal value, as the isopter that normally runs at 12° has 0.4 log unit lower luminance.

In practice this goes as follows. On the chart showing the normal kinetic sensitivity curve one looks for the stimulus luminance going with the isopter chosen for the calculation of the concentric contraction (in this case a luminance of 10 asb of the Tübinger perimeter). The position where this luminance level intersects the normal sensitivity curve is the normal position of the isopter in this meridian (22°) (Fig. 6). The distance (g.r.s.) between the intersection (ΔLg) of the stimulus luminance and the true position of the isopter, and the normal sensitivity curve, indicates the concentric contraction.

In a similar manner the intensity of a defect can be determined by means of kinetic perimetry. From the difference between the position where an isopter should run and that in which the isopter or the edge of the defect is found, the reduction of sensitivity in log units can be calculated. From this figure the number of log units concentric contraction is subtracted.

When the examination procedure as described in the preceding chapters is followed the results of kinetic perimetry need not be used for the calculation of the intensity.

Distribution of intensity in a defect.

The degree of general reduction of sensitivity is uniform by definition, at least within the limits of intra-individual variation. The intensity of a defect, on the other hand, is often far from uniform. The intensity in various parts of a defect may differ widely. The most extreme form of this is the sieve-like defect, in which great differences in intensity occur in adjacent positions. Defects of this kind also occur in glaucoma. Often defects of great intensity ($>$ 1.0 log unit) are found in areas of slight intensity ($<$ 0.5 log unit).

The marginal gradient of a defect has long been known as an important diagnostic and prognostic sign. When we determine the intensity of a defect we always do it at the deepest point. We register whether there are marked variations in intensity or whether the defect is uniform, whether the margins are sloping or steep, etc.

In the following chapter examples will be given demonstrating the localization of a defect, the general reduction of sensitivity and the calculation of intensity.

CHAPTER XI

THE EXAMINATION PROCEDURE IN PRACTICE; EXPERIENCES WITH
THE MULTIPLE STIMULUS METHOD FOR THE DETECTION OF
GLAUCOMATOUS DEFECTS

Examination procedure
  Research procedure
  Duration of the examination
  Organization
Glaucomatous defects
  Early defects in the opposite hemifield
Demonstration of 18 visual fields with glaucomatous defects
Results of the comparative study
  Number and position of stimuli in the Visual Field Analyser
  Comparative study of threshold measurements
Conclusion

This chapter consists of two parts. In the first part 18 examples of visual fields from glaucoma patients are shown. The purpose of this is, in the first place, to illustrate the examination procedure. In the second place these examples show the appearance of glaucomatous defects as found with meridional static perimetry, especially early glaucomatous defects. In the third place the possibilities and limitations of the Visual Field Analyser in the detection phase become apparent.

The second part deals with the results of a comparative visual field study in 1372 eyes, where again the function of the Visual Field Analyser as multiple stimulus method in the detection phase is the point at issue.

EXAMINATION PROCEDURE

In Chapter V and at the end of Chapter VIII a conclusion is drawn about the optimum examination procedure in the detection and the assessment phases. This conclusion is based on our experience in practice with various examination methods.

The examination procedure used in our research programme differs in some respects from the optimum procedure described.

Research procedure.

The examination procedure consisted of an examination with the Visual Field Analyser (thus multiple stimulus: 46 positions) and kinetic perimetry of the periphery and the blind spot: phase IA. If necessary this examination was supplemented by the examination of 72 fixed positions within the 30° parallel with single stimulus static perimetry: phase IB.

The main differences between this procedure and the optimum procedure described above is that in phase IB *single* stimulus static perimetry is used instead of multiple stimulus static perimetry, and that a total of 118 positions within the 25° parallel is examined instead of 150 positions within the 30° parallel. The single stimulus method was chosen for phase IB because we wished to compare it with the multiple stimulus method. The smaller number of positions was only chosen in order to limit the duration of the examination. If a multiple stimulus method is available for phase IB, 150 positions can be examined in a reasonable length of time. Phase IB was carried out with the Tübinger perimeter or the Double Projection Campimeter.

In the detection phase an indication must be found as to whether visual field defects are present or not. If this indication has already been obtained from phase IA it is unnecessary to carry out an additional phase IB. This applies to each part of the visual field separately. If defects are only found in the nasal part

TABLE I

Duration of the examination using the research procedure
and the routine procedure

Phase I	Research ms/ss	Routine ms
IA	4′–10′	4′
Kinetic periphery	10′	10′
IB	24′	8′
Total	±40′	22′

of the visual field in phase IA it is a sensible procedure to supplement the examination of the paracentral and temporal areas with phase IB.

On the basis of the data from phase I a choice must be made concerning the further investigation in phase II. The larger the defect the easier this choice will be. With static perimetry the exact intensity and limits of a defect usually along a meridian are established. Kinetic perimetry provides a survey of the topography of a defect showing its characteristic shape and position. The appearance of glaucomatous defects in classical kinetic perimetry is well known. However, the typical appearance of these defects in meridional static perimetry has not yet received the attention it deserves.

In cases of partial fibre bundle defects, i.e. every defect which does not extend from the blind spot to the nasal horizontal meridian, the attempt is made in phase II to define the defect:
1. where it is maximum;
2. where it is relative;
3. where it has not yet penetrated (e.g. patient 7).

In this way a record is made of how large the defect is for maximum luminance and how far it has advanced cecofugally or cecopetally. Increased intensity in the relative part of the defect and the appearance of new relative defects are indications of progression.

Duration of the examination.

In Table I the examination time for the detection phase per eye is given, in the first column as in our research programme (phase IB with single stimulus static perimetry) and in the second column as it can be when, in routine clinical examination, the whole detection phase is performed with multiple stimulus static perimetry. As has already been explained, phase IB is only carried out when in phase IA no defects have been found in one or both halves of the visual field. The complete detection phase will only be carried out when the patient reacts accurately and can stand the longer duration of the examination.

The times given in the column Routine-ms are based on pure detection, i.e. significant reductions in sensitivity are recorded ($\geqslant 0.4$ log unit) without further investigation of the intensity of the defect.

This time schedule sketches, on the one hand, the importance of the distinction between the two phases and, on the other hand, the time saved by the multiple stimulus method. When phase IA furnishes enough information, the duration of the detection phase is only 14 minutes. The duration of the assessment phase is dependent on the number and structure of the defects found in the detection phase. In addition, the comprehension, reactions and staying power of the patient decide how detailed this phase can be. In an average case, i.e. when the defects are not too complicated, the assessment phase for one eye takes about 30 minutes. In special cases this may be prolonged to 60 minutes. Thus a complete examination in our research programme, when there were defects in the visual field, took at least 45 minutes per eye. If necessary the examination was performed in two sessions. In the routine procedure which has been developed from our research programme, complete examination of a visual field *with defects* takes a minimum of 45 minutes and a maximum of 82 minutes per eye. These times apply to visual field examination in patients who react well. In a number of patients it is impossible to perform an extensive examination like this.

The duration of the examination is also dependent on the size of the areas in the visual field where the perception is still intact. When only a small central area remains, the duration will be appreciably shorter than the times given above. When the perception in one half of the visual field is almost completely lost the duration of the examination is shortened proportionally.

Organization.

An examination procedure as described above can only be realized in practice with the help of a well-organized department.

The Visual Field Department of the University Eye Clinic in Amsterdam is manned by 4 full-time specialized technical ophthalmic assistants and one perimetrologist. Each technician has had careful training in the theory, technique and pathology of visual field examination.

Every patient comes by appointment. $1\frac{1}{2}$ hour is reserved for one session. In this length of time a large proportion of the patients can be completely examined; the remaining patients return for a supplementary examination. All the results are discussed in a weekly meeting of technicians and perimetrologist, after which a report is written.

The organization of the Visual Field Department has been especially mentioned here, because some people may wonder whether what is described in this study can really be put into practice. With a well organized perimetric department this is indeed possible.

GLAUCOMATOUS DEFECTS

It is not the purpose of this study to give an extensive exposition on glauco-

231

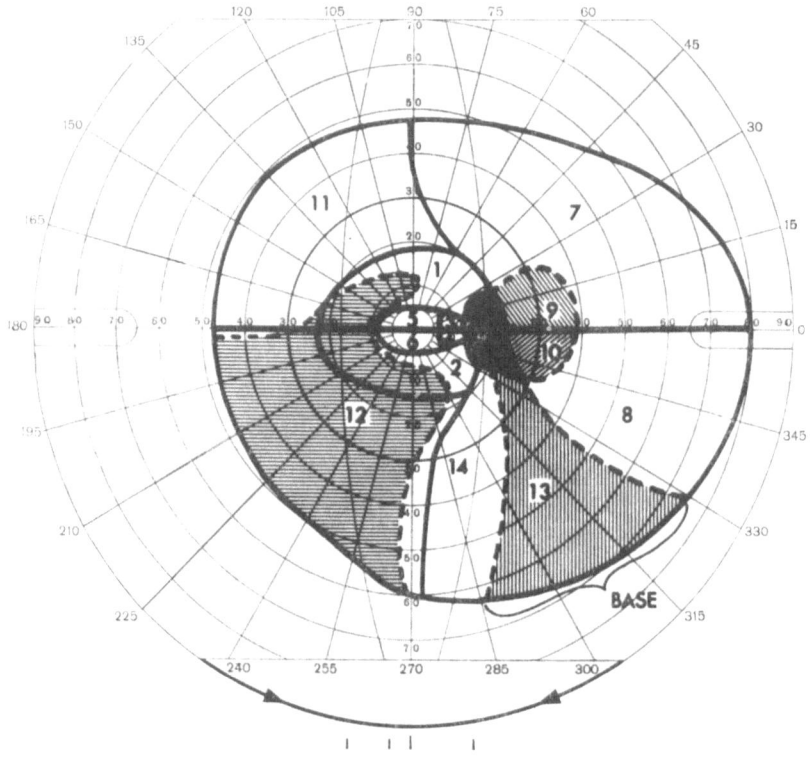

Fig. 1

Nerve fibre bundle scotomata

   1 and 2 : arcuate scotoma
   3 and 4 : juxtacecal scotoma
   5 and 6 : (hemi) centrocecal scotoma
   7 and 8 : supero- and inferotemporal sector defects
   9 and 10: temporal juxtacecal scotoma
  11 and 12: break-through of defects to nasal periphery
         13: inferotemporal wedge-shaped sector defect

matous visual field defects. Descriptions have been given by DUBOIS-POULSEN, FRANÇOIS & VERRIEST (kinetic perimetry), AULHORN & HARMS, DRANCE and co-workers and HEILMANN (static perimetry) (Fig. 1)[1]. Two types of early glaucomatous visual field defects, however, deserve special consideration.

The first type is the relative wedge-shaped scotoma (w.s.s.), which may appear

[1] Figure after FRANÇOIS & VERRIEST, 1954; DUBOIS-POULSEN, 1952–1969; AULHORN & HARMS, 1967; DRANCE et al., 1967–1972; HEILMANN, 1972.

anywhere in the 30° visual field. Nearly all partial fibre bundle defects end in a wedge-shaped scotoma, as is shown in the examples given here. Isolated wedge-shaped scotomata, however, are also found, without a defect for maximum luminance in the same bundle pathway (patient 1). The detection of a wedge-shaped scotoma is important because it is probably one of the earliest signs of reduction of light sensitivity due to glaucoma. Threshold examination is essential for the detection of wedge-shaped scotomata. They may be reversible[2].

The second type is the small, more or less isolated defect for maximum luminance, which can also appear anywhere in the 30° visual field. The second type of defect has been described by AULHORN & HARMS, who have by far the greatest experience with static perimetry of glaucomatous defects. The first type of defect has received little or no attention in the literature and it seems justified to stress its importance.

A distinction is often made between paracentral defects, defects in the Bjerrum area and nasal steps. The reason for the distinction between the paracentral area and the Bjerrum area is that the Bjerrum area has so long been considered to be the most important site for glaucomatous visual field defects. In the group of 1372 visual fields examined by us, paracentral defects were frequently found, a fact which is in agreement with the findings of AULHORN & HARMS[3]. The early defects can appear anywhere in the 30° visual field, although it is our impression that glaucomatous defects frequently develop along the nasal part of the horizontal meridian (e.g. patient 7) and spread cecopetally. When a defect develops along the nasal horizontal meridian this is expressed in kinetic perimetry as a relative nasal step. In this case a nasal step indicates that early defects are developing on one side of the horizontal meridian.

These early defects do not usually appear in the extreme nasal periphery, but in the paracentral area, the Bjerrum area or the adjacent peripheral visual field. For this reason a *peripheral* nasal step is not an early sign of glaucoma. In this study isolated peripheral nasal steps, i.e. without demonstrable defects in the 30° visual field, were not found. The nasal step in the paracentral and intermediate visual field, on the other hand, can be an early sign of glaucomatous visual field defects.

Recently DRANCE[4] has called attention to the defects which arise from lesions in the nerve fibre bundles fanning out towards the temporal visual field (see also Fig. 1).

---

[2] GREVE, Dublin 1972.

[3] AULHORN & HARMS, 1967.

[4] DRANCE, 1972; BRAIS & DRANCE, 1972.

Early defects in the opposite hemifield.

Early glaucomatous defects also occur in the half of the visual field opposite to an extensive defect (e.d.o.h.: early defects in the opposite hemifield; cf. patients 15, 16, 17). It does not take much time to find an extensive defect, whereas the complete detection phase is needed to discover the early defects in the opposite hemifield. The detection of the early defects in the opposite hemifield is important because progression can be most easily demonstrated in these defects (cf. patient 15).

When investigating glaucomatous defects the two halves of the visual field divided by the horizontal meridian must be regarded as separate entities in which different types of defects can occur.

Eleven of the 18 visual fields demonstrated here have defects in one half of the visual field. These include very early defects and a few cases in a transitional stage between early defects and fully developed fibre bundle defects, with threatened break-through to the nasal periphery. In 7 cases there are defects in both halves of the visual field, some of which are very early defects.

In the commentary on these visual fields the type of defect will be mentioned, but most attention will be paid to the practice of the detection phase. All the visual fields shown here are from patients with glaucoma simplex.

Guide to the figures of Chapter XI.

V.F.A.:	if no threshold value is indicated at a stimulus position, this stimulus is seen at the value indicated in the lower right hand corner. (L.O.S.: level of sensitivity). This has only been done in order to avoid too many figures.
	In the IB-phase this is impossible because the stimuli are not supposed to be seen at the same threshold level.
	The blind spot has been drawn on the VFA-chart only for orientation. Stimulus positions on the VFA are indicated by the letter and meridian e.g. J255.
	● indicates no perception.
IB-phase:	the actual threshold values as measured with the Tübinger perimeter are indicated; a localized reduction of sensitivity is indicated with a ＊; no perception is indicated with a ●; the threshold value of the central positions is indicated in the lower right hand corner.
g.r.s.:	general reduction of sensitivity.
'flattening':	indicates a flatter sensitivity curve; the central sensitivity is more decreased with respect to the normal sensitivity curve than the peripheral sensitivity.
max. L.:	indicates maximum luminance.
ecc.:	indicates eccentricity.
cecofugal:	means progression of a fibre bundle defect away from the blind spot.
cecopetal:	means progression of a fibrebundle defect towards the blind spot.

If a small defect is located on the border of two topographic units the one with the lower number has been indicated.

On each kinetic chart the meridians chosen for static perimetric examination are indicated by a dotted line.

In the diagram of static perimetry the normal sensitivity curve is drawn.

For reading the figures a transparant plastic sheet indicating the topographical units is provided with this monography.

Pat. no.: 1   age 73   OS

DESCRIPTION

Detection	IA25	g.r.s.	0.6–0.8 lu
		sup.	defects of 0.6 lu (TS 14), 1.0 lu (TS 16) and 0.8 lu (TS 24)
		inf.	no defects
	IA periphery		no defects
	IB	sup.	defect of < 1.2 lu (NS 21) surrounded by relative defects; relative superotemporal defects
		inf.	defect of varying intensity (NI 21)
Assessment	SP	g.r.s.	0.3 and flattening
		sup. 15	no significant defects
		45	relative defect at 19° with small defect of 1° Ø of max. L.
		90	w.s.s. defect of 1.0 lu
		120	extensive relative reduction of sensitivity
		150	w.s.s. defect of 0.9 lu
		inf. 315	defect of max. L. at 20°
	KP		no defects with classical isopterperimetry

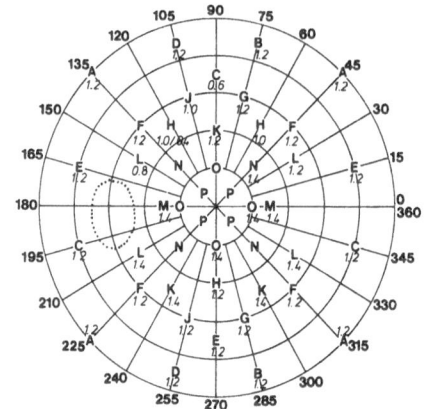

FOVEA: 2.0

L.O.S.: 1.6

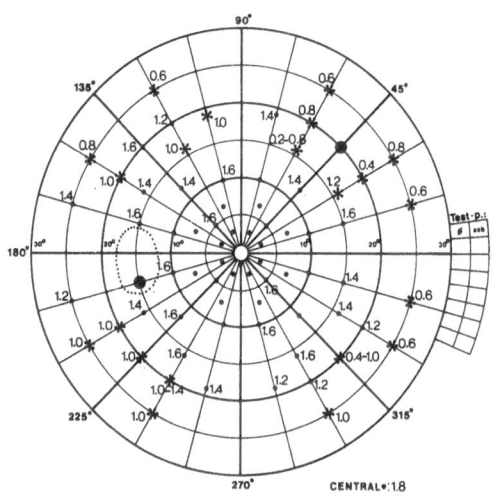

CENTRAL●:1.8

238

150°
120°
90°
45°
315°
15°
40
35
30
25
20
15
10
05
asb
0,32
1
3,2
10
32
100
320
1000
30°
20°
10°
0°
90°
135°
45°
180°
225°
270°
315°
Test-p.

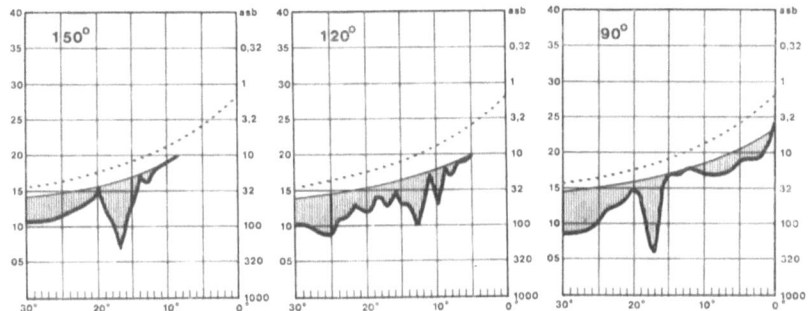

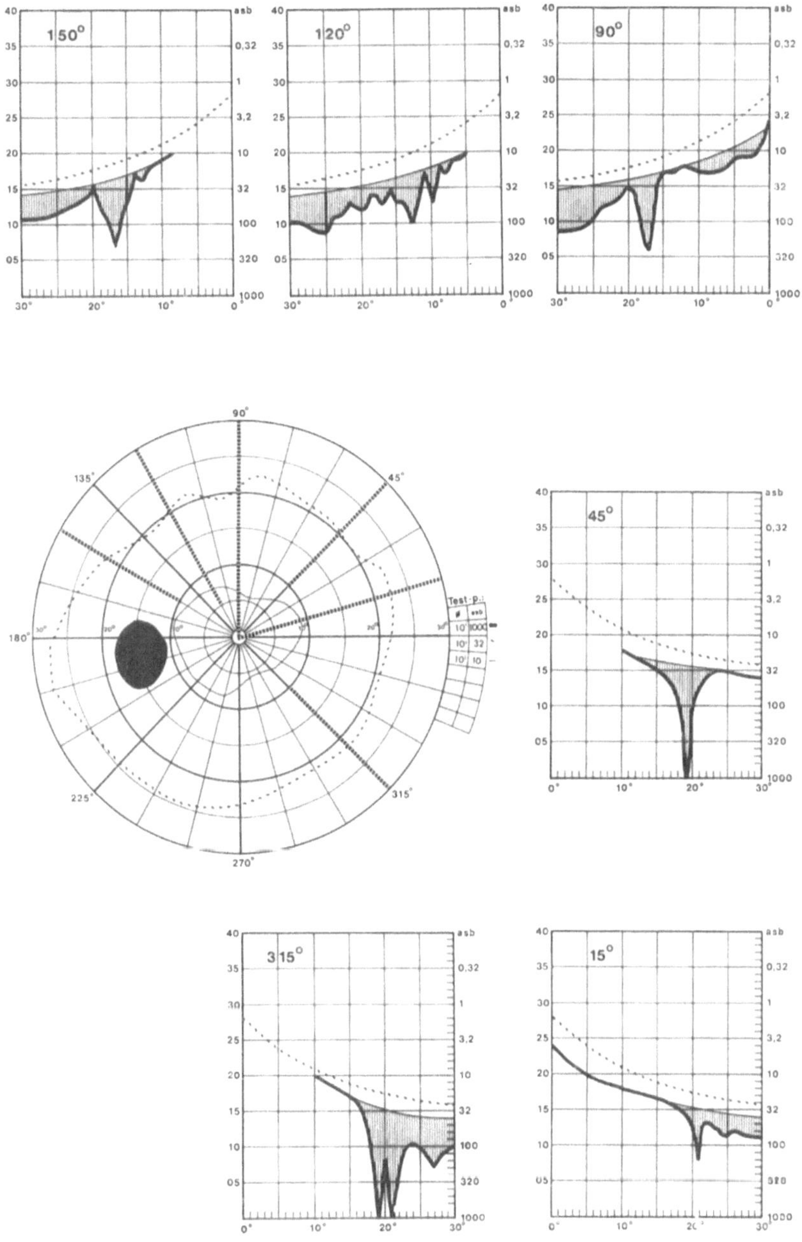

Patient no.1. Comment.

This visual field is a good example of early glaucomatous defects. In the detection phase it became apparent that early defects were to be found in the upper and lower halves of the visual field. The defect in the 45° M could be an angio-scotoma in a wedge-shaped scotoma. The defects in this visual field are the earliest in the series of visual fields shown here. The defects found are nearly all wedge-shaped scotomata. Examination of the 345° M would have been helpful in determining the significance of the defect in the 315° M.

In other visual fields to be demonstrated here many wedge-shaped scotomata will be seen, some of which do not form part of a defect of greater intensity (cf. patient 13, upper half of visual field).

Kinetic perimetry gave no indication of the existence of defects. The Visual Field Analyser revealed some of the defects: the supero-temporal wedge-shaped scotomata were found; the supero-nasal and infero-nasal defects were completely missed. These were discovered in phase IB. Where the smallest defect for max. L is located the Visual Field Analyser has no stimulus position.

Pat. no.: 2   age 75   OD

DESCRIPTION

Detection	IA25	g.r.s. sup. inf.	0.4–0.6 lu 0.4 lu reduction in Bjerrum – area defect for max. L. at NI 17
	IA periphery		no defects
	IB	sup. inf.	slight depression in Bjerrum – area defect for max. L. at NI 22
Assessment	SP	g.r.s. sup. 75 inf. 195 210 225 240 255 270 285	0.5 lu no significant defects no significant defects w.s.s. of 1.5 lu defect for max. L. defect for max. L. two defects w.s.s.of 0.7 lu relative defect of 0.3 lu
	KP	sup. inf.	no defects small isolated defect at NI 16, 17, 18 for max. L.

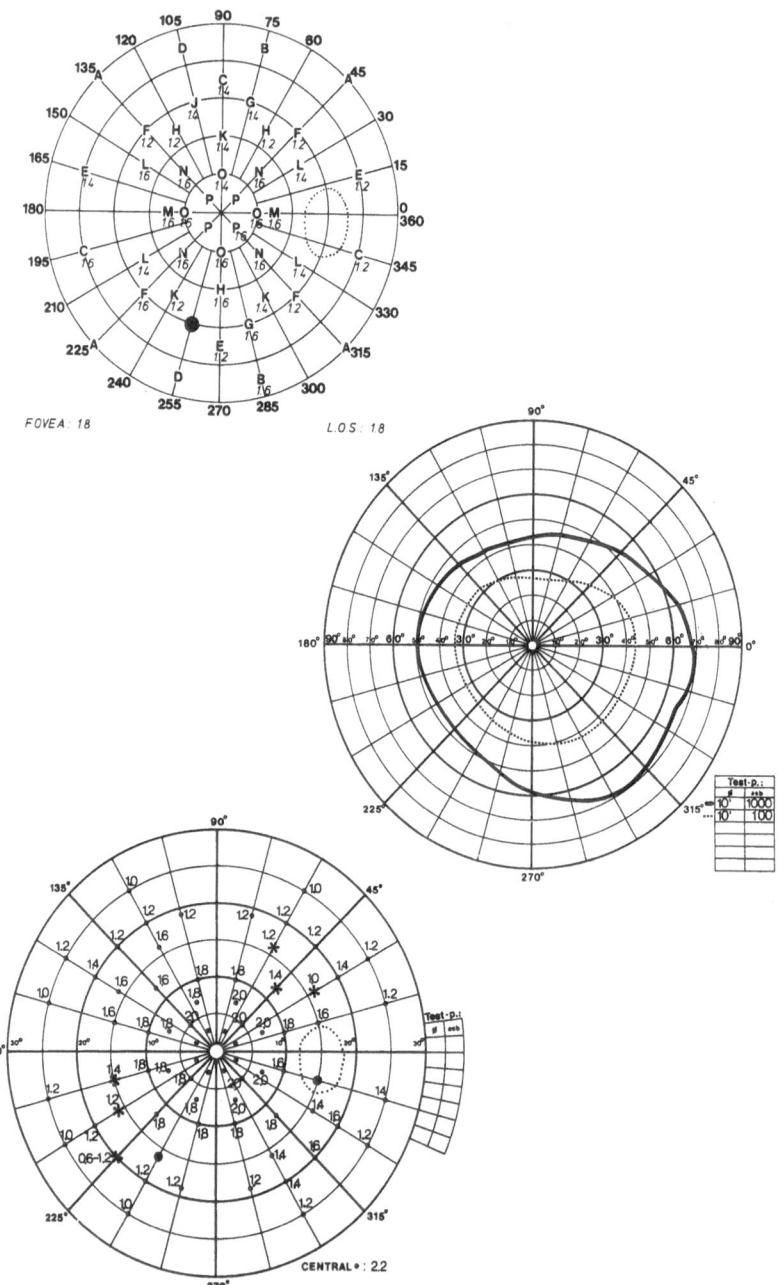

FOVEA: 18

L.O.S: 18

CENTRAL ●: 2.2

242

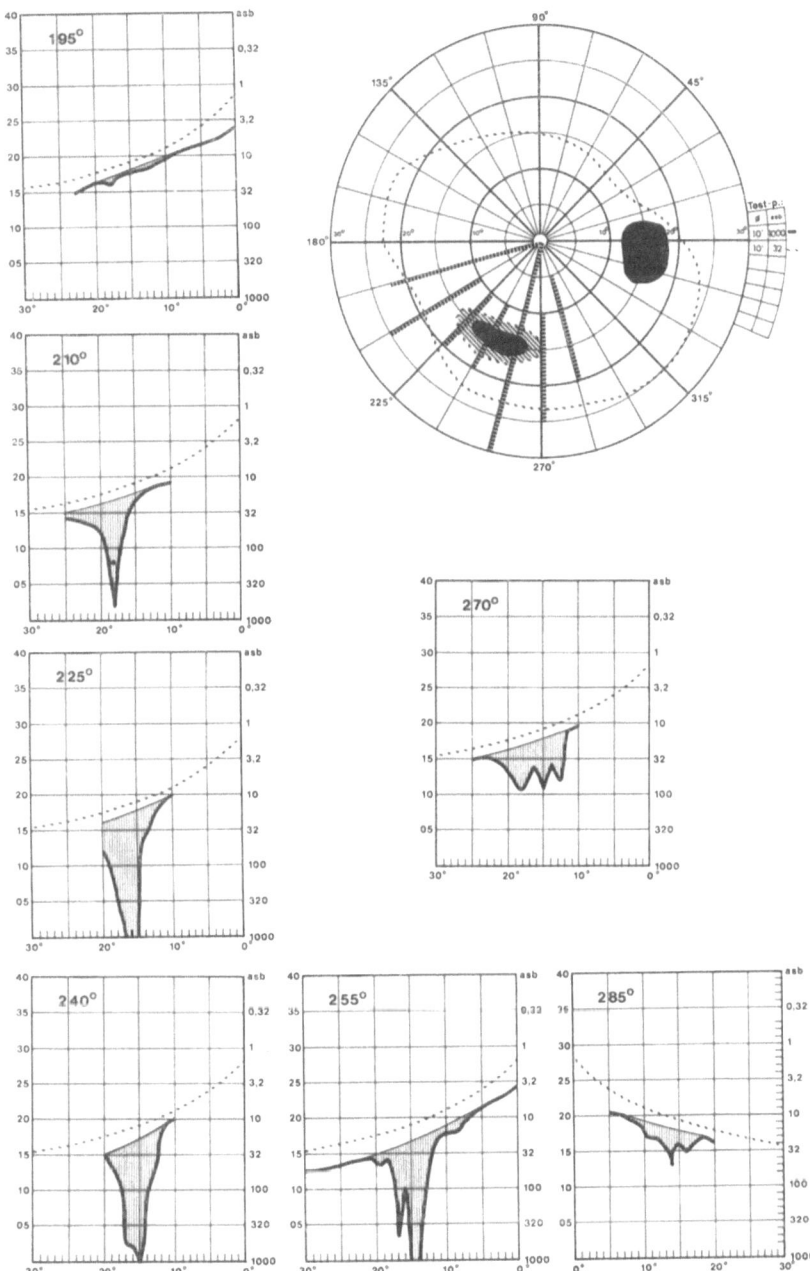

This is an example of an early type II defect: an isolated defect for max. L. In the detection phase the Visual Field Analyser had the good luck to discover this small defect, as it is exactly located at stimulus position J 255 of the Visual Field Analyser.

If the defect had been located 3° more peripherally the Visual Field Analyser would have missed it.

In this case phase IB gives no new information.

A series of static curves gives a good picture of the structure of this type of defect. Unlike other visual fields shown in this chapter the deepest point of the defect lies on the 240° M and there is no connection with the horizontal meridian or the blind spot. Both cecofugally and cecopetally the defect ends in a wedge shaped scotoma. In this way the extent of the defect has been recorded in all directions, both the part for max. L. and the relative extensions.

This visual field also shows that there is often no reason to perform static perimetry along a whole meridian; portions of 10° are sufficient.

Pat. no.: 3   age 60   OD

DESCRIPTION

Detection	IA25	g.r.s.	0.4 lu
		sup.	relative paracentral defects (NS 4, 9; TS 4 TS 12); relative defects in Bjerrum – area (NS 14, 16)
		inf.	no defects
	1A periphery		no defects
	IB	sup.	relative paracentral defect with nucleus for max. L. at TS 8; defect for max. L. at TS 22; relative defects at NS 7, 20 and 25
		inf.	no defects
Assessment		g.r.s.	flattening
		15	defect for max. L.
		60	defect for max. L.; relative defect of 0.3 lu
		120	w.s.s. of 1.3 lu
		135	w.s.s. of 0.8 lu
		150	relative defect of 0.3 lu
		165	several w.s.s.
	KP	sup.	paracentral and superotemporal defect for max. L.

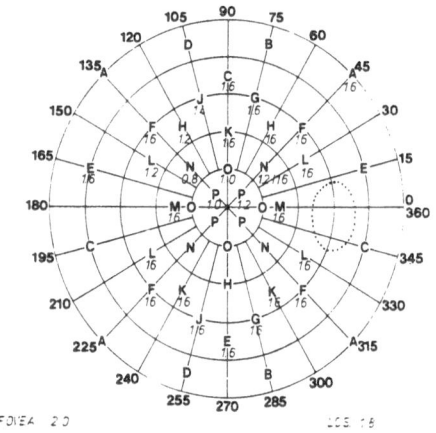

FOVEA 2.0   LOS 1.8

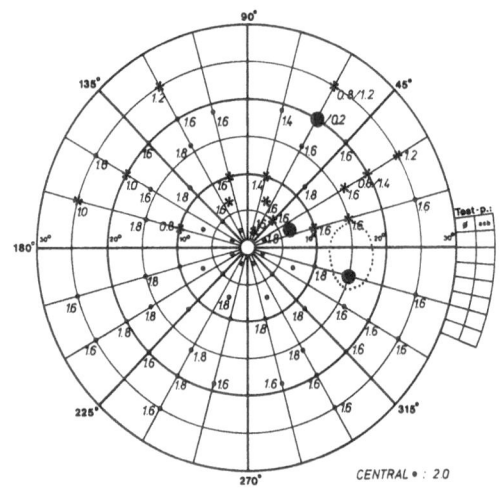

CENTRAL • : 2.0

246

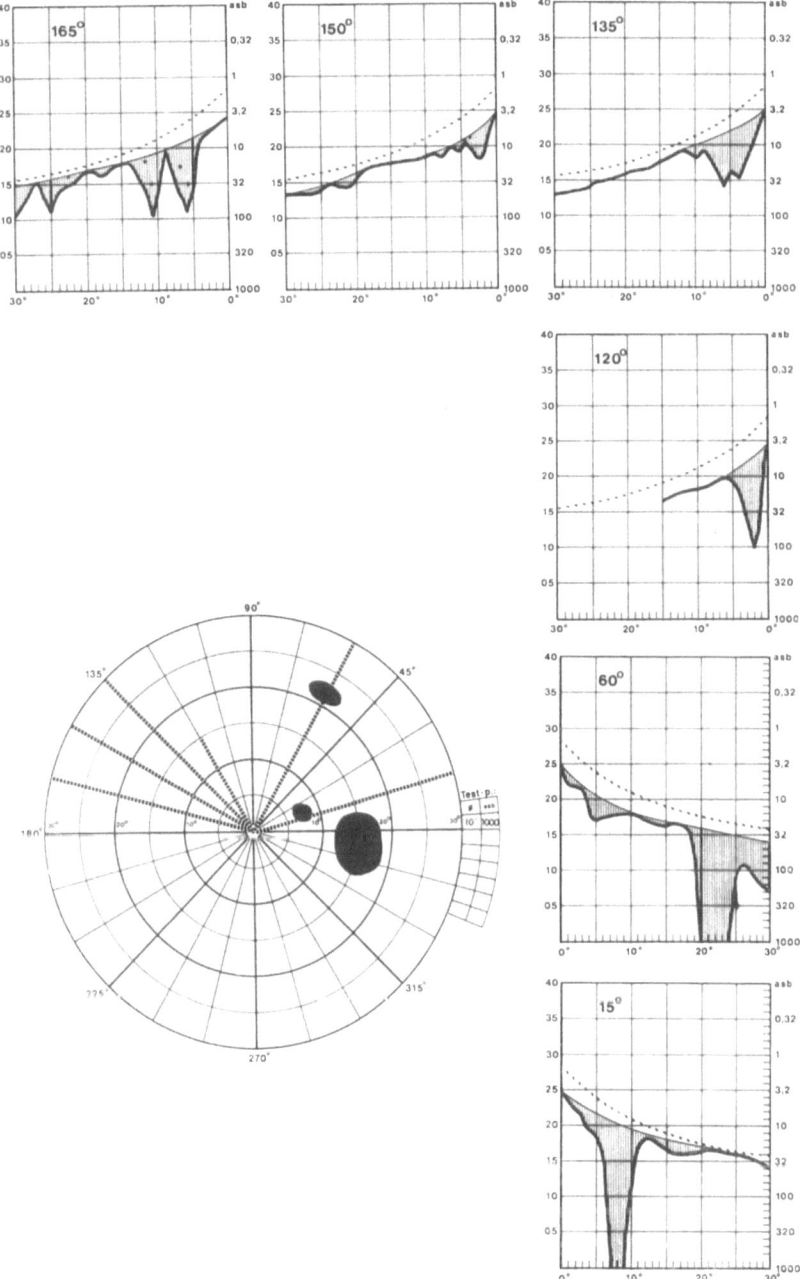

Patient no. 3. Comment.

This visual field is an example of a very early paracentral defect which to a large extent is still relative. In phase IA the nucleus for max. L. was missed because this falls exactly between 2 stimulus positions. The same applies to the defect for max. L. at TS 22. No indication of this defect was found in phase IA; this shows clearly the importance of phase IB.

The paracentral defect is an incomplete fibre bundle defect. In the 15° meridian a defect for max. L. is found, whereas in the 60° M only a slight relative defect (0.3 lu) can be demonstrated.

In the 135° M the intensity found with the Visual Field Analyser is greater than that found in phase II. The threshold value of stimulus position E 165 of the Visual Field Analyser was rightly found to be high, as appears from results of phase II in the 165° M.

Kinetic perimetry was only carried out with a stimulus of max. L. on the basis of the particulars obtained with static perimetry.

Pat. no.: 4   age 58   OD

DESCRIPTION

Detection	IA25	g.r.s.	0.8 lu
		sup.	relative defects at TS 16, 17
		inf.	defects for max. L. at TI 6 and 9; relative defects at TI 15
	IA periphery		no defects
	IB	sup.	no defects
		inf.	not examined
Assessment	SP	g.r.s.	flattening
		60	no defects
		75	no defects
		185	small relative paracentral defect (0.5. lu)
		195	relative paracentral defect (0.4 lu)
		210	relative paracentral defect (0.3 lu)
		225	w.s.s. of 1.3 lu
		240	w.s.s. of 1.1. lu
		270	paracentral defect for max. L.
		315	paracentral defect for max. L and w.s.s. at 15° ecc
		330	2 w.s.s. at 7° and at 15° ecc
	KP	sup.	no defects
		inf.	paracentral defect for max. L.

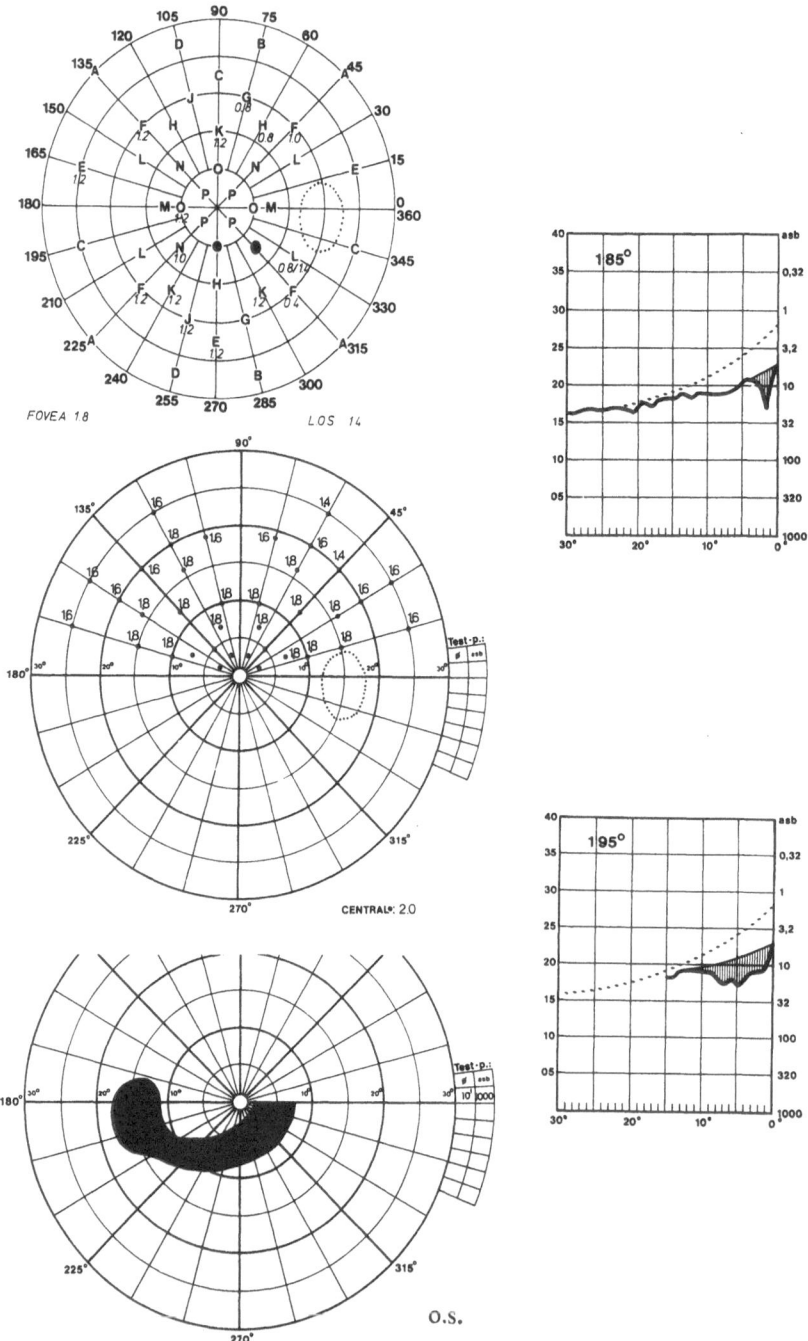

FOVEA 1.8 LOS 14

CENTRAL: 2.0

O.S.

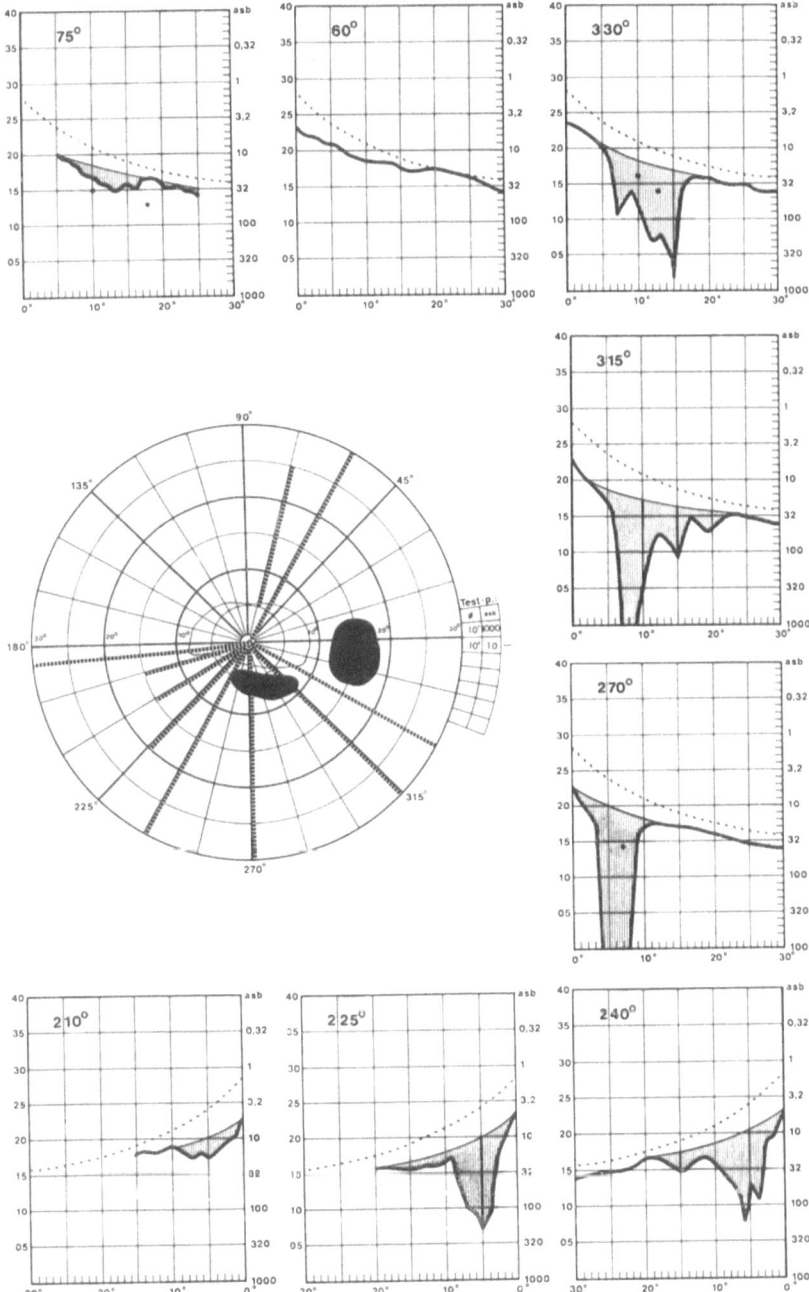

This visual field is a good example of an early isolated paracentral defect. The other eye (OS) has a similar defect at a more advanced stage. The left eye shows how the right eye will develop further. The Visual Field Analyser showed relative defects in the upper half of the visual field; in phase IB no further defects found. These two relative defects (H 60 and G 75) are probably caused by angio-scotomata. In the lower half of the visual field the Visual Field Analyser has shown exactly (as far as this is possible with the limited number of stimulus positions) which defects are present. It would have been correct to carry out a supplementary IB phase in the lower half of the visual field also, particularly between 10° and 30°. The examiner has compensated for this omission by examining a large number of meridians in phase II.

The paracentral defect begins (330° M) and ends (240° M) in wedge-shaped scotoma, as is the case with nearly all partial fibre bundle defects. The relative defect can be traced as far as the horizontal meridian (225° M, 210° M, 195° M, 185° M).

It is clear that this paracentral defect has developed somewhere within the 10° parallel between the 270° and 315° M. and that it will extend cecopetally and cecofugally. The progression can be followed on the basis of these data. In the 15° parallel a wedge-shaped scotoma was found alongside the paracentral defect (315° and 330° M).

This visual field also shows that a paracentral defect may occur without nasal depression.

Pat. no.: 5   age 56   OD

DESCRIPTION

Detection	IA25	g.r.s.	0.6 lu
		sup.	no defects
		inf.	relative defects at NI 6 and NI 9
	IA periphery		no peripheral nasal step; nasal step for intermediate isopter
	IB	sup.	no defects
		inf.	defects for mac. L. at NI 4, NI 11 and TI 11, relative nasal defects.
Assessment	SP	g.r.s.	flattening
		195	defect for max. L. at 6° ecc.; several w.s.s.
		225, 270	
		315, 330	defect for max. L.
	KP		small partial paracentral fibre bundle defect.

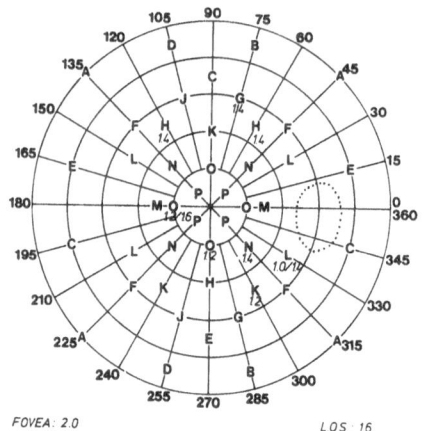

FOVEA: 2.0

LOS : 16

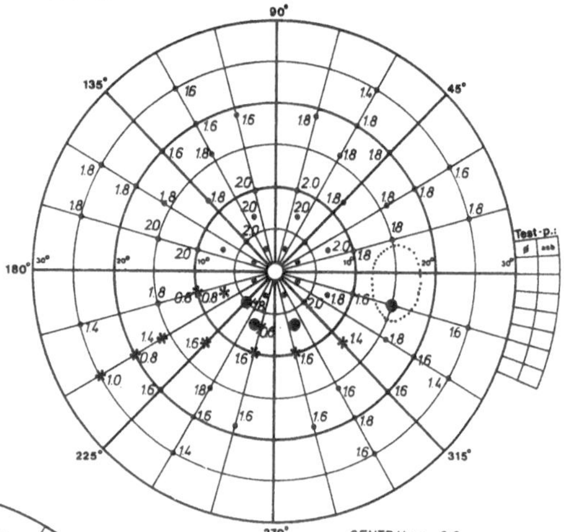

CENTRAL • : 2.2

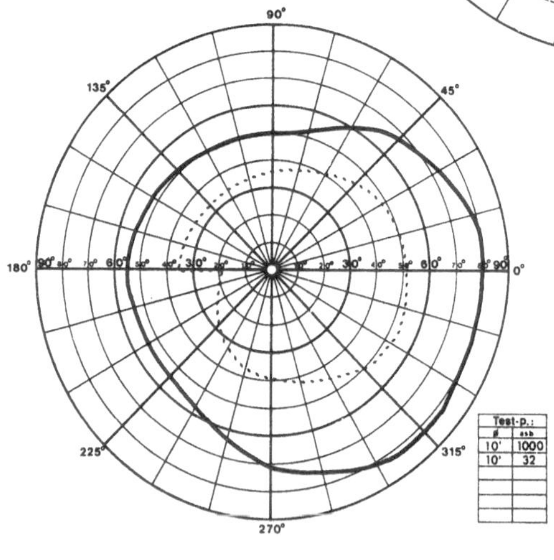

Test-p.:	
#	asb
10'	1000
10'	32

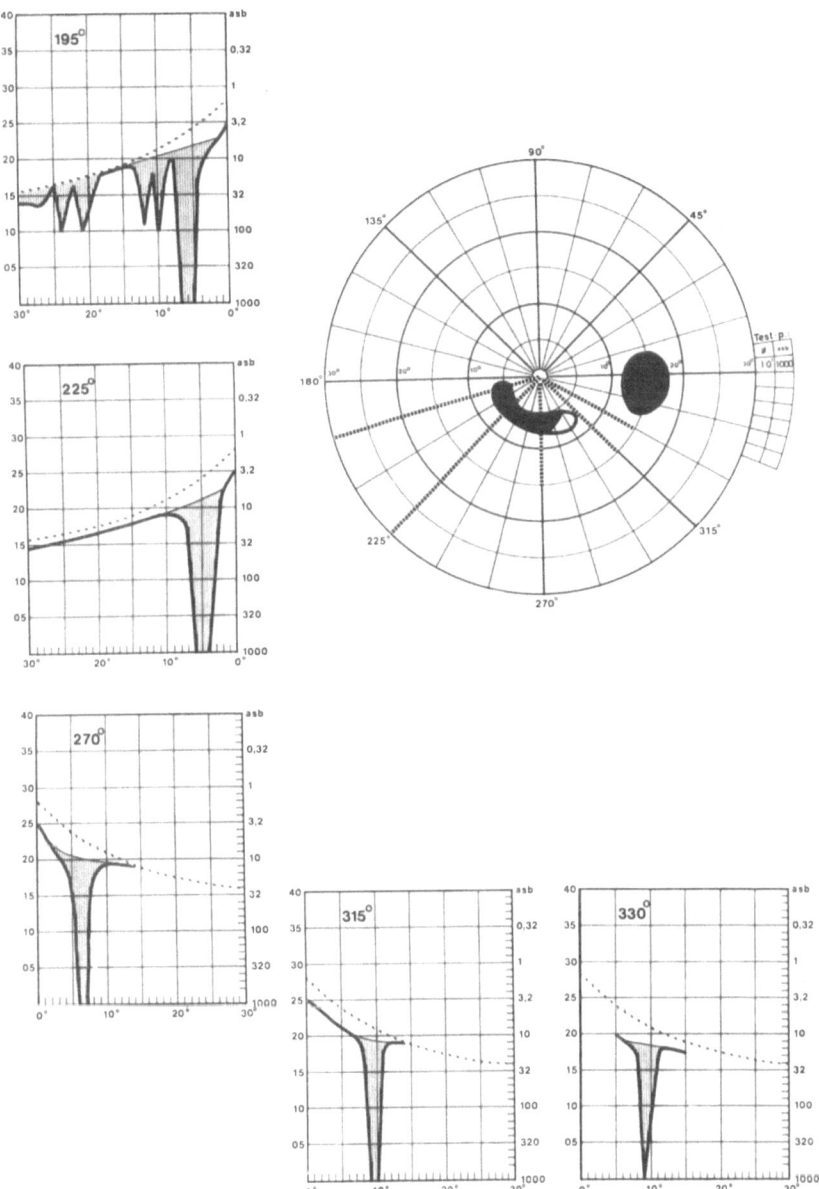

This visual field shows an absolute, but very narrow, paracentral defect with an incipient nasal depression. The nasal depression cannot be demonstrated in the peripheral visual field. In phase IA the paracentral defect falls exactly between the Visual Field Analyser stimulus positions. Only the O 180, O 270 and N 315 positions fall on the edge of the defect; the N 225 position falls exactly in an area of normal sensitivity. The stimulus positions of the IB phase fall exactly in the defect.

There is slight nasal loss of sensitivity, which is not shown by the Visual Field Analyser, but is discovered in the IA periphery phase. The paracentral defect would never have been discovered with KP; the cecopetal extension could not be recorded kinetically.

This visual field demonstrates:

1. an early paracentral fibre bundle defect of very small diameter (2°);
2. the usefulness of the IB phase, as this defect falls between the Visual Field Analyser stimuli;
3. a nasal depression without a peripheral nasal step.

Even the small relative defects found with the Visual Field Analyser deserve attention.

Pat. no.: 6   age 67   OD

DESCRIPTION

Detection	IA25	g.r.s.	0.6 lu
		sup.	defect for max. L. at TS/NS 6 and a defect of 0.4 lu at TS 9; defect of 0.6 lu at NS 19; relative depression in Bjerrum – area (0.4 lu)
		inf.	relative defects at TI 14 and TI 15 (0.4 lu)
	IA periphery	sup.	small nasal step
	IB	sup.	defect for max. L. at NS 5, at TS 4 and at NS 25; relative defects at TS 21, 22, 23
		inf.	no defects
Assessment	SP	g.r.s.	0.3 lu
		45	defect for max. L. of 3° Ø and w.s.s. at 18° ecc.
		60	defect for max. L. and w.s.s.
		75–90	deep defect reproduced
		135	w.s.s. of 1.5 lu
		165	defect for max. L. beginning at 17° ecc.; at several isolated locations the stimulus is sometimes seen.
	KP		relative superior nasal step, superotemporal depression, paracentral defect.

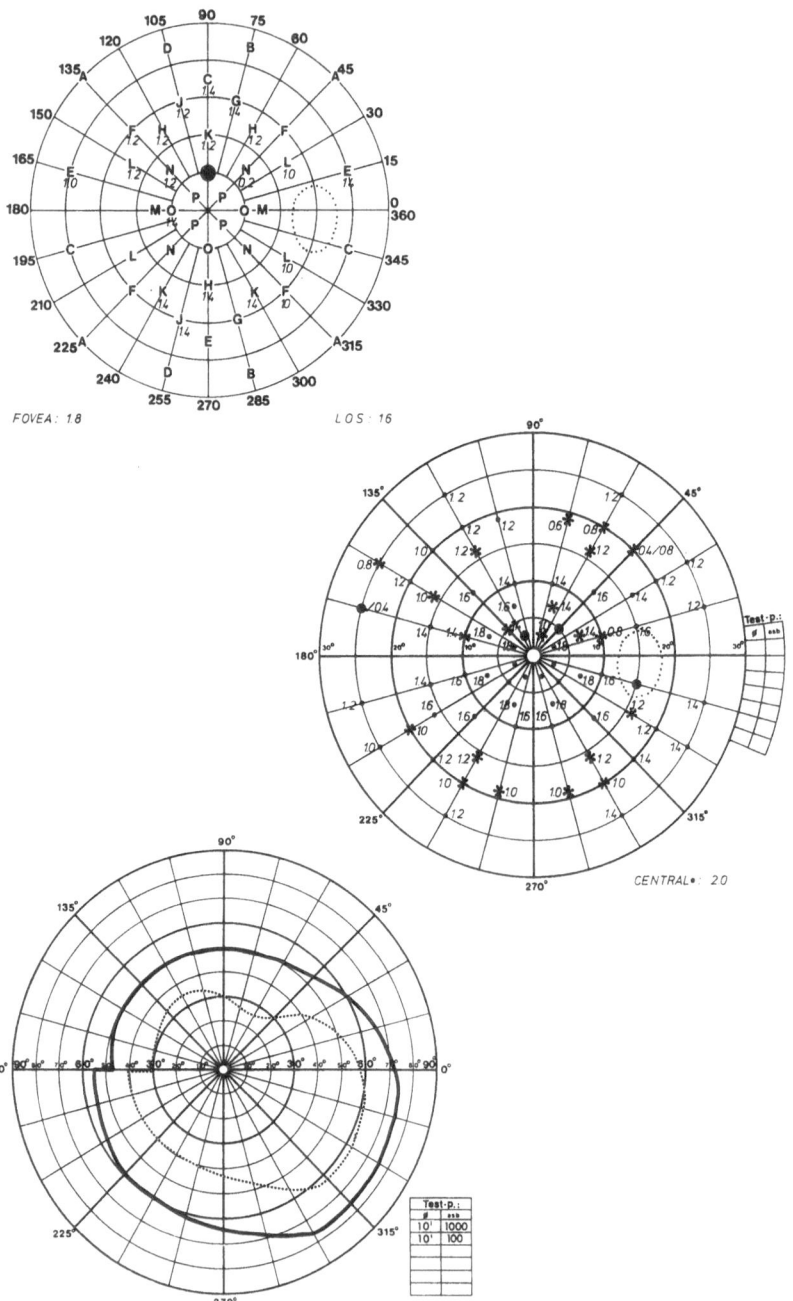

FOVEA: 1.8   LOS: 16

CENTRAL•: 20

258

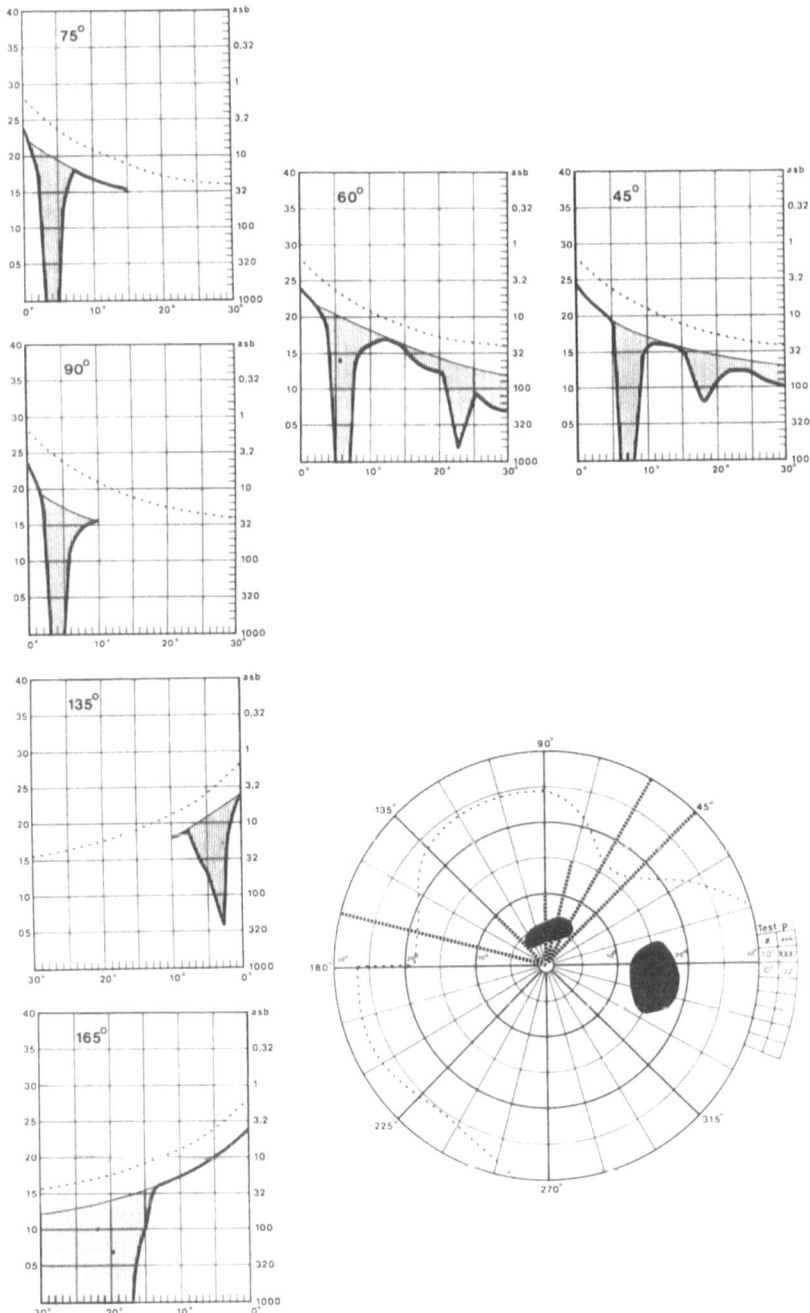

In phase IA a paracentral defect is detected with the Visual Field Analyser, a nasal defect is also indicated (E 165). In phase IB the paracentral defect is confirmed and it appears that there is a nasal defect for max. L. This illustrates again that the Visual Field Analyser has too few stimulus positions in the nasal visual field for adequate glaucoma detection. This is also true for the superotemporal area. In the IB phase a relative superotemporal defect was found. There are thus three early glaucomatous defects:

1. paracentral partial fibre bundle defect;
2. nasal defect;
3. superotemporal relative defect.

The paracentral defect is found in phase II to end in a relative wedge-shaped scotoma. In the 75° M the defect lies just between 2 stimulus positions of the IB phase. In the nasal defect there is some residual perception in a few positions, which explains the rather high threshold value for E 165 on the Visual Field Analyser.

The superotemporal wedge-shaped scotoma, an expression of functional loss in the fibre bundles which fan out downwards, was completely missed by the Visual Field Analyser as there are no stimulus positions at this point.

Kinetic perimetry revealed a nasal step with a relative extension in the central visual field. There is discrepancy here between the great reduction of sensitivity recorded by static perimetry (165° M) and the small nasal step. This is an observation which we have made many times: early nasal defects are often difficult or impossible to detect with kinetic perimetry although they can be easily demonstrated with static perimetry.

Pat. no.: 7   age 68   OD

DESCRIPTION

Detection	IA25	g.r.s.	0.8 lu
		sup.	no defects
		inf.	defects for max. L. at NI 19 and NI 15; relative defects in Bjerrum – area.
	IA periphery		peripheral nasal step
	IB	sup.	no defects
		inf.	not examined
Assessment	SP	g.r.s.	flattening
		195	defect for max. L. from 13° ecc. outwards
		210	the same defect
		225	defect splits up into two separate defects
		240	two defects; one at 15° ecc. for max. L. and one at 23° ecc. (0.9 lu)
		255	w.s.s.
		270, 285	relative cecopetal end of defect.
		315	no pathological defect, but typical angio-scotoma.
	KP		typical nasal defect.

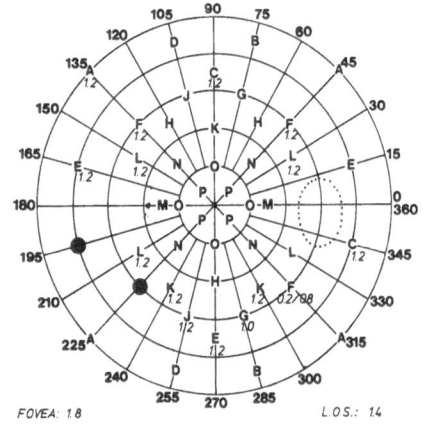

FOVEA: 1.8   L.O.S.: 1.4

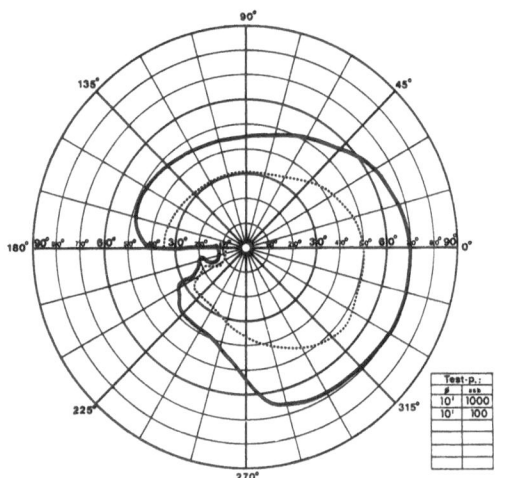

Test-p.:	
∅	asb
10'	1000
10'	100

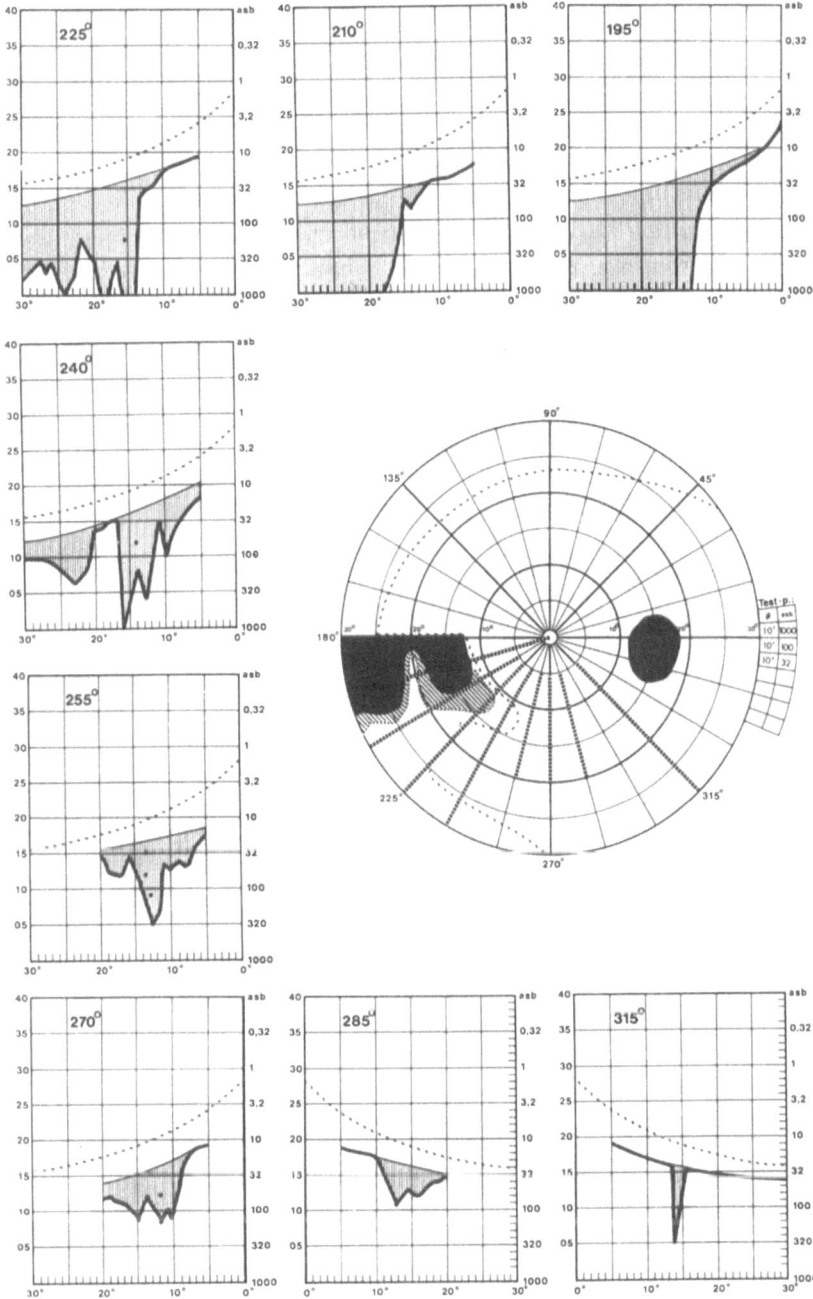

Patient no. 7. Comment.

This visual field is shown as a typical example of nasal depression without further defects. Like the preceding visual field it demonstrates the limitations of kinetic perimetry. There is also considerable variation in the kinetic results.

The intensity of the nasal defect decreases cecopetally.

The Visual Field Analyser in phase I recorded the defect adequately. Only the relative extension (wedge-shaped scotoma) of the nasal defect in the 270° M is not clearly shown. The low threshold value of stimulus position F 315 is probably due to an angioscotoma.

Pat. no.: 8   age 72   OD

DESCRIPTION

Detection	IA25	g.r.s.	0.4 lu
		sup.	no defects
		inf.	defects for max. L. at NI 19 and 14; relative defect at NI 3; NB. P 225 at 1.6.
	IA periphery		nasal step
	IB	sup.	no defects
		inf.	nasal defect for max. L.; defect for max. L at NI 4; relative defect at NI 11
Assessment	SP	g.r.s.	flattening
		195	defect for max. L.; w.s.s. of 0.8 lu at 5°
		225	2 defects for max. L.
		240	w.s.s. of 1.1 lu
		270	w.s.s. of 0.7 lu
		285	no defects
		300	no defects
	KP		nasal step.

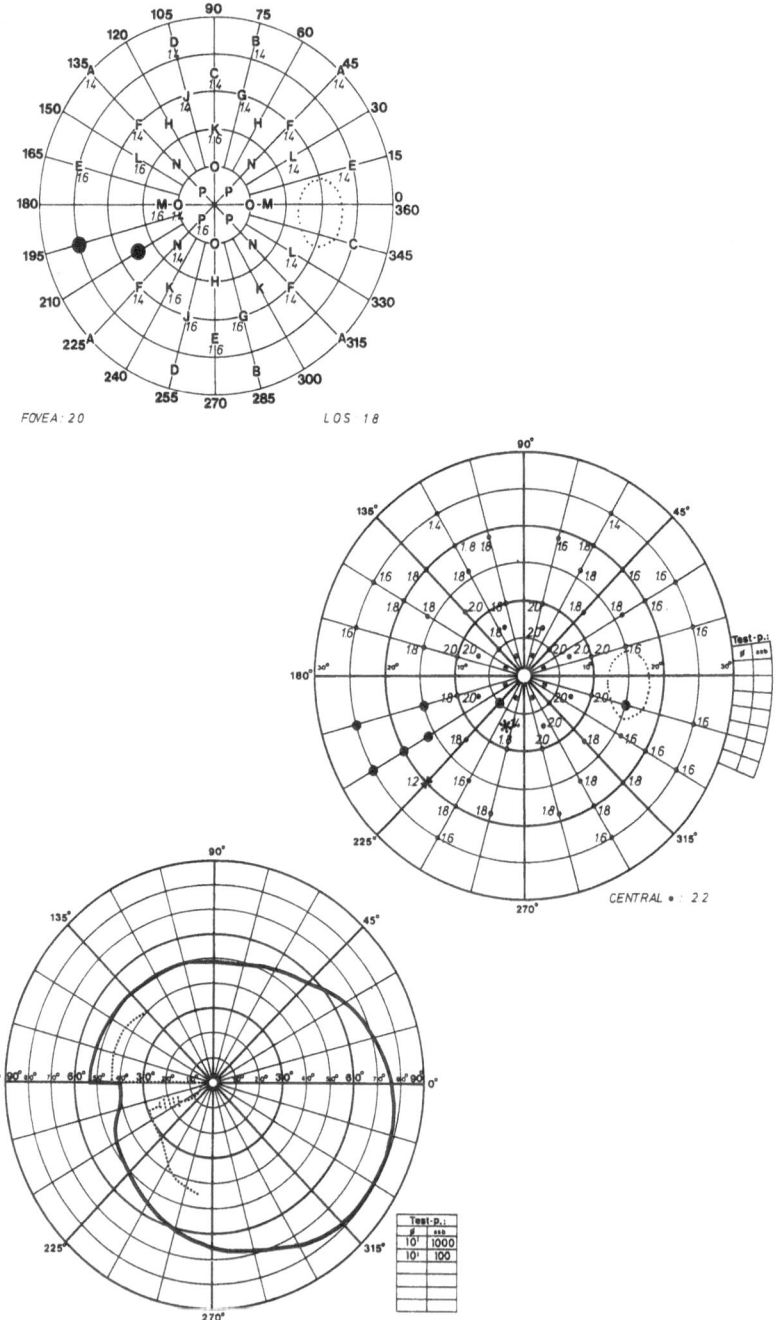

FOVEA: 20   LOS 18

CENTRAL ● : 22

Test-p.:
∅	asb
10'	1000
10'	100

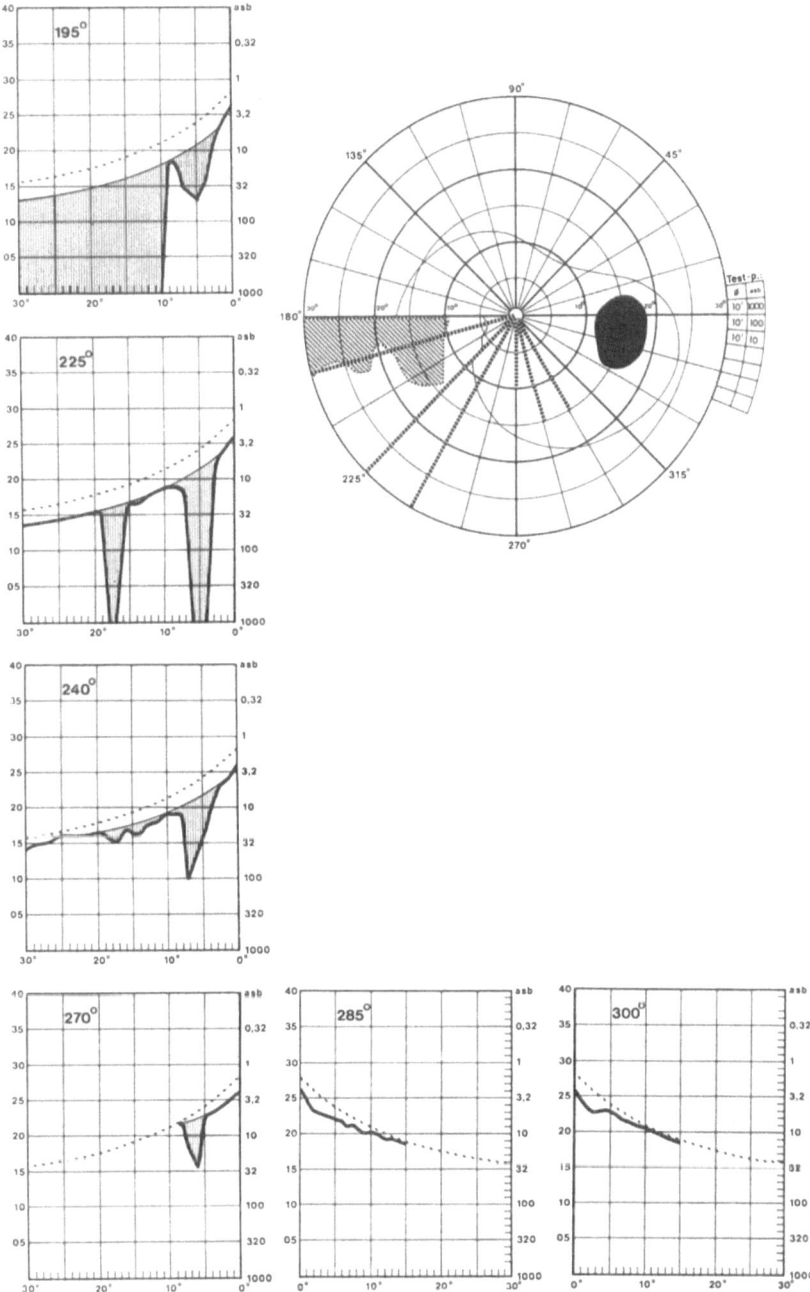

In the IA phase the Visual Field Analyser clearly shows a nasal defect. The paracentral defect, however, is hardly indicated (cf. pat. 5); the only indication might be the threshold value of stimulus position O 180:1.4. On repeat examinition with the Visual Field Analyser P 225 was not seen at all. The peripheral nasal step corresponds to the Visual Field Analyser findings.

The paracentral defect for max. L. was discovered in the IB phase. It falls exactly between 2 stimulus positions of the Visual Field Analyser (P and N 225). This paracentral defect is a classical example of an early defect (as has also been demonstrated in other patients; cf. pat. 3) with a nucleus for max. L. which extends cecopetally (240° and 270° M) and cecofugally (195° M) as a relative wedge-shaped scotoma. Stimulus position O 270 of the Visual Field Analyser again falls just outside the wedge-shaped scotoma in this meridian. With kinetic perimetry with max. L. neither the nasal defect nor the paracentral defect were found; a relative nasal step was recorded.

This visual field demonstrates:

1. an early paracentral glaucomatous defect, with a transition to a wedge-shaped scotoma on both sides;
2. the importance of complete detection.

The limits if both defects are registered: the large nasal defect cannot be found 240° M; the extension of the paracentral defect has disappeared in the 285° M.

Pat. no.: 9   age 65   OS

DESCRIPTION

Detection	IA25	g.r.s.	1.0 lu
		sup.	paracentral defect for max. L. (NS 1) superonasal defect of varying intensity
		inf.	no defects (K 240 was checked: angio-scotoma)
	IA periphery		slight peripheral superonasal depression
	IB	sup.	paracentral defect for max. L. and superonasal defect
		inf.	no defect
Assessment	SP	g.r.s.	0.5 lu; flattening
		15	paracentral defect for max. L.; w.s.s. and sievelike nasal defect
		45	paracentral defect, w.s.s. and sievelike nasal defect
		90	paracentral defect for max. L. and second defect for max. L. at 13° ecc.
		135	paracentral defect.
	KP		paracentral defect and superonasal area of great variation.

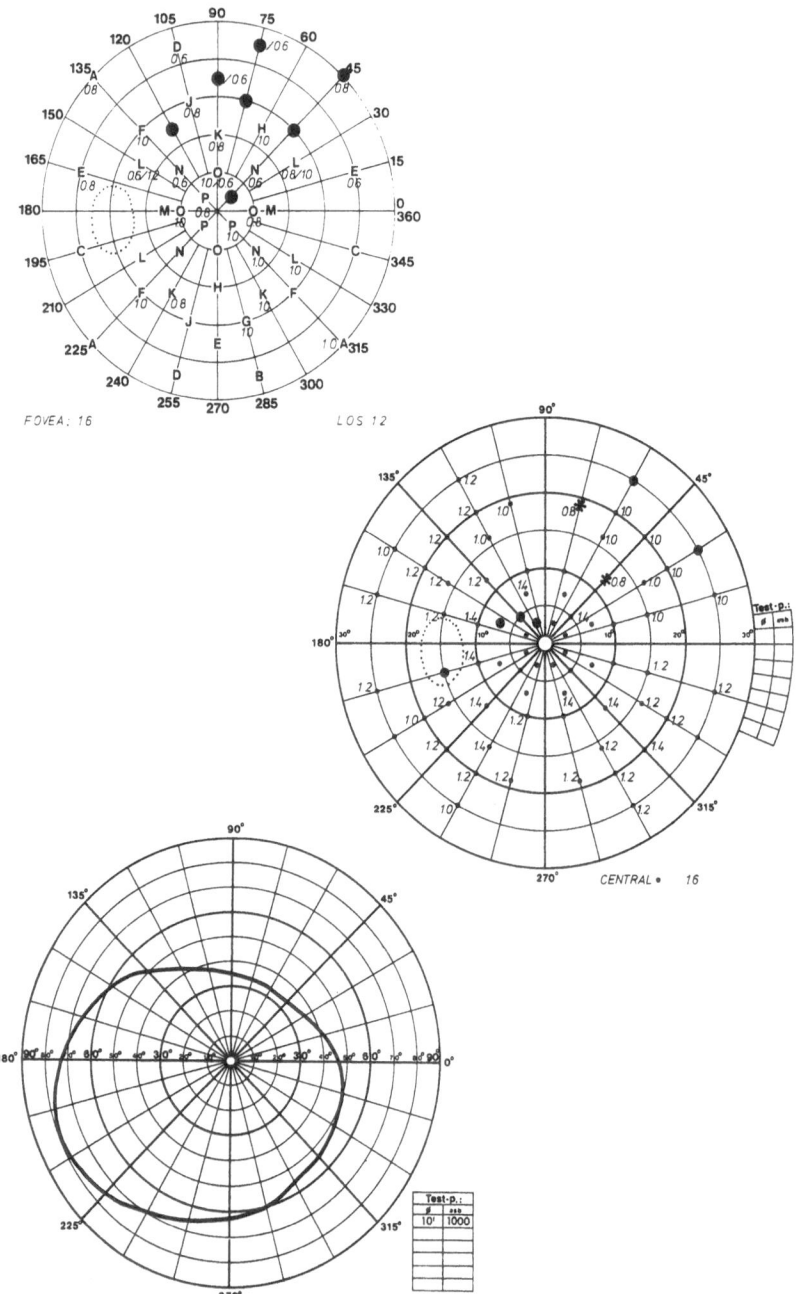

FOVEA: 16   LOS 12

CENTRAL • 16

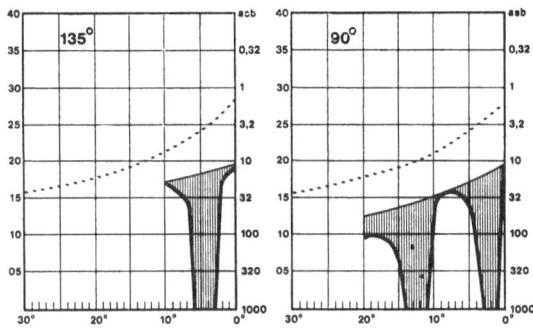

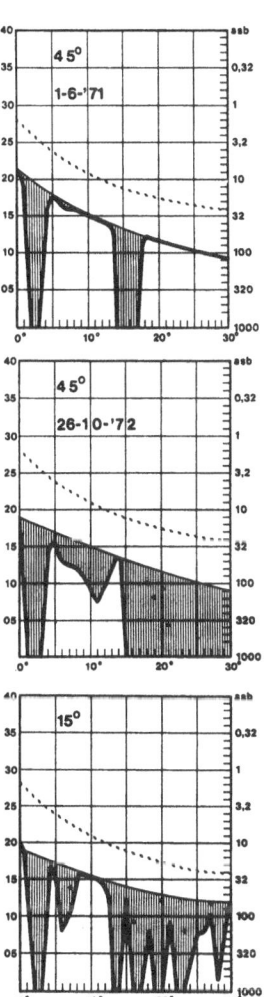

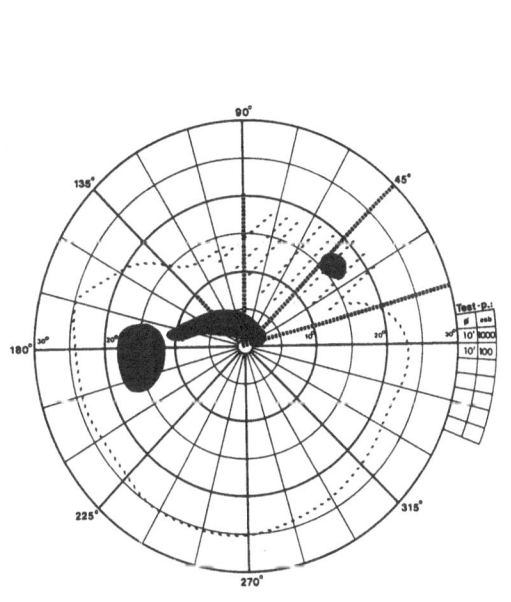

271

This visual field is an example of a transitional stage between an early defect (complete paracentral fibre bundle defect with nasal depression, cf. pat. 8) and a larger fibre bundle defect with breakthrough to the nasal periphery.

The Visual Field Analyser recorded the defects correctly. As well as indicating the paracentral defect (P 45) the Visual Field Analyser showed a large, variable superonasal defect. The picture presented by the Visual Field Analyser is much more serious than the impression given by the results of KP. This defect is so large that it cannot be missed by the Visual Field Analyser.

During the examination of this visual field we had the impression that defects were more easily discovered using the short presentation times of the Visual Field Analyser than with the longer presentation times of the Tübinger perimeter. Some of the defects found in phase II would not have been discovered without the help of the Visual Field Analyser. The IB phase did not contribute to the detection in the upper half of the visual field; in the lower half the absence of defects was confirmed.

In the 15° M and the 45° M there are typical sieve-like defects. One year earlier the sieve-like defect in the 45°M had not been there. On KP great variation was found in this area.

Pat. no. 10   age 65   OD

DESCRIPTION

Detection	IA25	g.r.s.	0.4–0.6 lu
		sup.	paracentral defect for max. L.; relative nasal defects and defects in Bjerrum – area
		inf.	no defects
	IA periphery		superior nasal step
	IB	sup.	not examined
		inf.	no defects
Assessment	SP	g.r.s.	flattening
		45	defects for max. L. at 5° and 11° ecc.
		90	defect for max. L. at 5° and second defect for almost max. L.
		135	2 defects for max. L. separated by small sensitivity peak (compare KP)
		165	two defects for max. L. with sievelike relative nasal defects.
	KP		fully developed paracentral bundledefect with second fragmented bundledefect; relative nasal depression.

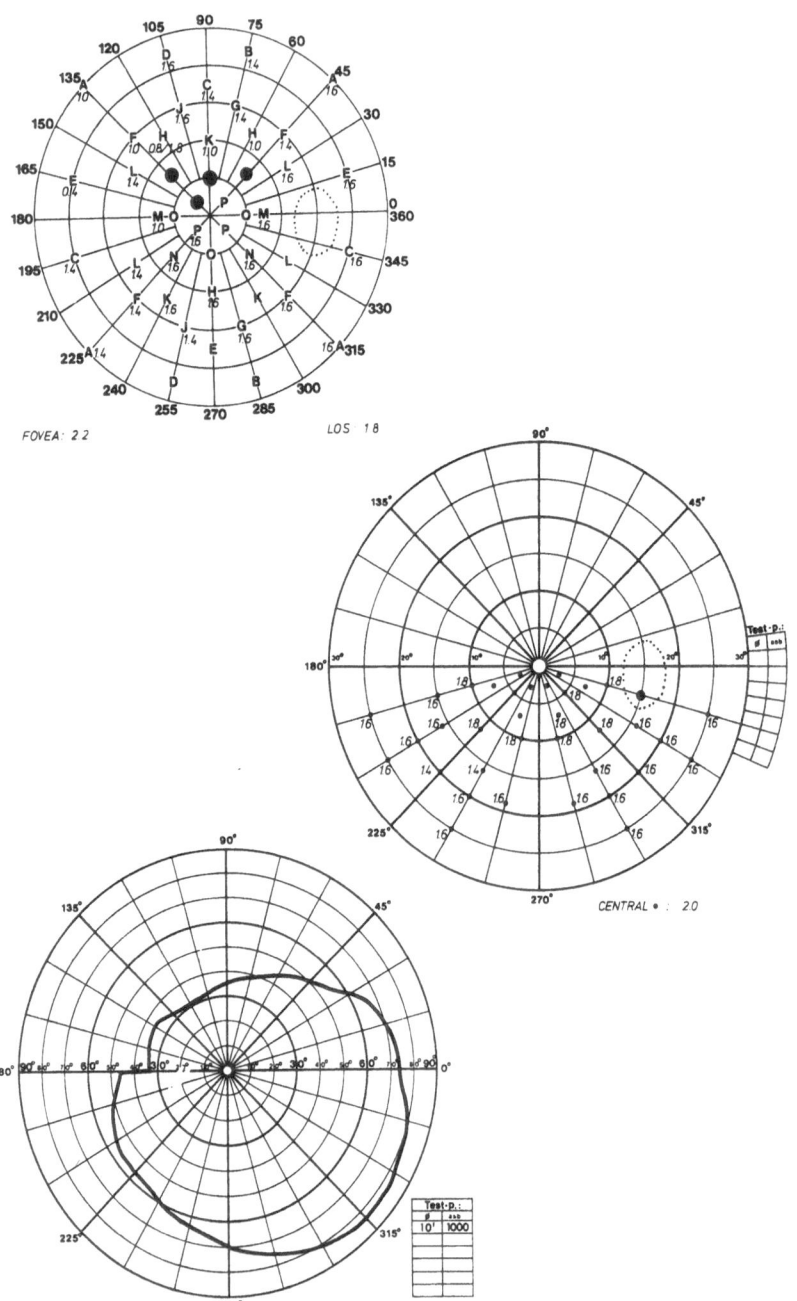

FOVEA: 2 2   LOS 1 8

CENTRAL • : 2 0

Test·p.:
| # | ab b |
| 10' | 1000 |

274

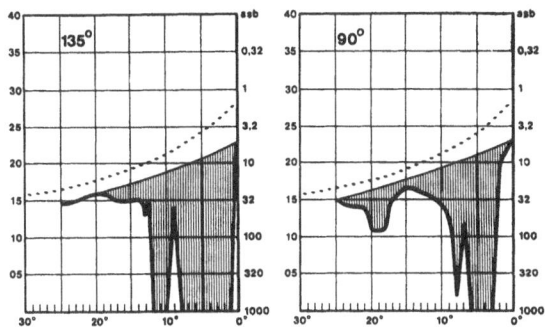

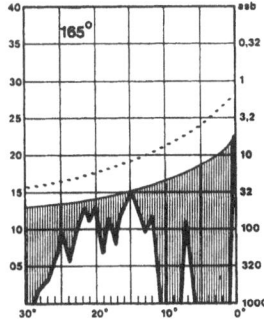

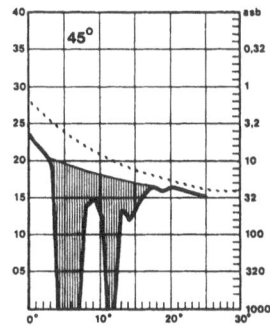

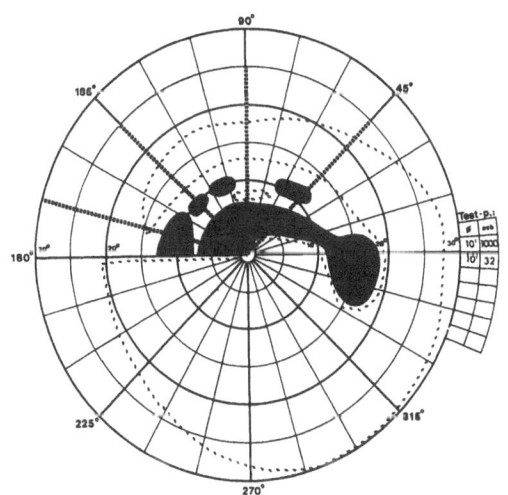

This is an example of a glaucomatous visual field which has passed the early stage. The defect began as an early paracentral fibre bundle defect (as pat. 6). The paracentral defect has extended cecopetally; a second adjacent fibre bundle has also fallen out, so that the defect has become wider. At the present stage a third fibre bundle defect is developing, which is still incomplete. Two such adjacent fibre bundle defects are also seen in patient 14. During the development of the paracentral defect a nasal depression has appeared.

The Visual Field Analyser in phase I provided sufficient evidence for the existence of the defects. The nasal constriction is indicated at stimulus position E 165. Here again more stimulus positions in the nasal area would be welcome. The threshold of the Visual Field Analyser stimulus positions are in agreement with the data from phase II. In this visual field a few examples are seen of stimuli which fall on the edges of a defect.

In phase IB the absence of defects in the lower half of the visual field was confirmed.

The good results obtained with kinetic perimetry of this defect have only been made possible on the basis of the data from static perimetry (phase II) and because the examiner has great perimetric experience and knows the possible course and development of glaucomatous visual field defects. Naturally a patient who gives accurate answers is a first essential.

Pat. no.: 11   age 69   OD

DESCRIPTION

Detection	IA25	g.r.s.	0.6 lu
		sup.	paracentral defects for max. L. and nasal defect for max. L. at NS 19
		inf.	defect for max. at NI 14; relative defect of 1.0 lu at NI 19
	IA periphery		peripheral nasal depression
	IB	sup.	paracentral and nasal defects for max. L.
		inf.	two nasal defects for max. L. with relative cecopetal extension
Assessment	SP	g.r.s.	0.3 and flattening
		45	paracentral defect for max. L.
		90	paracentral defect for max. L.
		135	small paracentral defect with relative extension to periphery
		165	larger defect for max. L.; sporadic perception at a few locations
		195	two defects for max. L.
		225	three relative defects at 6°, 10° and 20° ecc. being the cecopetal extension of the defect in the 195° meridian
	KP	sup.	paracentral defect and second defect along nasal horizontal meridian; almost complete relative fibre-bundle defect:
		inf.	nasal depression; between 7° and 30° ecc. area of variation for max. L.; no real defect for max. L. can be found.

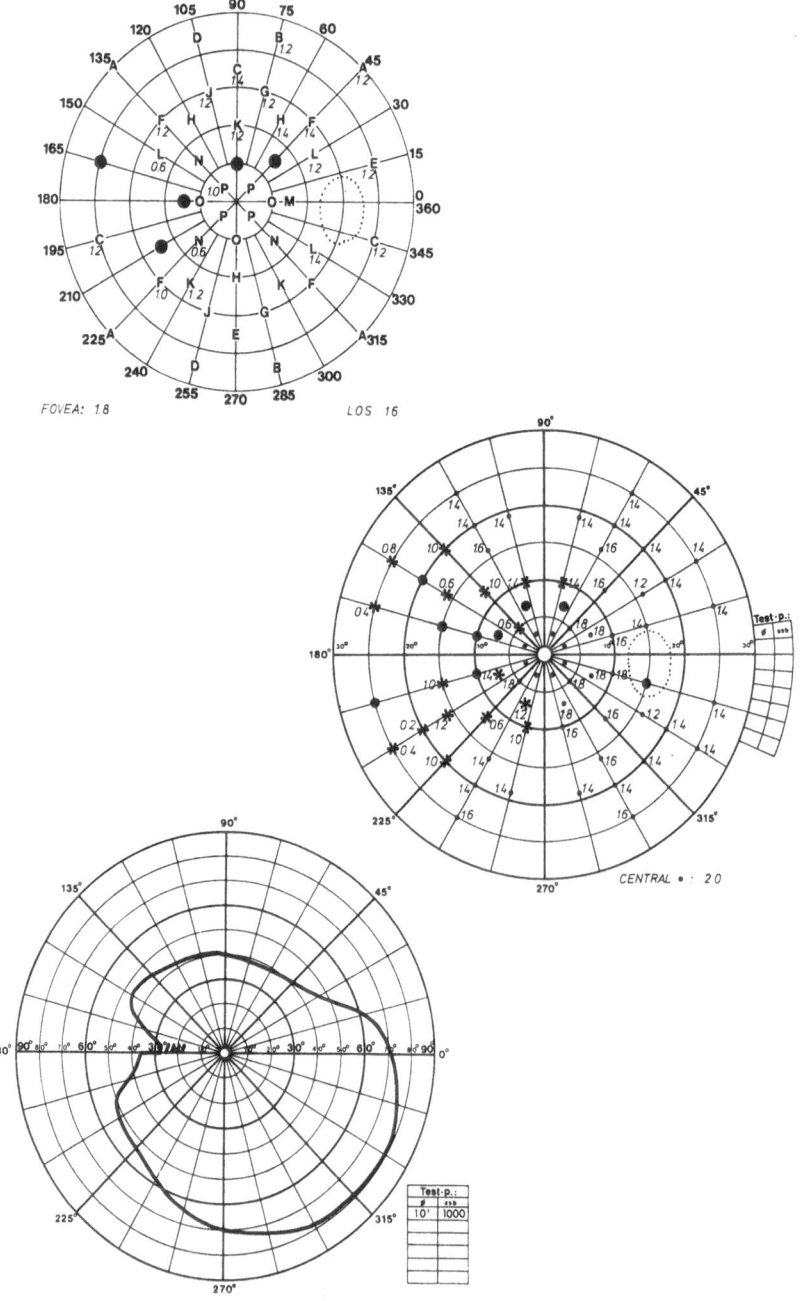

FOVEA: 1.8   LOS 16

CENTRAL ● : 2 0

278

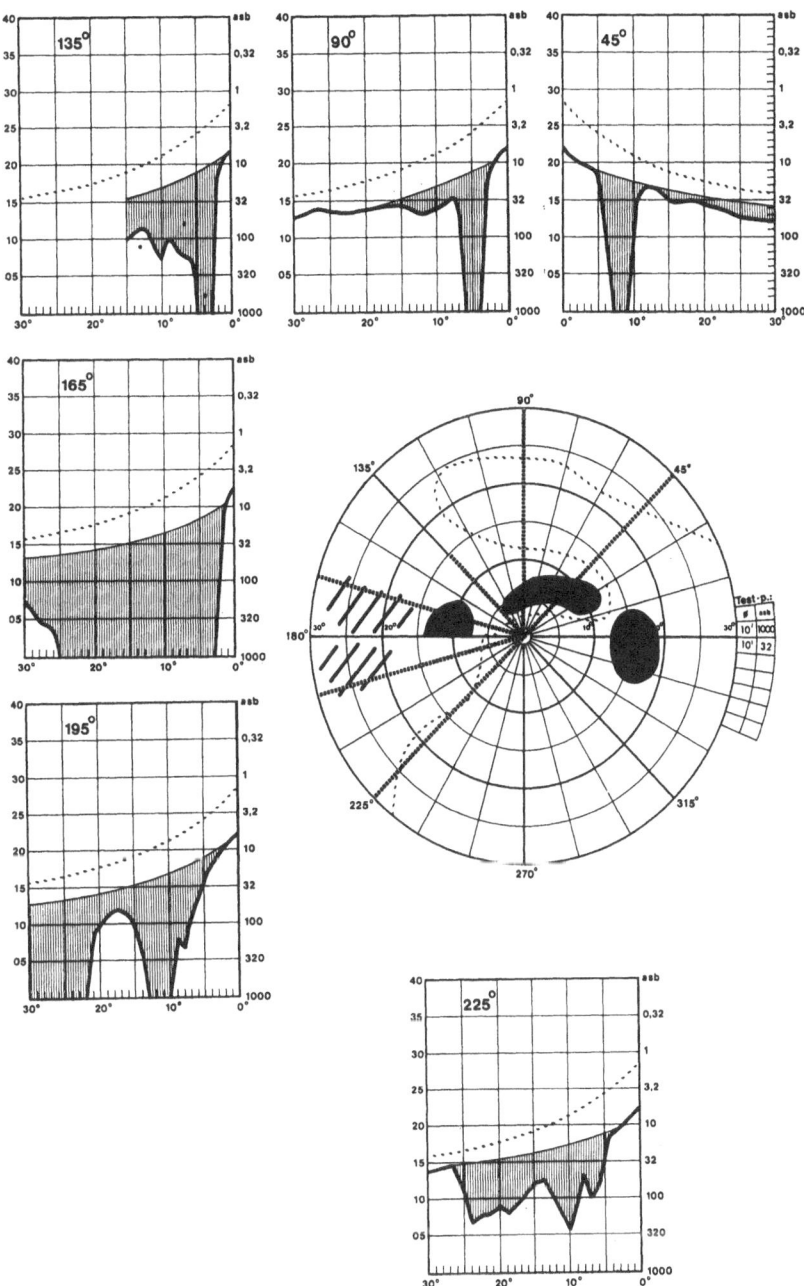

Patient no. 11. Comment.

In this case is a very narrow paracentral fibre bundle defect which in the 165° M is seen to be part of a larger nasal defect. The development of new cecopetal defects may be expected. That this is the case appears from the 135° M where new relative defects were found alongside the paracentral defect, while this has not yet occurred in the 90° M. In the lower half of the visual field various fibre bundle defects are present, as appears from the results in the 195° M and the 225° M. The relative defects in the 225° M in phase I correspond exactly with the findings in phase II. In follow-up examinations deterioration can be assessed in particular in the 225° M.

The defects shown here have been reproduced exactly on repeat examination. This visual field demonstrates that defects must be looked for in the whole 30° visual field and not in a restricted area. Both relative defects and defects for max. L. should be detected.

The IB phase gave no new information in this case; the Visual Field Analyser found all the defects in the IA phase. The paracentral defect lies exactly at 5° eccentricity in the 90° M so that stimulus position O 90° falls in the defect. Examples of defects have been given where a similar paracentral defect falls exactly between the stimulus positions. The findings of the Visual Field Analyser are confirmed in phase II. In other words, where the Visual Field Analyser registered normal sensitivity, normal sensitivity was found in phase II and where the Visual Field Analyser registered a defect this could also be reproduced in phase II. A discrepancy was again found between the extensive static defects and the limited kinetic defects.

Pat. no.: 12   age 59   OD

DESCRIPTION

Detection	IA25	g.r.s.	0.4 lu
		sup.	large nasal defect for max. L.; paracentral defect; centrocecal defect of 1.6 lu
		inf.	large nasal defect with relative cecopetal extension
	IA periphery		large nasal defect for max. L.
	IB		not necessary
Assessment	SP	g.r.s.	mainly flattening of sensitivity curve
		45	small defect at 12° ecc. (probably angio-scotoma), relative paracentral defect at 1° ecc.
		90	small relative paracentral defect at 2°; small paracentral defect for max. L. at 5°; defects at 18° and 26° ecc.
		135	three defects for max. L.; relative sieve-like defect between 6° and 19° ecc.
		165	defect for max. L. with sporadic perception
		225	two defects for max. L.
		270	w.s.s. of 0.6 lu at 17° ecc.
		315	no defects; the area around stimulus position P was carefully explored; close to this position a small relative defect was detected.
	KP		nasal and centrocecal defect.

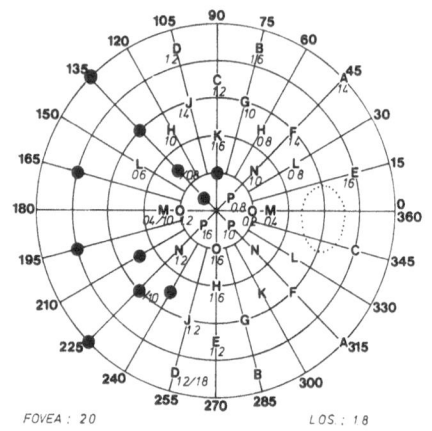

FOVEA : 20   LOS. : 1.8

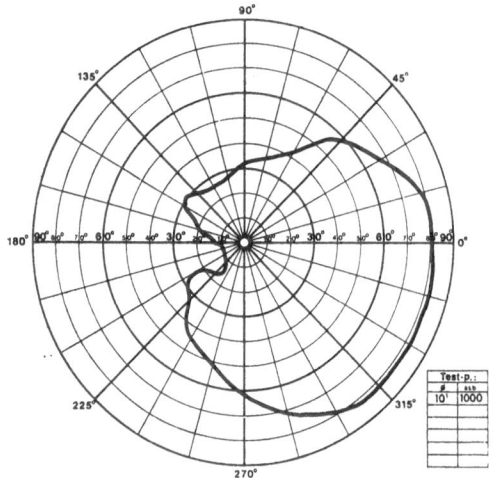

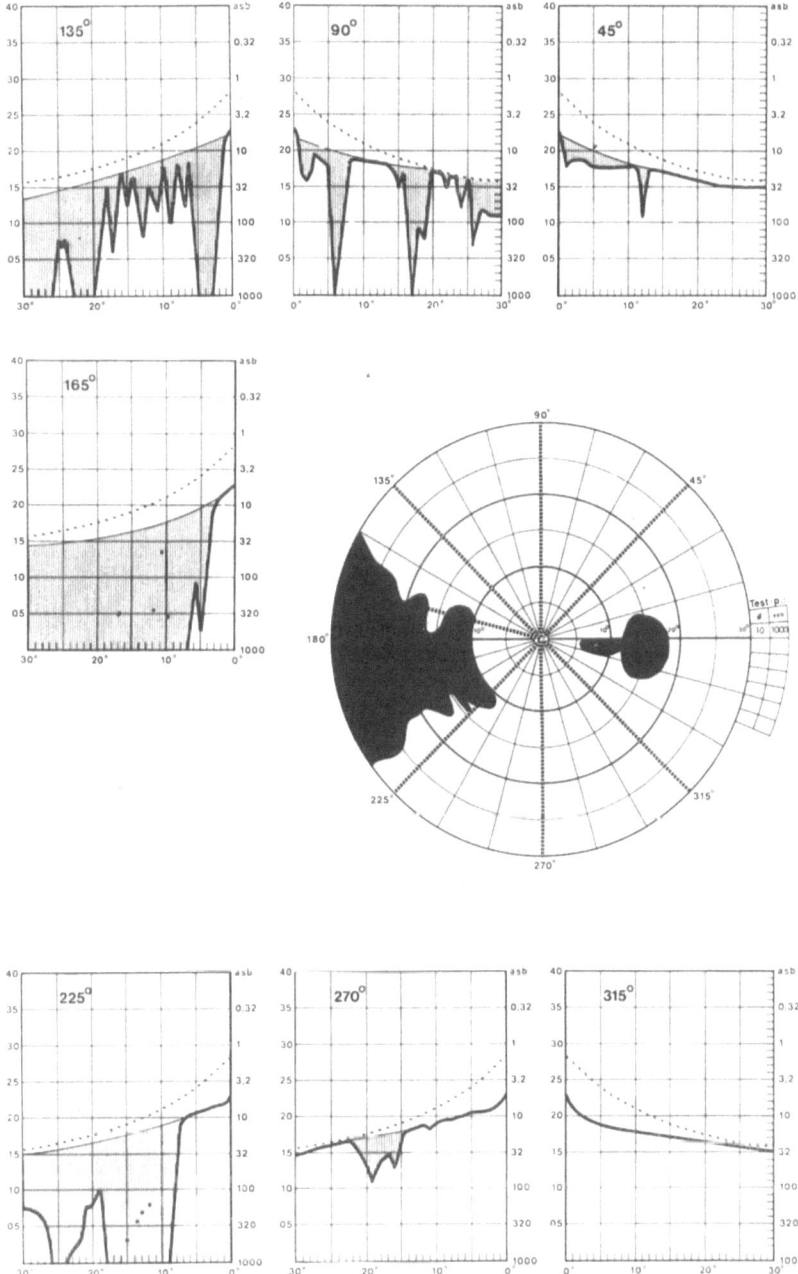

This visual field shows, in addition to the classical nasal defects, a paracentral defect and a centrocecal defect. All the defects were discovered in the IA phase so that an additional IB phase was unnecessary.

In the 90° M a defect was discovered at 5° with the Visual Field Analyser, which in phase II was found to be very small and which could only be reproduced with difficulty. The reason for this is probably the longer presentation time used in phase II. This phenomenon occurs regularly.

The defect at 16° eccentricity may well be a wedge-shaped scotoma of 0.9 lu with a superimposed angioscotoma of 0.9 lu. This does not apply to the defect at 5°. In our experience the blood vessels at 5° eccentricity are too small to cause an angioscotoma of any significance. Further examination of the 90° M shows that between 8° and 15° eccentricity the light sensitivity is still intact (K 90° = 1.6). The sieve-like defect in the 135° M is a type of defect which is quite often found in association with nasal defects like these. It is probably the expression of incipient loss of function in a number of adjacent fibre bundles. The fact that, at stimulus position F 135, no light perception is recorded with the Visual Field Analyser can be explained by the fact that, in a sieve-like visual field very large differences in sensitivity can exist side by side, which are difficult to record even with the help of single stimulus static perimetry.

In the lower half of the visual field there is a nasal defect similar to that in the upper half. In the 270° M only one wedge-shaped scotoma can be found as cecopetal extension of the nasal defect.

The centrocecal defect can be registered better with circular static perimetry than with meridional static perimetry.

Pat. no.: 13   age 69   OS

DESCRIPTION

Detection	IA25	g.r.s.	0.6 lu
		sup.	relative defect of 1.0 lu and 0.8 lu at NS 12 and TS 8; defect of 0.6 lu at TS 9
		inf.	defect for max. L. at 10° ecc.; small defect of varying intensity at NI 1; relative nasal defects.
	IA periphery		no defects
	IB		not examined
Assessment	SP	g.r.s.	0.5 lu
		45	no significant defects (0.3 lu)
		75	w.s.s. of 0.8 lu
		90	same w.s.s. as in 75° M (0.6 lu) and w.s.s. of 0.3 lu at 14° ecc.
		105	w.s.s. of 0.6 lu
		135	w.s.s. of 0.7 lu and typical angioscotomata
		225	defect for max. L.
		240	defect for max. L. with relative extension to periphery
		315	paracentral w.s.s. and two defects for max. L. with relative peripheral extension N.B.: After careful examination of the paracentral area a small defect for max. L. was discovered at $1\frac{1}{2}$° ecc. corresponding with the defect of phase IA (P) (see kinetic field)
		320	small relative defect of 1.1 lu at 3° ecc.
		330	paracentral w.s.s. of 0.9 lu
	KP	inf.	partial cecofugal arcuate scotoma for max. L.

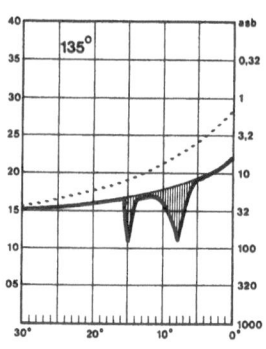

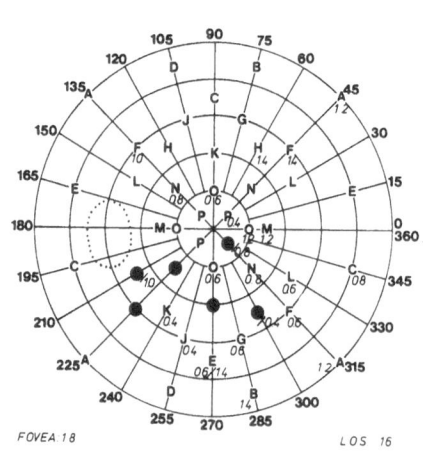

FOVEA 18   LOS 16

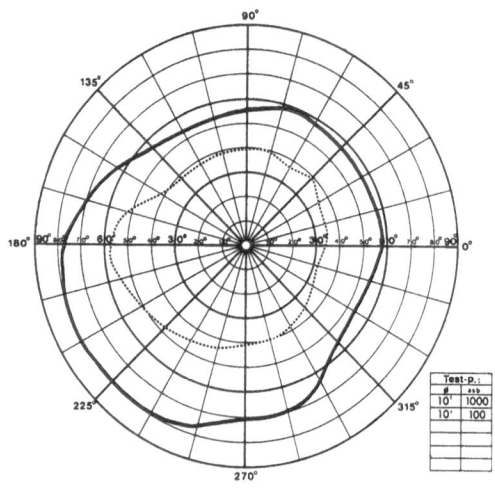

Test-p.:	
#	asb
10'	1000
10'	100

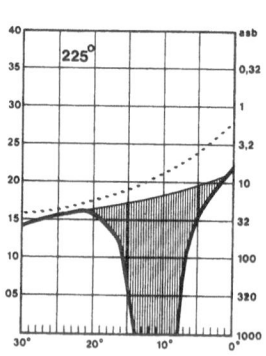

286

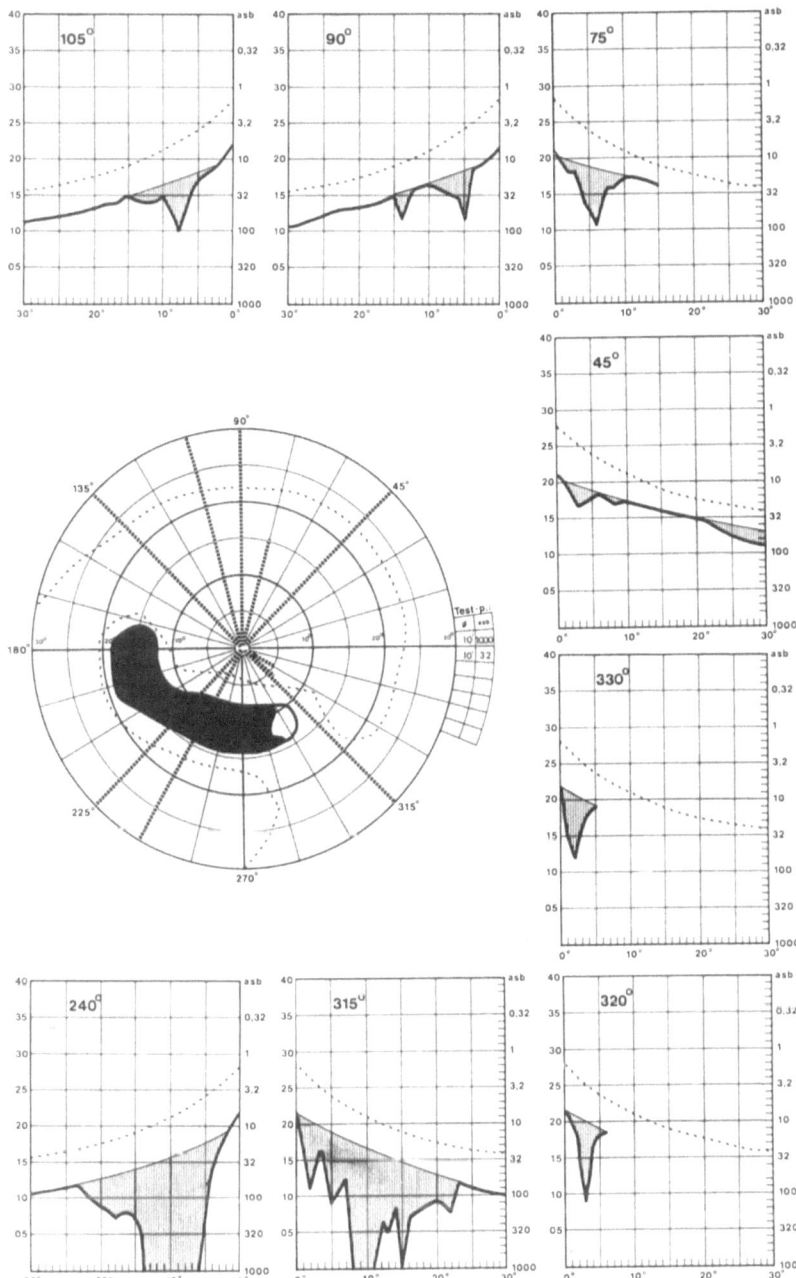

This visual field demonstrates 2 types of glaucomatous visual field defects. In the first place there is a cecofugal fibre bundle defect in the lower half of the visual field which has not yet reached the horizontal meridian. In the second place, in both halves of the visual field there are early defects in the form of paracentral wedge-shaped scotomata. This is a good demonstration of the fact that wedge-shaped scotomata not only occur in the Bjerrum area but also in the paracentral area. These defects were reproduced exactly in an examination performed 6 months later. They follow the course of the fibre bundles (cf. pat. no. 3).

The various defects were found in phase IA. Supplementary IB detection in the upper half of the visual field would have been advisable. The Visual Field Analyser findings correspond with the findings in phase II. In the upper half of the visual field O (0.6 in 90° M) and N (0.8 in 135° M) correspond with the wedge-shaped scotomata. The measurement of 1.0 lu at F (135° M) was probably due to an angioscotoma. In the lower half of the visual field stimulus position F(225° M) falls on the edge of the defect. In the 135° M the fibre bundle defect has split into two parts. The wedge-shaped scotomata in this meridian are evidence of the fact that the fibre bundles which supply the area adjacent to the defect for max. L. are already suffering from the raised intraocular pressure. The recorded complete loss of function at stimulus P (315 M) was confirmed: in this position there is a very small defect of great intensity. Such defects are very difficult to record on account of the physiological nystagmus. Small defects like this are sometimes found in the paracentral area.

Pat. no.: 14   age 44   OS

DESCRIPTION

Detection 11-9-1971	IA25	g.r.s.	0.4 lu
		sup.	defects for max. L. following the course of fibre bundles
		inf.	idem
	IA periphery		small peripheral nasal depression; large relative depression
	IB		not examined
Assessment 11-9-1971	SP	g.r.s.	0.3 lu
		45	small defect (2° Ø) for max. L.; area of varying sensitivity between 10° and 20° ecc.
		135	defect for max. L. (4° Ø)
		225	two small defects separated by a sensitivity peak of 1° Ø
		315	two defects separated by a small sensitivity peak
	KP	sup.	fibre-bundle defect not yet fully developed; new defect starting at NS 19, 25; nasal area of variation
		inf.	two separate fibre-bundle defects fully developed.

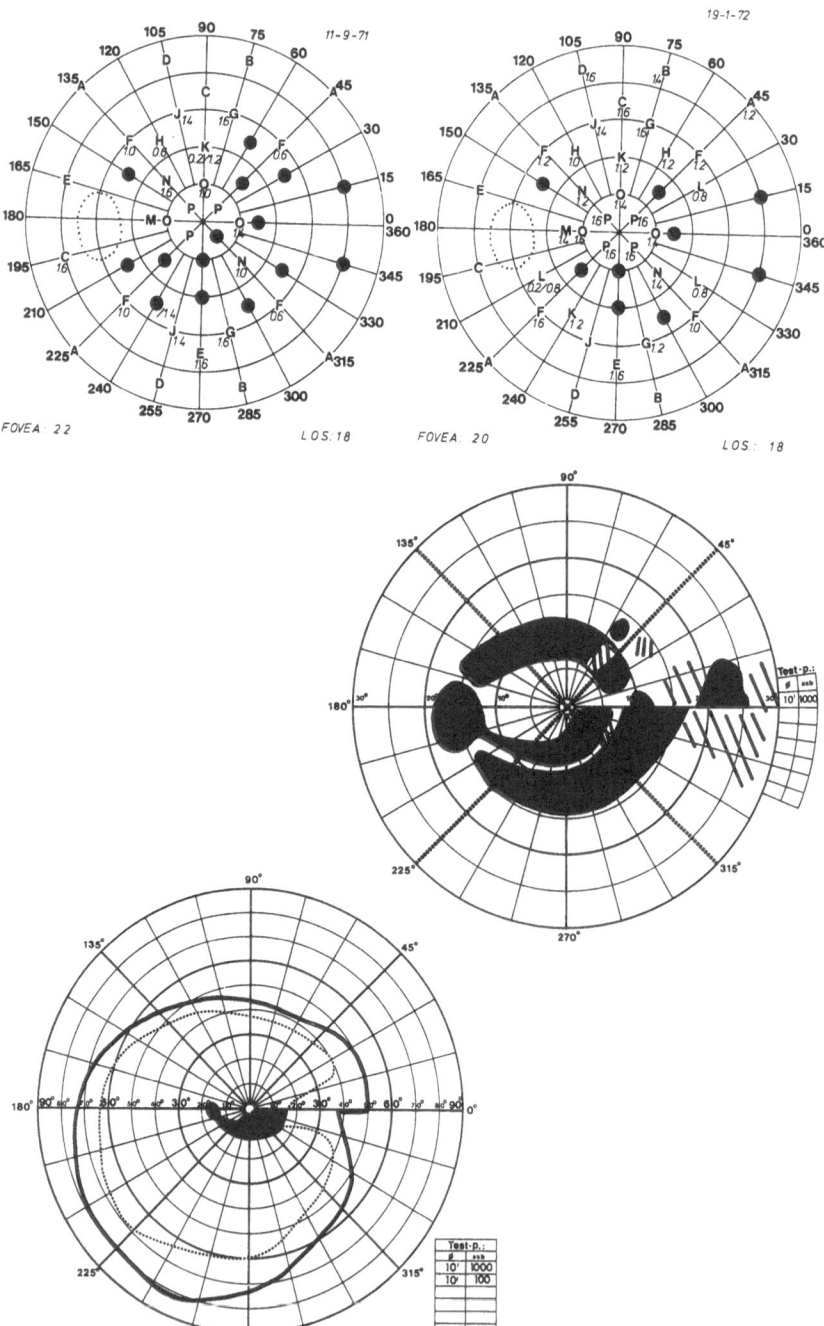

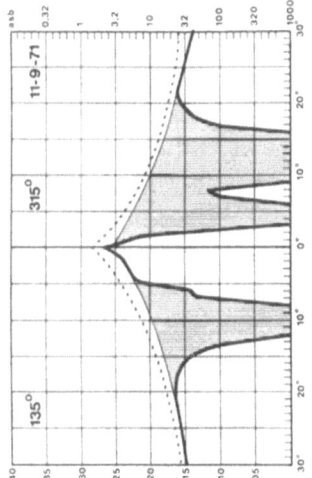

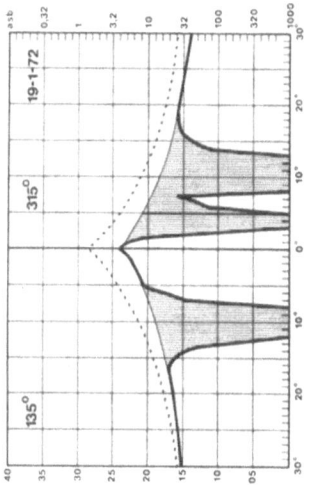

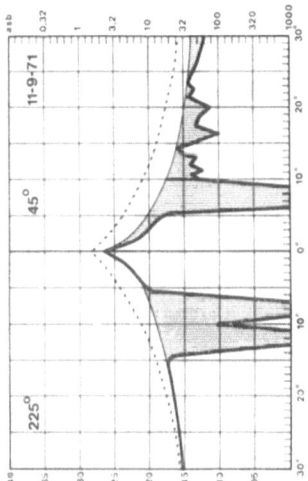

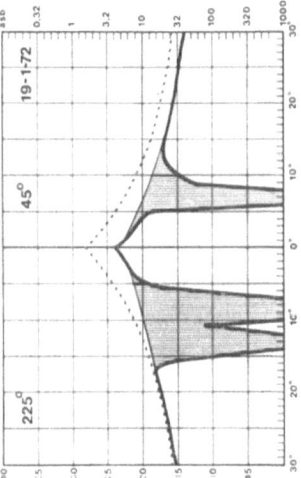

Patient no. 14. Comment.

This field is a perfect example of typical glaucomatous defects. In the lower half of the visual field two fibre bundle defects run close together with a clearly demonstrable area of perception between. The defects were indicated in the IA phase; it was not necessary to supplement this with a IB phase.

The measurements from the IA phase correspond with the measurements from phase II. The two stimulus positions where variable measurements were obtained (K 90 and K 240) fall on the edges of the defects. The stimulus position N (315° M), where a defect of 0.8 lu is recorded, falls exactly between the two fibre bundle defects. Along the nasal horizontal meridian an area of variable sensitivity was found with kinetic perimetry.

This patient was operated on shortly after the examination recorded here. The visual field examination has been repeated 3 times since the operation. The result of a repeat examination (19.1.72) is given. These results show how well the results of static perimetry can be reproduced even when the examinations have been performed by different examiners. When we compare the Visual Field Analyser results of 11.9.71 and 19.1.72 slight improvement seems to have taken place. In phase II it appears that the curve of the 225° M is unchanged. This is in agreement with the Visual Field Analyser findings. The change at F 225 from 1.0 to 1.6 must be ascribed to the proximity of the edge of the defect. On the 135° M the defect at 5° eccentricity is reproduced exactly; the defect between 9° and 15° eccentricity has become a little narrower. Stimulus position F 315 has changed from 0.6 to 0.1 and position L 330 has improved from no perception to 0.8 (edge of defect). In the 45° M the defect for max. L has been reproduced exactly but the wedge-shaped scotoma has disappeared. Stimulus position F 45 has changed from 0.6 to 1.2. The defect (19.1.72) in the 135° M lies between two Visual Field Analyser positions, as does the defect in the 315° M (between N and F). Stimulus P 315 falls on the edge of the defect.

In the above examples two possible reasons are given for changes in the threshold values of the Visual Field Analyser stimuli obtained at different examinations:

1. a genuine change in sensitivity can have taken place;
2. the stimulus position can lie at the edge of a defect and can have just fallen in the defect in the first examination and just outside it in the repeat examination or vice versa. A network of stimulus positions, as presented in the detection phase, is not suitable for following up minute changes in glaucomatous defects. The Visual Field Analyser should not be the only source of information when progression of glaucomatous defects is to be established. For this purpose the greater spatial accuracy of phase II (degree by degree) is needed, by means of which the edges of defects can be better evaluated.

Pat. no.: 15   age 74   OS

DESCRIPTION

Detection 3–10–1972	IA25	g.r.s.	0.6–0.8 lu
		sup.	large defect for max. L.; variation of stimuli P
		inf.	defects of 0.4 lu in Bjerrum – area and a defect of 0.6 lu at NI 1 (P)
	IA periphery	sup.	absolute nasal depression with step; breakthrough of bundle defect for max. L. to nasal periphery.
	IB	sup.	not examined
		inf.	defects for max. L. at NI 4 and NI 8
Assessment 3–10–1972	SP	g.r.s.	flattening
		sup.	defect for max. L. between 2° and 12°
		225	w.s.s. defect of 1.1. lu
		255	small defect of 3° Ø for max. L.
		315	defect of 4° Ø for max. L.
		352,5	defect of 7° Ø for max. L.
	KP	sup.	see detection
		inf.	small partial arcuate scotoma

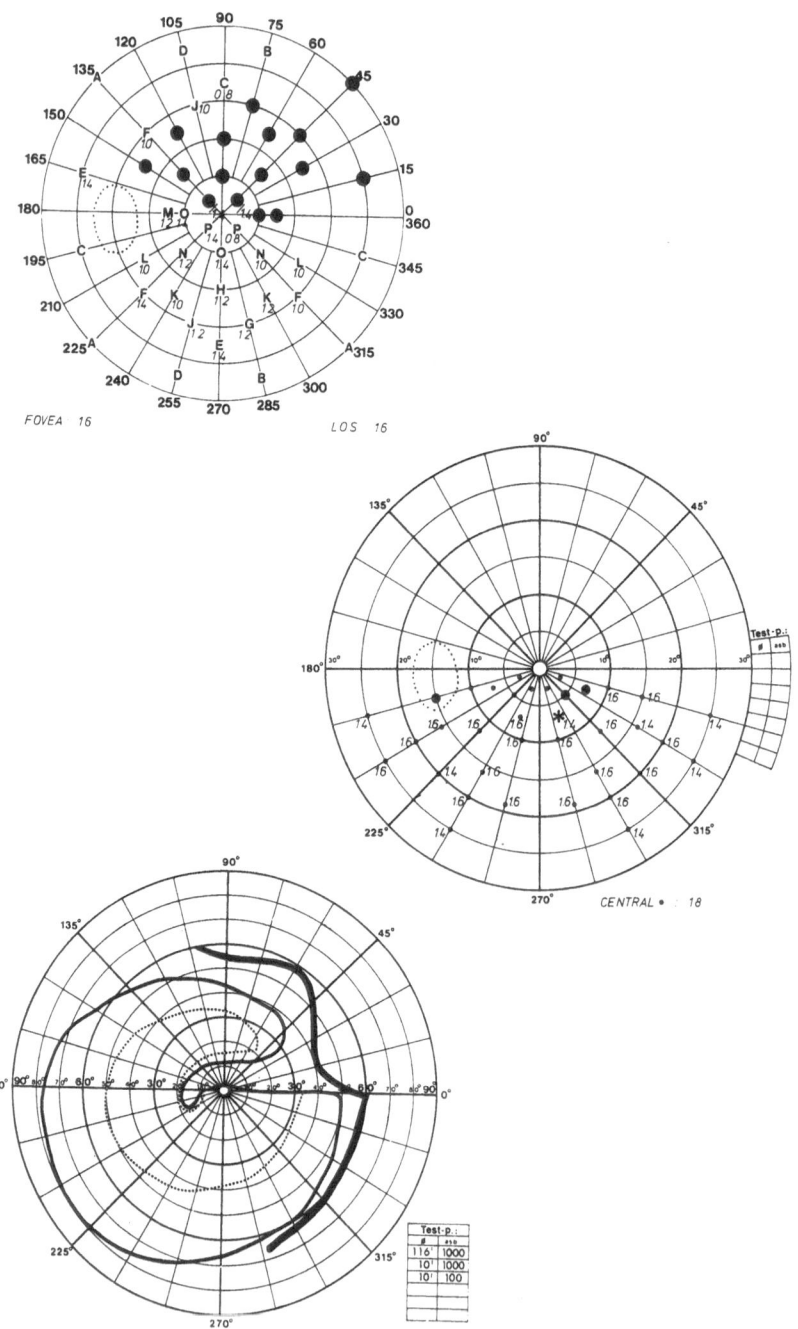

FOVEA 16

LOS 16

CENTRAL • : 18

294

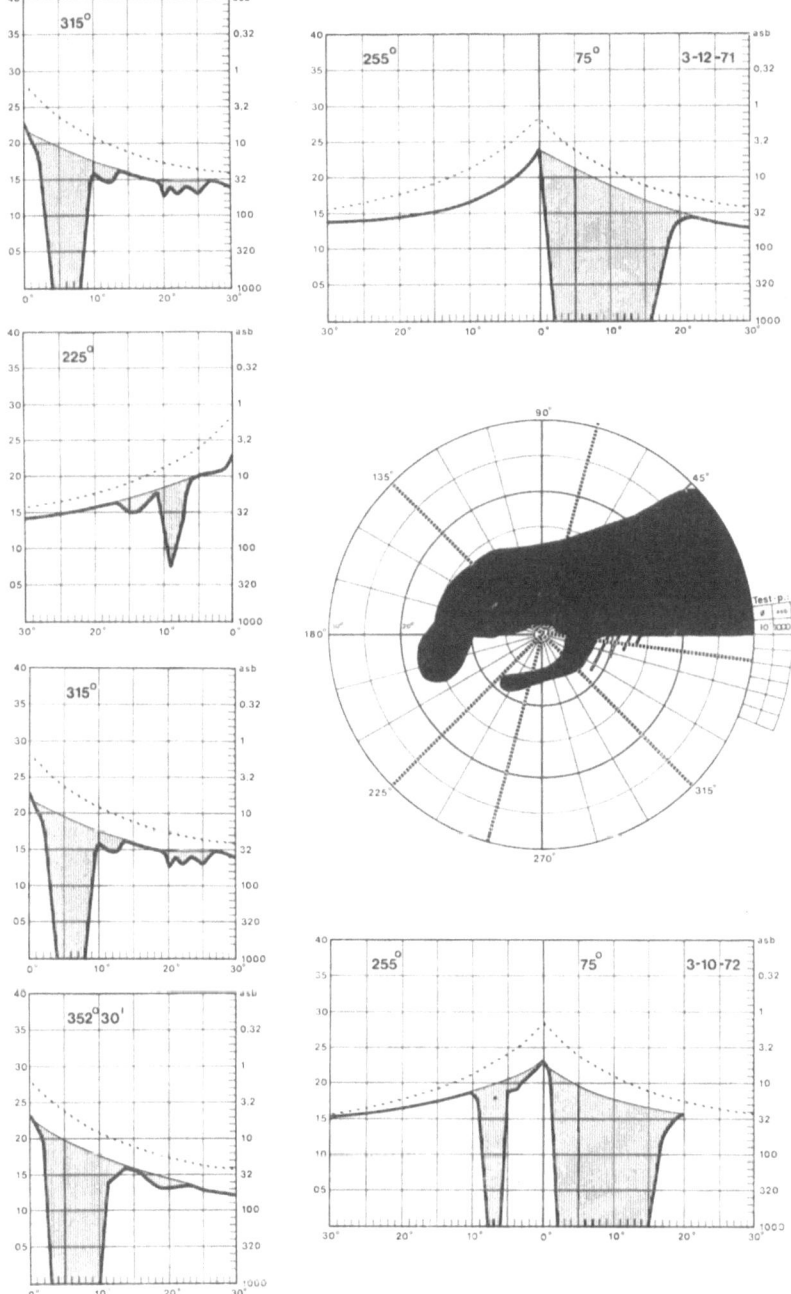

In the detection phase the large fibre bundle defect in the upper half of the visual field was naturally found; further detection in the upper visual field was not necessary.

The intensity of the defect, which was registered by both stimuli P (45° M and 135° M), varied from max. L. to 'no defect'. This is another example of the large degree of variation in measurements which results when a stimulus falls on the edge of a steep defect. A large degree of variation nearly always means that the examination is being performed on the edge of a defect and has nothing to do with the reliability of the patient.

In the lower half of the visual field, in addition to reduced sensitivity in the Bjerrum area, a relative defect (P = 0.8) was found at NI 1. In phase IB it appeared that in this area defects for max. L. were present.

This visual field shows how important it is to look for an early defect in the other hemifield. Stimulus position P of the Visual Field Analyser must have fallen on the edge of the defect; in phase IB the stimulus fell exactly in the defect. On repeat examination stimulus position P fell exactly in the small defect: no perception for max. L. This illustrates the usefulness of phase IB.

In the 225° M (phase II) a relative defect of 1.1 lu was found. This defect is the relative cecopetal extension of the narrow arcuate scotoma in the lower half of the visual field. This defect has its maximum intensity in the 255° M. In an examination performed a year earlier (3.12.71) no defects were found on this meridian.

When the 225° M from phase II is compared with the results of phase I it appears that this defect was completely missed in phase I. The reason for this is that there are no stimulus positions at the location of the defect, either in phase IA or in phase IB. The same applies to the 255° M, where a defect with a diameter of 3° was found; here again there are no stimulus positions in phase I at the location of the defect.

Even the examination of 118 positions thus does not garantee that defects with a diameter of 3° will be found. The fact that this is to be expected has been discussed in Chapter V.

The defect in the 352° 30′ M was not found in phase IA (Visual Field Analyser). This illustrates our objection to the small number of stimulus positions which the Visual Field Analyser has in the nasal visual field, that is so important for glaucoma.

The narrow arcuate fibre bundle defect would never have been discovered with kinetic perimetry. Even when the defect had been found by means of static perimetry it was difficult to define it with kinetic perimetry. This paracentral defect is not accompanied by peripheral nasal depression (see 185° M, patient 4).

Pat. no.: 16   age 60   OS

DESCRIPTION

Detection	IA25	g.r.s.	0.2–0.4 lu
		sup.	large defect for max. L.
		inf.	relative defects at NI 9, 12, 14, 19 and TI 14, 16
	IA periphery		only examined with stimulus of max.L. see phase II
	IB	sup.	not examined
		inf.	defects for max. L. at NI 11, TI 11, relative nasal defects.
Assessment	SP	g.r.s.	none
		225	w.s.s.
		240	relative defect of 0.3 lu
		247,5	defect for max. L.
		255	w.s.s.
		270	deep (1.8 lu) relative defect at 9° ecc.
		300	defect for max. L.
		315	defect for max. L. and small w.s.s.
		345	defect for max. L. and several w.s.s.
	KP	sup.	large absolute fibre-bundle defect with breakthrough to nasal periphery
		inf.	relative arcuate scotoma with two nuclei for max. L.

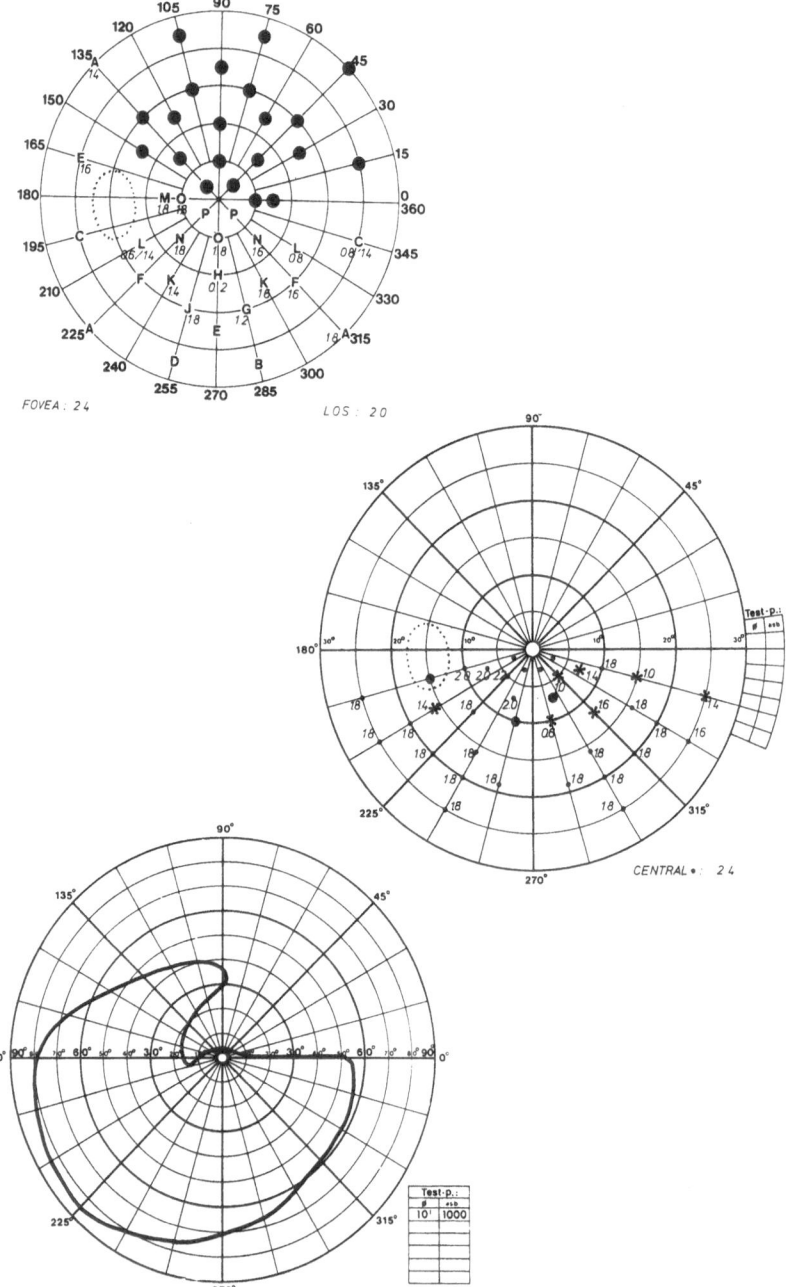

FOVEA : 24

LOS : 20

CENTRAL • : 24

298

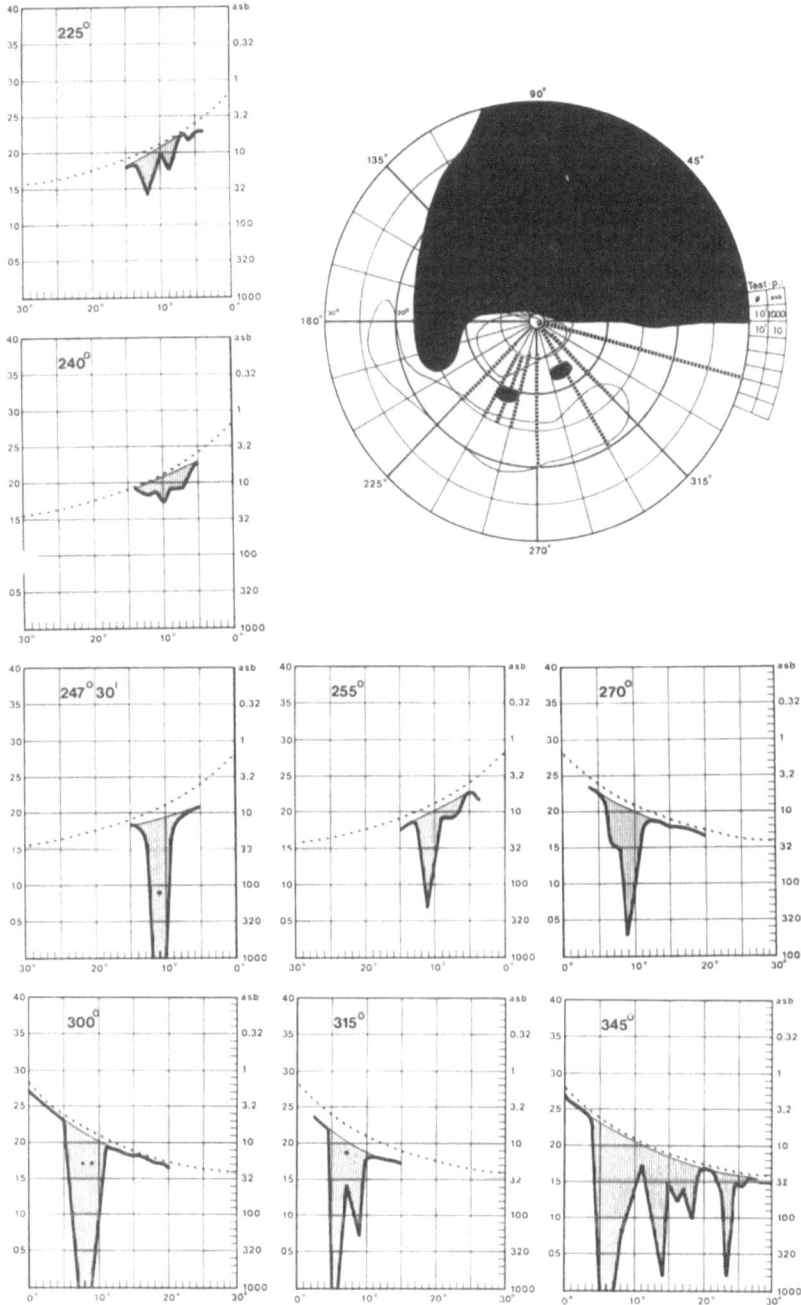

Patient no. 16. Comment.

This case resembles the preceding case in many respects; it is also an example of early defect in the other hemifield. The perception in the upper half of the visual field has to a large extent disappeared due to an absolute fibre bundle defect with breakthrough to the nasal periphery.

In the lower half, on the other hand, early defects were found. The two halves of a glaucomatous visual field must be examined and assessed separately.

The paracentral defect is expressed in phase IA as a relative defect, although its intensity is nearly maximum. This is again a very narrow defect which falls between the Visual Field Analyser stimulus positions. The Visual Field Analyser has provided all the information possible, bearing in mind the limited number of stimulus positions. In this case stimulus position H 270 falls exactly in the defect. Stimulus position L 330 indicates that one of the defects from the 345° M has already extended further cecopetally. We are concerned here with an incomplete cecopetal paracentral fibre bundle defect. At the 315° M a second fibre bundle defect is developing alongside the defect for max. L. One of these two defects is seen again on the 255° M.

The difference between this case and patient 15 is that here there is an accompanying nasal defect (cf. patient 6).

Pat. no.: 17   age 60   OS

DESCRIPTION

Detection	IA25	g.r.s.	0.4 lu
		sup.	small paracentral defect for max. L.
		inf.	large fibre bundle defect for max. L.
	IA periphery		inferior nasal step
	IB		not examined
Assessment	SP	45, 135	paracentral defect for max. L.
		225, 311	large defects for max. L.
	KP		inferior arcuate scotoma with peripheral nasal step; the superior paracentral defect was not examined with kinetic perimetry.

Patient no. 17. Comment.

Some examples have been shown where the Visual Field Analyser failed to some extent to detect paracentral defects for max. L. (i.e. the Visual Field Analyser only indicated relative defects). This visual field is an example of an early defect in the other hemifield which was completely detected by the Visual Field Analyser in phase IA, so that phase IB in the paracentral area was unnecessary. This paracentral defect is also slightly larger than some of those demonstrated previously ($\emptyset = 4°$). Note how close to the centre the defect is situated.

Nasal and superotemporal defects were not excluded with certainty in this detection phase.

In this case the two oblique meridians were examined in phase II.

Supplementary examination of the 15° meridian would have been desirable to discover whether there were any early nasal defects. From other examples it has become apparent that the number of stimulus positions of the Visual Field Analyser on the nasal area is insufficient for adequate detection.

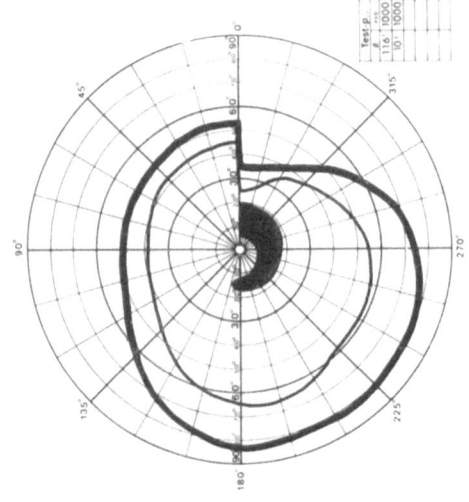

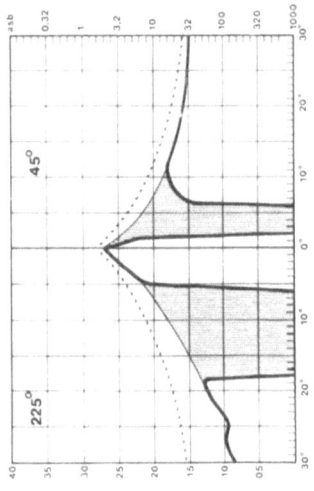

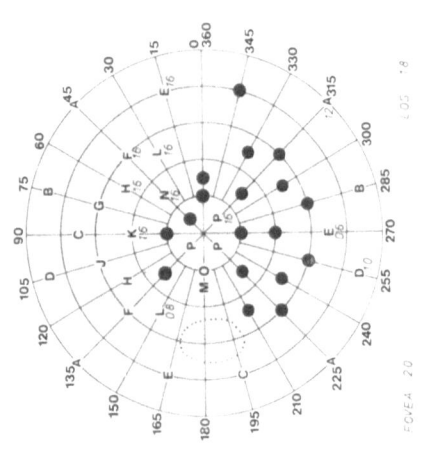

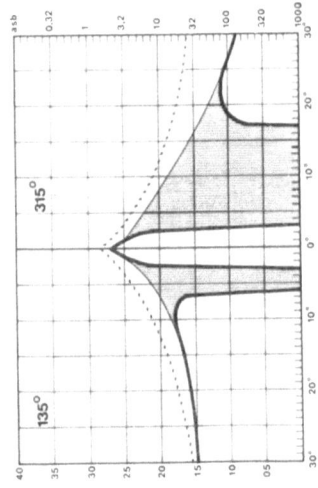

Pat. no.: 18   age 71   OD

DESCRIPTION

Detection	IA25	g.r.s.	0.6 lu
		sup.	no defect
		inf.	large fibre-bundle defect for max. L.
	IA periphery		fibre-bundle defect for max. L. with breakthrough to nasal periphery
	IB	sup.	no defects
Assessment	SP		not necessary

Patient no. 18. Comment.

This visual field has been included as an example of a visual field in which one half is almost completely eliminated while in the other half no defects were found in phases IA and IB. After phase IA a supplementary phase IB in the lower half was naturally unnecessary.

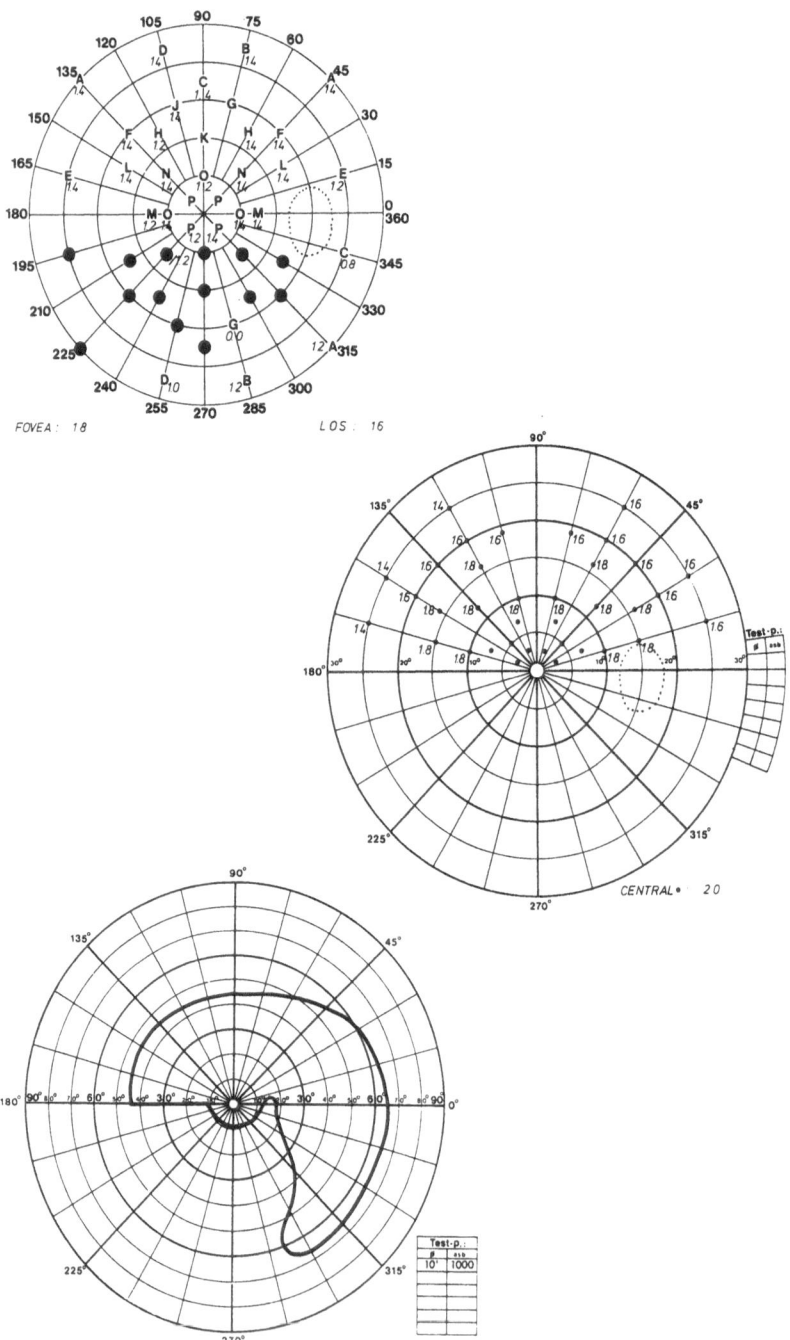

FOVEA : 18

LOS . 16

CENTRAL • 20

304

In the first part of this chapter a number of examples are given of the results of examination with the Visual Field Analyser in the detection phase. In the commentary on these individual cases the possibilities of the Visual Field Analyser, some reasons why defects can be missed with the Visual Field Analyser, and reasons for discrepancies between the results obtained with the Visual Field Analyser and with the Tübinger perimeter, were pointed out.

In this second part the results of a comparative study of the visual fields of 1372 eyes with raised intra-ocular pressure will be discussed. The point at issue is, to what extent the Visual Field Analyser, as the best representative of the multiple stimulus method, misses defects which can be found by single stimulus static perimetry, or vice versa.

This question has to be divided into two subsidiary questions: a distinction must be made between defects missed by the Visual Field Analyser because *the number and position* of the stimuli is insufficient, and defects missed because *threshold measurements with multiple stimulus presentation* might not reveal the same intensity of defects as single stimulus presentation. To find the answer to the second part of this question is the object of our study.

In the first place a short description will be given of those cases among the 1372 eyes examined with the Visual Field Analyser in which defects were missed. Subsequently, on the basis of 1001 positions, an exact comparison of threshold measurements with the multiple stimulus method on the one hand and with the single stimulus method on the other hand will be made. The study was performed on 1372 eyes from 716 patients with raised intra-ocular pressure[5].

TABLE II

Subdivision of the visual fields of 1372 eyes of patients with intra-ocular hypertension

	number		% of total	% of defects
no defects or g.r.s.	355		26	
complete arcuate scotoma or larger	715		52	70
small defects	241	1017	22	30
e.d.o.h.	61			
total	1372		100	100

---

[5] In some patients only one eye was examined.

These were all patients from the University Eye Clinic of the Wilhelmina Gasthuis, Amsterdam. Patients who were not suitable for quantitative perimetry were not included in the study.

The subdivision of the defects by type is shown in Table II.

The group 'no defects or g.r.s.' comprises the visual fields in which no localized defects could be found, either with the Visual Field Analyser, or in phase IB, or when checked in phase II.

The group 'complete fibre bundle defects or larger' speaks for itself. *These extensive defects were detected by the Visual Field Analyser in 100% of cases.*

The most interesting group for the demonstration of the results obtained with the Visual Field Analyser in the detection phase, is the group of small defects, which includes the early defects in the opposite hemifield. The partial fibre bundle defects and isolated scotomata, whether of relative or maximum intensity, belong to this group. This group includes both defects which are found in only one half of the visual field and defects which are found in both halves.

Number and position of stimuli in the Visual Field Analyser.

In 17 of the 302 cases with small defects (241 small defects + 61 e.d.o.h.) a defect in the visual field was completely missed by the Visual Field Analyser. These 17 defects were mainly nasal defects with occasionally a temporal defect outside the 15° parallel (see patient 3).

In Chapter VIII, in anticipation of the results given here, the question of the number and position of the stimuli in the Visual Field Analyser has already been discussed. Summarizing, the situation is as follows:
1. the stimuli in positions O and M on the horizontal meridian are useless for the examination of glaucomatous defects;
2. there are too few stimuli in the whole nasal area between the 135° meridian and the 225° meridian;
3. there are too few stimuli in the whole area between the 15° parallel and the 24° parallel.

In addition to these three points, the density of the stimuli in the Visual Field Analyser, as has been pointed out in Chapter VIII, is insufficient for the detection of small defects.

The 17 cases of missed defects must be regarded as examples, and cannot be used to calculate a percentage.

It was not our original intention to investigate the lacunae between the examination positions in the Visual Field Analyser. In the course of the study, however, it became apparent that false-negative results with the Visual Field Analyser should not be ascribed to the multiple stimulus presentation but to the deficiency of stimulus positions. From the more detailed examinations (phase IB) carried out later, it has become apparent that a number of small defects can be missed on account of insufficient spatial accuracy. It must be emphasized that very small defects can be found with the Visual Field Analyser when they fall on the positions of stimuli.

Comparative study of threshold measurements.

The only way to decide whether the threshold values found with multiple stimulus static perimetry are the same as those found with single stimulus static perimetry is to compare the intensity of a defect at a given position in the visual field, as measured with both methods.

The data from the examination with the Visual Field Analyser and the data from phase II are available for a comparison of this kind. For this purpose 1001 positions which were examined both with the Visual Field Analyser and with the Tübinger perimeter were evaluated. Only visual fields with defects are included. In a visual field with defects areas of normal light sensitivity also exist, so that data about normal light sensitivity as well as about the intensity of defects were obtained. For each position the light sensitivity or the reduction of light sensitivity (intensity) was expressed in log units, as described in Chapter X. Thus, both for the Visual Field Analyser and for the Tübinger perimeter, an intensity value is available for each position.

When comparing the intensity values of defects which have been examined with the Visual Field Analyser and with the Tübinger perimeter, differences in intensity can be found for the following reasons:
1. difference in presentation: multiple stimulus – single stimulus;
2. difference in adaptation level;
3. difference in presentation time: temporal summation;
4. difference in stimulus size: spatial summation;
5. angioscotomata;
6. type of defect;
7. reconstruction of the individual sensitivity curve;
8. normal variation of threshold measurements;
9. imperfections in the Visual Field Analyser;
10. inadequate examination.

Adaptation level, presentation time and stimulus size have been discussed in Chapter IV. The great difference in presentation time between the Visual Field Analyser and the Tübinger perimeter, in particular, could lead to differences in defect intensity. Differences in adaptation level and stimulus size will scarcely affect the results.

Angioscotomata are, in the Bjerrum area, a cause of differences in intensity which deserves consideration (see Chapter VII).

The type of defect is an important factor in producing differences in intensity in the results of examination with the Visual Field Analyser and the Tübinger perimeter, as has been seen in the examples in the first part of this chapter. This factor is mainly of importance in sieve-like defects and in defects with steep edges. In both these cases, repetition of the measurement can result in great differences in intensity, when in the first measurement the stimulus falls just within the defect and in the following measurement just outside it. This reason for a difference in intensity is mentioned separately. The reconstruction of the supposed normal sensitivity of a given position in a defect, from the surrounding normal parts of the visual field as examined with the Tübinger perimeter cannot always be performed with an accuracy of 0.1 log unit. This implies that the

TABLE III

Results of the comparative study of threshold measurements performed with the Visual Field Analyser and Tübinger perimeter (see text).

	1001					
	541		460			
	0 – 0	0 – +	+ – + +	+ + – +	+ – 0	+ – +
	486	55	34	48	81	297
0.4–0.6		34	17	26	52	
0.8–1.0		11	9	14	14	
⩾ 1.2		10	8	8	15	
explained by defect type		38 = 60%	31 = 83%	41 = 84%	48 = 60%	
other explanation		17	3	7	33	
0.4–0.6		14			26	
0.8–1.0		1			6	
⩾ 1.2		2			1	
		3/541			7/460	

intensity of defects is accurate within a range of $\pm$ 0.1 log unit, or sometimes even more, especially when the defect is large.

The intra-individual variation is normally approximately 0.2 log unit. In a defect this variation can be greater, so that even when the examination is repeated using exactly the same method a different intensity may be found. Starting from the normal intra-individual variation of 0.2 log unit, differences in intensity of 0.3 log unit can be expected between the results obtained with the Visual Field Analyser and the Tübinger perimeter. In the threshold comparison, therefore, only differences of 0.4 log unit and higher are noted.

As has been described in chapter VIII differences of 0.4 or 0.6 log unit between the threshold of some positions of the Visual Field Analyser and the general level of sensitivity occur in normal subjects. If differences of 0.4–0.6 log unit are found in the intensity of defects as measured with the Visual Field Analyser and the Tübinger perimeter, this cannot be ascribed to the multiple stimulus presentation unless it occurs more frequently than in the examination of normal subjects.

The results of the threshold comparison are given in Table III. The results are subdivided into 6 groups:

0 — 0 : both Visual Field Analyser and Tübinger perimeter no defect;
0 — + : Visual Field Analyser no defect; Tübinger perimeter defect;
+ — ++: Visual Field Analyser defect; Tübinger perimeter defect of greater intensity;
++ — + : Visual Field Analyser defect of greater intensity than Tübinger perimeter;
+ — 0 : Visual Field Analyser defect; Tübinger perimeter no defect;
+ — + : Visual Field Analyser and Tübinger perimeter defect of the same intensity.

The differences in intensity are subdivided into three groups:

0.4 — 0.6 log unit;
0.8 — 1.0 log unit;
$\geqslant$ 1.2 log unit.

Of the 1001 positions examined the Visual Field Analyser detected no defect in 541 cases. In 55 of these 541 cases a defect was found on examination with the Tübinger perimeter. 38 of these cases (60%) could be explained by the type of defect. In 14 of the remaining 17 cases (3% of the total 541) the difference was 0.4–0.6 log unit. In view of the list of possible explanations for the existence of a difference in intensity these differences may be expected.

In 3 cases a difference of 0.8 log unit or more was found, for which no direct explanation could be given. The most probable causes are angioscotomata and inadequate examination.

In 460 cases a defect was found with the Visual Field Analyser. In 252 cases the intensity of the defect was the same as that found with the Tübinger perimeter. In 45 cases this was a maximum intensity for both the Visual Field Analyser and the Tübinger perimeter.

In 34 cases a lower intensity was recorded with the Visual Field Analyser than with the Tübinger perimeter, and in 48 cases a greater intensity. A striking fact is that, in both the cases of lower and of greater intensity, the same high percentage (82% and 84%) can be explained by the type of defect. This means that the chance that a difference in intensity will be to the disadvantage of the Visual Field Analyser is the same as the chance that it will be to the advantage of the Visual Field Analyser. This is to be expected if the threshold measurements with the multiple stimulus method and the single stimulus method are equivalent.

The remaining 3 cases of lower intensity on examination with the Visual Field Analyser and the 7 cases of greater intensity with the Visual Field Analyser are too small in number to carry any weight.

In 81 cases a defect was found on examination with the Visual Field Analyser which could not be reproduced on examination with the Tübinger perimeter. It is again noticeable that the same percentage (60%) as in the (0 — +) group can be explained by the type of defect.

In 33 cases another explanation must be sought (33 is 7% of the total of 460 cases). In 26 of these 33 cases the difference is not more than 0.4–0.6 log unit. The same considerations apply here as for the (0 — +) group. The 7 cases with a difference in intensity of more than 0.8 log unit may be explained by angioscotomata or inadequate examination.

CONCLUSION

False-positive (+ — 0 group) and false negative (0 — + group) results do occur on examination with the Visual Field Analyser.

In many cases the difference in intensity is in the range of 0.4–0.6 log unit. The frequency of these differences, however, does not exceed that of normal subjects. Differences of 0.8 log unit or more can generally be explained by the type of defect.

From these results it appears that the light sensitivity of positions without defects and with a glaucomatous defect, when measured with multiple stimulus static perimetry, is the same as the light sensitivity measured with single stimulus static perimetry, with only a few exceptions.

This is in accordance with the results of comparative multiple stimulus and single stimulus measurements as described in Chapter VIII.

Multiple stimulus static perimetry is a rapid method of detecting visual field defects. It only differs from the classical single stimulus static perimetry in that, thanks to the simultaneous presentation of stimuli, more information is obtained per unit of time.

CHAPTER I

The purpose of this study is to investigate the present possibilities for routine examination of the visual field in a large eye clinic. Much attention has been paid to static perimetry. Static perimetry can be subdivided into examination with single stimuli and examination with multiple stimuli. The place of multiple stimulus presentation has been especially considered. The study is mainly concerned with glaucomatous visual field defects and consists of an extensive survey of the literature, our experiments and the examination of 1372 visual fields of patients with intraocular hypertension.

It is hoped that this study will be a guide to those who wish to specialize in the difficult subject of visual field examination.

CHAPTER II

Visual field examination is a method of determining the *function* of the visual system. The specific function under examination is the *differential light sensitivity*. Visual field examination is one of the psychophysical methods of examination: a physically defined stimulus is presented, received and integrated. The subject is asked to react to the stimulation.

The physical factors involved are discussed in the first part of this chapter. A conclusion is drawn regarding the standardization of instruments for visual field examination.

The factors belonging to the realm of visual physiology are considered in the second part of this chapter, as far as these are needed to understand the principles

312

of visual field examination. Adaptation level, spatial and temporal interaction, local adaptation, movement and fixation are the most important factors involved.

The significance of the adaptation level for the differential light sensitivity, as appears from the literature, is summarized here:

1. Isolated activity of the cone system or the rod system is only certain when the retinal illumination is either very high or very low;
2. In the intermediate area of retinal illumination it is probable that combined action of the two receptor systems is responsible for the light sensitivity;
3. At the low photopic and mesopic constant adaptation level there is little difference in sensitivity between the cone and the rod system, as is shown by the dark adaptation curve;
4. It is not possible to define the mesopic level sharply. In visual field examination we define the mesopic level as the adaptive condition in which the light sensitivity in the area within the 30° parallel is uniform;
5. The differential light sensitivity reaches a maximum at the photopic level. Above about 315 asb (100 cd/m²) no further change in the differential sensitivity occurs when the background luminance is increased. The differential sensitivity decreases as the background luminance decreases;
6. Under different adaptive conditions both the light sensitivity and the topography of the light sensitivity within the 30° parallel change;
7. In adaptometry there is an 'equivalent background' corresponding to each point of time after the end of the pre-adaptation. In this way adaptometry is directly comparable to adaptoperimetry;
8. For visual field examination it is important to know that an adaptation time of 5–10 minutes is needed for photopic adaptation levels, and that at least 30 minutes are needed for scotopic adaptation levels.

Spatial interaction is one of the most essential neural processes on which the difference threshold is based. From the literature it is concluded that:

1. Spatial interaction is greater in the periphery of the visual field than in the centre;
2. Spatial interaction decreases as the eye becomes more adapted to light;
3. Spatial interaction varies with the colour of the stimulus;
4. Spatial interaction is greater when the presentation time is shorter.

Some electrophysiological findings concerning the receptive field are discussed in relation to the psychophysical concept of spatial interaction.

The differences in temporal interaction between the centre and the periphery of the visual field are much smaller than the differences in spatial interaction.

Temporal interaction is slightly stronger in the peripheral visual field. Temporal interaction decreases when the eye is more adapted to light.

Perception of a stimulus of long duration at threshold level is limited by local adaptation.

Perception of a moving stimulus probably involves different cortical units from those concerned with the perception of a static stimulus.

The different types of physiological fixation nystagmus are well known. Our measurements of the fixation nystagmus under the conditions of visual field examination show that the amplitude in the horizontal direction is about 30 minutes. The torsional nystagmus causes a displacement of the lower margin of the blind spot of 4 degrees of arc i.e. varying between the 193° and 199° meridian.

CHAPTER III

In this chapter the fundamental principles of static and kinetic perimetry are considered. In the three-dimensional representation of the visual field (the island of vision in the sea of darkness) static perimetry provides a vertical section and kinetic perimetry a horizontal section. The differences between these methods of examination are set out. Kinetic perimetry is a relatively rapid method. This rapidity is the result of the movement of the stimulus. This movement however introduces a factor of variation that is *not* involved in static perimetry. As the stimulus follows a certain path over the retina successive lateral spatial summation arises. This phenomenon is dependent on the local gradient. On account of the movement the results of kinetic perimetry are dependent on the reaction time of the patient and the examiner.

For these reasons the accuracy of kinetic perimetry, both with regard to the detection of defects and the assessment of defects, is limited. Therefore static perimetry should always be an integral part of every routine examination of the visual field.

CHAPTER IV

On the basis of the perimetric literature and our own experiments the optimum conditions for routine visual field examination are discussed.

At present there is no reason to change the low-photopic adaptation level that is provided by the background luminances of the Goldmann and Tübinger perimeters. The value of mesopic adaptation levels is probably limited where glaucomatous defects are concerned.

A stimulus size of 6'–10' as provided by the Goldmann and Tübinger perimeters is to be preferred to larger sizes.

Reasons for this choice are:

1. Pathological changes in spatial interaction usually result in reduced inhibition; this means that the intensity of a defect is greater with a small stimulus than with a large stimulus;

2. The accuracy with which a defect can be recorded becomes greater as the stimulus size becomes smaller;

3. The minimum stimulus size is limited by the contrast transfer function of the eye, which is approximately 6' at the fovea;

4. The intra- and inter-individual variation is not much affected by differences in stimulus size;

5. The influence of ametropia on the threshold level of small stimuli can be eliminated by the use of correcting lenses.

From our own experiments we concluded that short presentation times are to be preferred to longer ones. 'Short' means shorter than the critical duration. The intra- and inter-individual variation of threshold measurements is not affected by changes in presentation time. Several other advantages of short presentation times are discussed.

As a preference for short presentation times has already been expressed the phenomenon of local adaptation does not play a part in static threshold measurements. The investigation of local adaptation time is very difficult. No useful information has been obtained about changes in local adaptation in glaucomatous defects.

CHAPTER V

In this chapter the principles of our examination procedure are expounded. The distinction between the two phases of visual field examination is emphasized:

1. Detection phase
2. Assessment phase

The place of kinetic and static perimetry in these two phases is discussed.

Detection phase.

The essential requirement for the detection phase is the even distribution of an adequate number of static stimuli within the 30° parallel. As a compromise between the time necessary for the examination of the statistically calculated optimum number of stimuli and an acceptable duration of the examination the *number of 150 positions* has been selected.

The threshold of these 150 positions is measured using the static method. The specific value of this detection phase can be ascribed to the distribution of the stimuli and the actual use of static threshold measurements. The use of supraliminal stimuli is unsatisfactory. In the detection phase the peripheral visual field and the blind spot are examined by means of kinetic perimetry. The efficiency of the detection phase is increased by first using a coarse grid of stimuli (phase IA). If necessary a subsequent examination with a finer grid of stimuli can be added (phase IB). In this connection the upper and lower halves of the visual field should be considered separately.

Assessment phase.

The assessment phase consists of combined kinetic and static perimetry. Static perimetry is performed on every patient unless there are specific reasons for not doing so. In the assessment phase the distribution of positions to be examined is completely different from that in the detection phase. The examination is performed with an accuracy of one degree along a meridian or parallel and provides a vertical section through a defect. Kinetic perimetry delineates the general topography of a defect while static perimetry reveals the intensity of a defect in one meridian. Static perimetry is indispensable in the following cases:

1. a defect in which areas of very different intensity are found close to each other (sieve-like defects);
2. small defects;
3. paracentral defects;
4. slowly progressing defects;
5. defects of low intensity.

All these defects may be found in glaucomatous visual fields. Static perimetry has given a new insight into the structure and development of glaucomatous defects.

CHAPTER VI

In this chapter a detailed description is given of the Goldmann perimeter, the Tübinger perimeter and the Double Projection Campimeter (developed in the University Eye Clinic, Amsterdam).

Chapter VII gives the *normal values* of kinetic and static visual field examination with the three above-mentioned instruments. The *inter*-individual variation of both the level and the shape of the normal sensitivity curve is discussed. The importance of the *intra*-individual variation is set out. The size of the luminance steps is considered (0.2 log unit for the detection phase; 0.1 log unit for the assessment phase). A defect is a significant reduction of sensitivity, i.e. larger than the intra-individual variation. With a normal range of measurements of 0.2 log unit, a defect of 0.3 log unit is significant from a statistical point of view.

The influence of *age* on the results of kinetic and static perimetry is discussed. Prolonged reaction time and opacities of the lens are the main causes of an apparent general reduction of sensitivity in old age.

The normal blind spot is described and special attention is paid to the flat pericecal gradient.

From our own measurements we concluded that angioscotomata are limited to the intermediate visual field and usually have a diameter of 1°. Their intensity is less than 1 log unit. They are funnel-shaped.

Some remarks about cartographic deformation are made.

Chapter VIII deals with the multiple stimulus method. Although descriptions of a few multiple stimulus instruments are available multiple stimulus static perimetry has not received the attention it deserves.

In the previous chapters it was concluded that the static method is to be preferred for the detection phase, particularly within the 30° parallel. The examination of 150 positions in the detection phase by means of static perimetry is time-consuming. The simultaneous presentation of a number of static stimuli saves a considerable amount of time. In this chapter and Chapter XI it is shown that this time is saved without loss of information. In the first part of this chapter some specific problems concerning multiple stimulus presentation are dealt with.

The application of the multiple stimulus method is limited to the detection phase as the gain of time – which is the only reason for its use – is not achieved in the assessment phase. The saving of time arises from the simultaneous threshold approach of the multiple stimuli. Simultaneous perception at threshold level of simultaneously presented stimuli is not the rule.

In multiple stimulus static perimetry threshold measurements are to be preferred to the presentation of supraliminal stimuli. Several theoretical possibilities of interaction between multiple stimuli are discussed. From our own experiments on normal subjects we concluded that, whatever the possibilities of interaction, they do not influence the level or the variation of multiple stimulus threshold measurements as compared to single stimulus threshold measurements.

It also appeared that 4 and 5 simultaneously presented stimuli can be recognized correctly at one glance. Under favourable conditions up to 8 stimuli can be counted correctly.

Some reasons for pseudo-variations of multiple stimulus threshold measurements are mentioned.

The possibility of specific problems with the multiple stimulus method in patients with a disturbance of higher perceptual function is considered (extinction phenomenon). This however does not apply to glaucomatous defects.

In the second part of this chapter a detailed description and critical discussion of the Visual Field Analyser are given, following a survey of some earlier instruments (HARRINGTON-FLOCKS, FINCHAM-SUTCLIFFE).

As special advantages of the Visual Field Analyser are listed:
1. ingenious presentation system for multiple stimuli;
2. one source of light for all stimuli;
3. variable stimulus luminance;
4. large range of stimulus luminance;
5. short presentation time;
6. built-in background illumination;
7. central light sensitivity can be examined;
8. easy to use.

As disadvantages are listed:
1. poor fixation control;
2. too few stimuli; choice of positions in some cases not suitable for glaucomatous defects;
3. choice of stimulus size does not completely compensate the sensitivity gradient; compensation by altering luminance is preferable;
4. the same strength of stimulus is used for the nasal and temporal intermediate visual field;
5. low background luminance (with reservations, see text);
6. no built-in standardizing method.

Special attention is given to the Xenon flash tube, and the number, position and size of the stimuli.

The method of examination with the Visual Field Analyser and the normal visual field are described. Again the importance of threshold measurements is stressed. Differences of 0.4 to 0.6 log unit in the threshold level of the stimuli of the Visual Field Analyser can be accounted for by normal variation of threshold measurements and imperfections in the size of the stimuli. These differences in normal subjects should be taken into account when the results of the examination with the Visual Field Analyser are compared with the results of examination with the Tübinger perimeter (see Chapter XI).

In the third part of this chapter the few publications which have appeared on the Visual Field Analyser are mentioned.

The ratio between the duration of the examination with the Visual Field Analyser and comparable kinetic and static examination is 4:9:12 (minutes).

When the results of examination with the Visual Field Analyser are compared with the results of classical kinetic or static perimetry a number of characteristics in which the Visual Field Analyser differs from these classical methods should be taken into account:

1. 46 fixed positions in the 25° field;
2. cartographic accuracy;
3. background luminance of 0.5 asb;
4. luminance steps of 0.2 log unit;
5. presentation time of 0.0003 s;
6. multiple stimuli.

In such a comparative study one is concerned with false positive and false negative results.

Two extensive investigations were carried out: a mass visual field investigation of 1832 subjects with supposedly normal eyes and a more detailed examination of 1372 eyes of patients with raised intraocular pressure. The mass investigation provided data on the reaction of normal subjects to multiple stimulus presentation. No problems were encountered. The reactions were quick and accurate. Counting stimuli was easier than the indication of their position. The number of false positive results was small (about 1%). The duration of the examination was short. In 2 percent of the total number of subjects visual field defects were detected. From this mass visual field investigation it also appeared that adequate screening of visual fields on a large scale is possible with the multiple stimulus method. The accuracy of the screening on the one hand and the duration of the examination on the other hand depend on the number of positions examined and whether threshold measurements are performed or not.

Based on the conclusions drawn in this and the preceding chapters the requirements for an optimum multiple stimulus method for routine visual field examination are formulated:

1. Static stimulation;
2. Threshold measurements;
3. Built into an existing perimeter;
4. 150 stimuli distributed over the visual field within the 30° parallel;
5. Subdivision into 2 phases with increasing accuracy;
6. A maximum of 4 stimuli;
7. Preferably irregular patterns;
8. Stimulus size about 10 minutes;
9. Compensation of the gradient by means of neutral density filters;
10. Luminance range of 3 log units;
11. Luminance steps of 0.2 log unit;
12. Short presentation time;
13. Photopic adaptation level;
14. Built-in standardization.

Consideration of these requirements suggests that the Visual Field Analyser is susceptible to improvement on a number of points.

At the end of this chapter Armaly's and Gloster's detection procedures are described. The reasons for preferring the multiple stimulus method with threshold measurements are stated.

CHAPTER IX

In this chapter the influence of pupil size, opacities of the lens, ametropia and accommodation on the results of visual field examination are discussed. It is stressed that the intensity of relative defects is usually not influenced by preretinal factors.

Increase of the pupil diameter beyond 2 mm does not influence the visual field. When the pupil diameter is less than 2 mm a general reduction of sensitivity may occur, especially if opacities of the lens are present.

The effect of generalized opacity of the lens is a general reduction of sensitivity which may be associated with mesopization of the sensitivity curve.

The influence of ametropia on the visual field is well known. We make a distinction between a central ametropia scotoma and a peripheral ametropia scotoma or refraction scotoma. The myopization due to miotics should be taken into account when examining glaucomapatients.

CHAPTER X

In this chapter the importance of an accurate description of defects is empha-

sized. The evaluation of defects should be based on:
1. topography (size, shape, localization);
2. intensity (degree and distribution of the reduction of light sensitivity).

After giving a definition of some of the current descriptive topographical terms a numerical topographical classification is proposed. The visual field is divided into 180 units which can be used to indicate the localization and size of a defect. This classification is used in chapter XI.

The intensity of a defect should be quantitatively expressed in tenths of a logarithmic unit reduction of sensitivity. An essential point in the determination of intensity is the differentiation between general reduction of sensitivity and localized reduction of sensitivity. The intensity of a defect is the difference between the threshold of a defect and the average normal threshold, with the general reduction of sensitivity subtracted from the difference.

CHAPTER XI

This chapter consists of two parts. In the first part eighteen examples of visual fields from glaucoma patients are shown. They are used to illustrate the examination procedure. These examples also demonstrate the appearance of glaucomatous defects, especially early glaucomatous defects, as found with meridional static perimetry. The main purpose of this section is to illustrate the possibilities and limitations of the Visual Field Analyser in the detection phase.

The second part deals with the results of a comparative study based on the results of examination of 1372 eyes of patients with intraocular hypertension, with the Visual Field Analyser and the Tübinger perimeter; again the function of the Visual Field Analyser as multiple stimulus method in the detection phase is at issue.

The difference between the research examination procedure and the optimum examination procedure (Chapter VIII) is described.

In phase II it is important to define the following aspects of a defect: where it is maximum, where it is relative and where it has not yet penetrated.

The duration of a visual field examination if no defects are present is 40 minutes per eye with the research procedure, but only 20 minutes with the optimum procedure. A complete examination if defects are present takes at least 45 minutes per eye. A good visual field examination which aims at detecting early glaucomatous defects and at early assessment of progression takes time. It is for the benefit of the patient that this amount of time is spent in practice.

This kind of extensive visual field examination can only be realized in practice with the help of a well-organized visual field department. The functioning of a visual field department depends on the presence of carefully trained specialized technical assistents. In our department 1½ hour is reserved for each patient.

In the introduction to the 18 examples given in this chapter two types of early glaucomatous visual field defects, as found with meridional static perimetry, are described. The first type is the relative wedge-shaped scotoma which may appear anywhere in the 30° visual field. The detection of this type of scotoma is important as it is one of the earliest signs (if not the earliest) of reduction of light sensitivity due to glaucoma. These relative defects are sometimes reversible. The second type is the small isolated scotoma for maximum luminance as described by AULHORN & HARMS (1967).

Early defects also occur in the half of the visual field opposite to an extensive defect. The value of the detection of these early defects is stressed.

After the eighteen examples the results of the comparative study are given. This study attempts to give an answer to the question whether the Visual Field Analyser, as the best representative of the multiple stimulus method, misses defects which can be found by single stimulus static perimetry, or vice versa.

This question is divided into two subsidiary questions; a distinction should be made between two possible reasons why defects are missed by the Visual Field Analyser:
1. the number and position of the stimuli are insufficient;
2. threshold measurements with multiple stimulus presentation do not yield the same result as with single stimulus presentation.

To give an answer to the first question the defects of 1372 eyes with raised intraocular pressure were studied. In 355 cases there was no localized defect. In 715 cases there was a complete arcuate scotoma or a larger defect. In both groups the results of the examination with the Visual Field Analyser were accurate, i.e. the Visual Field Analyser indicated no defect in the first group and a defect in the second group.

In 241 cases we found small defects and in 61 cases we found a small defect in the visual field half opposite to a large defect. In these 302 cases 17 defects were missed by the Visual Field Analyser due to the absence of a stimulus position at the site of the defect.

This emphasizes the necessity of an adequate number and distribution of stimulus positions in the detection phase, if one is attempting to detect early glaucomatous defects.

To answer the second part of the question formulated above, a comparative study of threshold measurements at 1001 positions was carried out. The values obtained with the Visual Field Analyser and the Tübinger perimeter for the intensity of a defect at a given position were compared.

322

As explained in Chapter VIII differences of 0.4–0.6 log units between threshold measurements with the Visual Field Analyser occur in normal subjects.

It follows that these differences can also be found in the comparative study of the intensity of defects. If the multiple stimulus and single stimulus method are equivalent with respect to threshold measurements, it is to be expected that the number of times a difference in intensity of 0.4–0.6 log unit is recorded in these patients will not exceed the number of times this is found in normal subjects.

A defect of 0.4–0.6 log unit was *not* indicated by the Visual Field Analyser at only 14 positions when it had been found by the Tübinger perimeter. At 26 positions a defect of 0.4–0.6 log unit was indicated by the Visual Field Analyser which could not be reproduced by the Tübinger perimeter. These figures, percentages of 1.4 and 2.6 respectively, do not exceed the figure found in normal subjects. Only 3 defects of 0.8 log unit intensity or more were not indicated by the Visual Field Analyser, while the Visual Field Analyser found 7 of these defects that could not be reproduced by the Tübinger perimeter. Differences in intensity of defects that could not be explained by the type of defect were only found at 10 positions.

The conclusion can be drawn from this chapter that, with a few exceptions, the light sensitivity in visual fields of patients with raised intraocular pressure as measured with multiple stimulus static perimetry is the same as the sensitivity measured with single stimulus static perimetry.

By using multiple stimulus static perimetry in the detection phase of visual field examination more information per unit of time is obtained. The multiple stimulus method is a welcome addition to the available methods of visual field examination.

REFERENCES

AGUILAR, M. & W. S. STILES. Saturation of the rod mechanism of the retina at high levels of stimulation. *Optica Acta* 1: *59–65* (1954).

ALPERN, Eye movements. In: Handbook of Sensory Physiology VII/4: Visual Psychophysics. ed. *D. Jameson, L. M. Hurvich*, Springer, Berlin, 303–330 (1972).

ARMALY, M. F. Refraction and stimulus value in perimetry. In: Symposium on Glaucoma. Tr. New. Orleans Acad. Ophthal. C. V. Mosby, St. Louis, 224–231 (1967).

—— Ocular pressure and visual field – a 10 year follow up study. *Arch. Ophthal.* 81: *25–40* (1969).

—— Size and location of the normal blind spot. *Arch. Ophthal.* 81: *192–201* (1969).

ASPINALL, P. Variables affecting the retinal threshold gradient in static perimetry. Master of Science. Thesis. Department of psychology. University of Edinburgh (1967).

AUERBACH, E. & H. M. BURIAN. Studies on the photopic-scotopic relationships in the human electroretinogram. *Amer. J. Opthal.* 40: *42–60* (1955).

AUBERT, H. Uber die Grenzen der Farbenwahrnehmung auf den seitlichen Teilen der Retina. *Graefes Arch. Ophthal.* 3: *38–67* (1857).

—— & R. FOERSTER. Untersuchungen über den Raumsinn der Retina. *Graefes Arch. Ophthal.* 3: *1–37* (1857).

AUBERT, L. Campimétrie et périmétrie en pratique courante. L'Année thérapeutique et clinique en Ophtalmologie. 11: *39–65* (1960).

AULHORN, E. Papillenveränderung und Gesichtsfeldstörungen bei Glaukom. *Ophthalmologica* 139: *279–285* (1960).

—— Entwicklung und Fortschritt in der Augenheilkunde. Fortb. kurs für Augenärtze, Hamburg, 701–706 (1963).

—— Über die Beziehung zwischen Lichtsinn und Sehscharfe. *Graefes Arch. Ophthal.* 167: *4–74* (1964).

—— Glaukomgesichtsfeld. *Ophthalmologica* 158: *469–487* (1969).

—— & H. HARMS & M. RAABE. Die Lichtunterschiedsempfindlichkeit als Funktion der Umfeldleuchtdichte. *Docum. Ophthal.* 20: *537–556* (1966).

—— & —— Early visual field defects in glaucoma. In: Glaucoma Tutzing Symp. ed. W. LEYDHECKER, Karger, Basel, 151–186 (1967).

—— & —— Visual perimetry. In: Handbook of Sensory Physiology VII/4: Visual Psychophysics. ed. D. JAMESON, L. M. HURVICH, Springer, Berlin, 102–145 (1972).

AUST, W. & J. L. MORLANG. Pilocarpinmyopie. *Klin. Mbl. Augenheilk.* 156 : *30–39* (1970).

AVERBACH, E. The Span of apprehension as a function of exposure duration. *J. Verb. Learn. Behav.* 2 : *60–64* (1963).

—— & A. S. CORIELL. Short-term memory in vision. *Bell. Syst. Techn. J.* 40 : *309–328* (1961).

BAIR, H. L. Some fundamental physiologic principles in the study of the visual field. *Arch. Ophthal.* 24 : *10–20* (1940).

BARLOW, H. B. Eye movements during fixation. *J. Physiol.* 116 : *290–306* (1952).

—— Summation and inhibition in the frog's retina. *J. Physiol.* 119 : *69–88* (1953).

—— Increment thresholds at low intensities considered as signal noise discriminations. *J. Physiol.* 136 : *469–488* (1957).

—— Temporal and spatial summations in human vision at different background intensities. *J. Physiol.* 141 : *337–350* (1958).

—— Dark and light adaptation: psychophysics. In: Handbook of Sensory Physiology VII/4: Visual Psychophysics. ed. D. JAMESON, L. M. HURVICH, Springer, Berlin, 1–28 (1972).

—— R. FITZHUGH & S. KUFFLER. Change of organisation in the receptive fields of the cats retina during dark adaptation. *J. Physiol.* 137 : *338–354* (1957).

—— & R. M. HILL. Selective sensitivity to direction of movement in ganglion cells of the rabbit retina. *Science* 139 : *412–414* (1963).

—— & J. M. B. SPARROCK. The role of afterimages in darkadaptation. *Science* 144 : *1304–1314* (1964).

—— R. M. HILL & W. R. LEVICK. Retinal ganglion cells responding selectively to direction and speed of image motion in the rabbit. *J. Physiol.* 173 : *377–407* (1964).

—— & W. R. LEVICK. The mechanism of directinally selective units in rabbits retina. *J. Physiol.* 178 : *477–504* (1965).

BARTLETT, W. R. Dark adaptation and light adaptation. In: Vision and Visual Perception. ed. C. H. GRAHAM, John Wiley & Sons, New York, 185–207, (1966).

BATTERSBY, W. S. Neural limitations of visual excitability VII. Nonhomonymous retrochiasmal interaction. *Amer. J. Physiol.* 206 : *1181–1188* (1964).

—— H. P. KRIEGER., M. POLLACK & M. B. BENDER. Figure-ground discrimination and the 'abstract attitude' in patients with cerebral neoplasms. *Arch. Neurol. Psychiat.* 70 : *703–712* (1953).

—— & I. WAGMANN. Neural limitations of visual excitability IV. Spatial determinants of retrochiasmal interaction. *Amer. J. Physiol.* 203 : *359–365* (1962).

—— & J. DEFAUBAUGH. Neural limitations of visual excitability: after-effects of subliminal stimulation. *Vision. Res.* 9 : *757–768* (1969).

—— & H. SCHUCKMAN. The time course of temporal summation. *Vision. Res.* 10 : *263–273* (1970).

BAUMGARDT, E. Quantic and statistical bases of visual excitation. *J. Gen. Physiol.* 31 : *269–290* (1948).

—— Les theories photochimiques classiques et quantiques de la vision et l'inhibition nerveuse en vision liminaire. *Rev. Opt.* 28 : *478–543/661–690* (1949).

—— Sur la sommation spatiale aux niveaux éléves de l'enchaînement rétinien. *J. Physiol. (Paris)* 45 : *24–29* (1953).

—— Visual spatial and temporal summation. *Nature* 184 : *1951–1952* (1959).

—— & B. HILLMANN. Duration and size as determinants of peripheral retinal response. *J. Opt. Soc. Amer.* 51 : *340–344* (1961).

BAY, E. Agnosie und Funktionswandel. Springer, Berlin, (1950).

—— Disturbances of visual perception and their examination. *Brain* 76 : *515–550* (1953).

BEASLY, H. The visual fields in aphakia. *Trans. Amer. Ophthal. Soc.* 63 : *364–416* (1965).

BECK, P. Variation of the blind spot with age. Thesis Bern. (1955).

BEDWELL, C. The design of instrumentation for the efficient investigation of the visual fields. *Amer. J. Optom.* 44 : *609–633* (1967).

BEGG, I. S., & S. M. DRANCE & V. P. SWEENEY. Ischaemic optic neuropathy in chronic single glaucoma. *Brit. J. Ophthal.* 55 : *73–91* (1971).

BENDER. M. B. & L. T. FURLOW. Phenomenon of visual extinction in homogenous fields and the psychologic principles involved. *Arch. Neurol. Psychiat.* 53 : *29–33* (1945).

—— & H. L. TEUBER. Phenomenon of fluctuation, extinction and completion in visual perception. *Arch. Neurol. Psychiat.* 55 : *627–658* (1946).

BENNET, A. G., J. L. FRANCIS & K. N. OGLE. Visual Optics and the Optical Space Sense. In: The Eye 4. ed. H. Davson, Academic Press, New York, (1962).

BERRY, V., S. M. DRANCE & R. L. WIGGINS. An evaluation of differences between two observers plotting and measuring visual fields. *Can. J. Ophthal.* 1 : *297–300* (1966).

BIERSDORF, W. R. Critical duration in visual brightness discrimination of retinal areas of various sizes. *J. Opt. Soc. Amer.* 45 : *920–925* (1955).

BIGGER, J. F. & B. BECKER. Cataracts and open angle glaucoma. The effect of cataract extraction on visual fields. *Amer. J. Ophthal.* 71 : *335–341* (1971).

BIRREN, J. E., R. C. CASPERSON & J. BOTWINICK. Age changes in pupil size. *J. Gerontology* 5 : *216–224* (1950).

BJERRUM, J. Ueber eine Zufügung zur gewöhnlicher Gesichtsmessung und über das Gesichtsfeld beim Glaukom. 10 Internat. M. Kongr. Berlin 66.

BLACKWELL, M. C. Contrast threshold of the human eye. *J. Opt. Soc. Amer.* 36 : *624–643* (1946).

BLACKWELL, H. R. Studies of psychophysical methods of measuring visual thresholds. *J. Opt. Soc. Amer.* 42 : *606–616* (1952).

Studies of the form of visual threshold data. *J. Opt. Soc. Amer.* 43 : *456–463* (1953).

—— Neural theories of simple visual discriminations. *J. Opt. Soc. Amer.* 53 : *129–160* (1963).

—— Luminance difference thresholds. In: Handbook of Sensory Physiology VII/4: Visual Psychophysics. ed. D. JAMESON, L. M. HURVICH, Springer, Berlin, 78–101 (1972).

BLAKEMORE, C. Binocular depth discrimination and the nasal temporal division. *J. Physiol.* 471–497 (1969).

BLOCH, A. M. Expériences sur la vision. *Compt. Rend. Soc. Biol.* 2 : *493–495* (1885).

BLONDELL, A. M. & J. REY. Sur la perception des lumières brèves à la limite de leur portée. *J. Physiol. (Paris)* 1 : *530–550* (1911).

BLUM, F. G., L. K. GATES & M. R. JAMES. How important are peripheral fields? *Arch. Ophthal.* 61 : *1–8* (1959).

327

BORNSCHEIN, H. Die absolute Lichtschwelle des menschlichen Auges. *Graefes Arch. Ophthal.* 151 : *446–475* (1961).

BOUMAN, M. A. & H. A. VAN DER VELDEN. The two-quanta hypothesis as a general explanation of the behaviour of the threshold values and visual acuity for the several receptors of the human eye. *J. Opt. Soc. Amer.* 38 : *575–581* (1948).

—— & G. VAN DER BRINK. On the integrate capacity of in time and space of the human peripheral retina. *J. Opt. Soc. Amer.* 42 : *617–620* (1952).

—— & —— Absolute threshold for moving point sources. *J. Opt. Soc. Amer.* 43 : *895–898* (1953).

—— & J. TEN DOESSCHATE. On the mechanism of dark-adaptation. *Vision. Res.* 1 : *386–403* (1961).

BOYNTON, R. M. & L. A. RIGGS. The effect of stimulus area and intensity upon the human retinal response. *J. Exper. Psychol.* 42 : *217–226* (1951).

—— & F. J. J. CLARKE. Sources of entoptic scatter in the human eye. *J. Opt. Soc. Amer.* 54 : *110–119* (1961).

—— Some temporal factors in vision. In: Sensory Communication, 37, ed. W. ROSENBLITH, Wiley, New York, 739–756, (1961).

BRAIS, P. & S. M. DRANCE. The temporal field in chronic simple glaucoma. *Arch. Ophthal.* 88 : *518–522* (1972).

BRINDLEY, G. S. The Bunsen-Roscoe law for the human eye at very short durations. *J. Physiol.* 118 : *135–139* (1952).

—— The summation areas of human colour-receptive mechanism at increment threshold. *J. Physiol.* 124 : *400–408* (1954).

BRINK, G. VAN DER. Retinal summation and the visibility of moving objects. Thesis Utrecht. (1957).

—— A note on visual facilitation. *Vision. Res.* 5 : *217–222* (1965).

—— Psychophysical experiments on visual addition and facilitation. in 'Performance of the eye at low luminances' ed. M. A. BOUMAN & J. J. VOS; Exerpta Medica Found. Amsterdam p. 23–40: (1966).

—— & M. A. BOUWMAN. Variation of integrative actions in the retinal system: an adaptational phenomenon. *J. Opt. Soc. Amer.* 44 : *616–620* (1954).

—— & G. A. REIJNTJES. Spatial and temporal facilitation in vision. *Vision. Res.* 6 : *533–551* (1966).

BROADBENT, D. E. Perception and communication. Pergamon Press. New York, (1958).

BROCA, A. & D. SULZER. La sensation lumineuse en fonction des temps. *J. Physiol. Path. gén.* 4 : *632–640* (1902).

—— & —— La sensation lumineuse en fonction des temps. *C. R. Acad. Sci.* 137 : *944–946/977–979/1046–1049* (1903).

BROWN, R. H. Complete spatial summation in the peripheral retina of the human eye, *Amer. J. Psychol.* 60 : *254–259* (1947).

—— The effect of extent in the intensity-time relation for the visual discrimination of movement. *J. Comp. Physiol. Psychol.* 50 : *109–114* (1957).

BROWN, J. Some tests of the decay theory of immediate memory. *Quart. J. Exp. Psychol.* 10 : *12–21* (1958).

BRUNETTE, J. R. & S. MOLOTCHNIKOFF. Calibration of flashtube photostimulators in electroretinography. *Vision. Res.* 10 : *95–102* (1970).

328

BUCHANAN, W. & J. GLOSTER. An automatic device for rapid assessment of central visual field. *Brit. J. Ophthal.* 49 : *57–70* (1965).

CARIFA, R. P. & F. W. HEBBARD. Involuntary eye movements occurring during fixation effects of changes in target contrast. *Amer. J. Optom.* 44 : *73–90* (1967).

CASSIDY, V. & W. HAVENER. Evaluation of a screening procedure in the detection of eye disease. *Arch. Ophthal.* 61 : *589–598* (1959).

CIBIS, P. Zur Pathologie des Lokaladaptation I und II. *Graefes Arch. Ophthal.* 148 : *1–93/216–258* (1948).

—— & H. MÜLLER. Lokaladaptometrische Untersuchungen am Projektionsperimeter nach Maggiore. *Graefes Arch. Ophthal.* 148 : *468–490* (1948).

CLARK, W. C. Relations between the thresholds for single and multiple light pulses in the human eye. Dissertation. University of Michigan (1958).

CLARKE, F. J. J. A study of Troxler's effect. *Optica Acta* 7 : *219–236* (1960).

—— Visual recovery following local adaptation of the peripheral retina (Troler's effect). *Optica Acta* 8 : *121–135* (1961).

—— & S. BELCHER. On the localization of Troxler's effect in the visual pathway. *Vision. Res.* 2 : *53–68* (1962).

MC. COLGIN, F. H. Movement thresholds in peripheral vision. *J. Opt. Soc. Amer.* 50 : *774–779* (1960).

COLLIER, G. Probability of response and intertrial association as function of monocular and binocular summation. *J. exp. Psychol.* 47 : *75–83* (1954).

CONREUR, L. & G. MEUR. Influence de la longueur d'onde du stimulus lumineux dans les phénomènes de sommation spatiale rétinienne. *Bull. Soc. Belge Ophtal.* 143 : *532–541* (1966).

COOPER, G. F. & J. G. ROBSON. Directionally selective movement detectors in the retina of the grey squirrel. *J. Physiol.* 186 : *116–117* (1966).

CORNSWEET, T. N. Determination of the stimuli for involuntary drifts and saccadic eye movements. *J. Opt. Soc. Amer.* 46 : *987–993* (1956).

CORTE, M. DE & G. LAVERGNE. La mesure de la fréquence critique de fusion au périmètre de Tübingen. *Bull. Soc. Belge Ophtal.* 110 : *593–596* (1969).

COTTON, J. The dependence of frequencies of seeing on procedural variables: II procedure of terminating series of intensity ordered stimuli. *J. Gen. Psychol.* 53 : *49–57* (1955).

CRAWFORD, B. J. The change of visual sensitivity with time. *Proc. Roy. Soc. (Lond).* B 123 : *69–89* (1937).

CRAWFORD, B. J. Visual adaptation in relation to brief conditioning stimuli. *Proc. Roy. Soc. (Lond).* B 134 : *283–302* (1947).

CRAWFORD, B. J. The Stiles-Crawford effects and their significance in vision. In: Handbook of Sensory Physiology VII/4: Visual Psychophysics. ed. D. JAMESON, L. M. HURVICH, Springer, Berlin, 470–483 (1972).

CRAWFORD, B. J. & M. J. PIRENNE. Steep frequency of seeing curves. *J. Physiol.* 126 : *404–411* (1954).

CRONE, R. A. Diplopia. Excerpta Medica, Amsterdam (1973).

DAENEN, P. & R. WEEKERS. Correction des amétropies pour l'étude du champ visuel. *Bull. Soc. Belge Ophtal.* 103 : *204–210* (1953).

—— Correction des ametropies pour l'étude du champ visuel. *Arch. Ophtal. (Paris).* 13 : *384–390* (1953).

329

DANNHEIM, F. Über die Untersuchung der Dunkelanpassung mit hellen und dunklen Prüfpunkten. Inaugural Dissertation. Tübingen (1967).

—— & S. M. DRANCE. Studies of spatial and temporal summation of central retinal areas in normal people of all ages. *Opthal. Res.* 2 : *295–303* (1971).

DAVY, E. The intensity-time relation for multiple flashes of light in the peripheral retina. *J. Opt. Soc. Amer.* 42 : *937–941* (1952).

DAWSON, H. The Eye, vol. 2, The visual Process, Acad. Press, New York, (1962).

DAY, R. M. & H. G. SCHEIE. Simulated progression of visual field defects of glaucoma. *Arch. Ophthal.* 50 : *418–433* (1953).

DEMAILLY, PH. Revue du glaucome. *Arch. Ophtal. (Paris)* 31 : *361–367* (1971).

—— L. LAPOZ & B. WENKER-BRISSET. L'analyse périmétrique quantitative de Friedmann; son intérèt dans le depistage des altération périmétriques débutantes du glaucome chronique à l'angle ouvert. *Arch. Ophtal. (Paris)* 33 : *109–122* (1973).

DITCHBURN, R. W. A new apparatus for producing a stabilized retinal image. *Optica. Acta.* 10 : *325–331* (1963).

—— & B. L. GINSBORG. Involuntary eye movements during fixation. *J. Physiol.* 119 : *1–17* (1953).

—— & B. FOLEY-FISHER. Assembled data in eye movements. *Optica Acta* 14 : *113–118* (1967).

DOESSCHATE, J. TEN. Perimetric charts in aequivalent projection allowing a planimetric determination of the extension of the visual field. *Ophthalmologica* 113 : *257–270* (1947).

DOWLING, J. E. The site of visual adaptation. *Science* 155 : *273–279* (1967).

—— & B. B. BOYCOTT. Neural connections of the retina: Fine structure of the inner plexiform layer. Cold Spring Harbor Symposia on Quantitative Biology 30 : *393–402* (1965).

—— & —— Organization of the primate retina: Electron microscopy. *Proc. Roy. Soc. Belge* 166 : *80–111* (1967).

—— & F. WERBLIN. Organization of the retina of the mudpuppy, Necturus maculosus I. Synaptic structure. *J. Neurophysiol.* 32 : *315–338* (1969).

DRANCE, S. M. The early field defects in glaucoma. *Invest. Ophthal.* 8 : *84–91* (1969).

—— The glaucomatous visual field, *Brit. J. Ophthal.* 56 : *186–200*, (1972).

—— V. BERRY & A. HUGHES. Studies in the reproducibility of visual field areas in normal and glaucomatous subjects. *Canad. J. Ophthal.* 1 : *14–23* (1966).

—— —— & —— The effects of age on the central isopter of the normal visual field. *Canad. J. Ophthal.* 2 : *79–82* (1967).

—— —— & —— Studies on the effects of age on the central and peripheral isopters of the visual field. *Amer. J. Ophthal.* 63 : *1667–1672* (1967).

—— C. WHEELER & M. PATULLO. The use of static perimetry in the early detection of glaucoma. *Canad. J. Ophthal.* 2 : *249–258* (1967).

—— —— & —— Uniocular open-angle glaucoma. *Amer. J. Ophthal.* 65 : *891–902* (1968).

—— see BEGG et al.

—— see ROCK et al.

—— see REED et al.

DUBOIS-POULSEN, A. Variations de la sensibilité et interactions nerveuses dans le champ visuel. *Ann. Oculist (Paris)*, 185 : *1025–1052* (1952).

—— Le champ visuel. Masson et Cie. Paris (1952).

—— Reproduction expérimentale du ressaut de Rönne et du scotome de Bjerrum. *Ann. Oculist. (Paris)*, 189 : *37–52* (1956).

—— La périmétrie à deux variables du laboratoire à la clinique. *Bull. Soc. Ophtal.* de *France.* (1957).

—— Seuils et périmétrie. L'année thérapeutique et clinique en ophtalmologie. (1960).

—— Etude critique des techniques d'examen de la vision péripherique. *Canad. J. Ophthal.* 1 : *24–35* (1966).

—— Discussion of the article of Aulhorn and Harms. In: Glaucoma, Tutzing Symp. ed. W. LEYDHECKER, Karger, Basel 176–179 (1967).

—— A. TIBI & A. MAGIS. De quelques facteurs de variation de la tache aveugle (Ametropies, accommodation, fixation binoculaire). *Ann. Oculist. (Paris)* 184: *17–40* (1951).

—— & C. MAGIS. Caractère non pathognomonique du scotome arciforme de Bjerrum et du ressaut nasal de Rönne. *Bull. et Mem. Soc. France d'Opht.* 66 : *115–125* (1953).

—— & —— Pathogénie du scotome de Bjerrum. *Ann. Oculist. (Paris)* 189 : *174–185* (1956).

—— & —— La notion de sommation spatiale en physio-pathologie oculaire. *Mod. Probl. Ophtal. (Basel)* 1 : *218–238* (1957).

—— & —— La dysharmonie photométrique dans le champ visuel des glaucomateux. *Doc. Ophthal.* 13 : *186–302* (1959).

—— & —— Discussion of HARMS and AULHORN's Article. *Doc. Ophthal.* 13 : *334–342* (1959).

—— & —— Les procédés d'examen de la fonction visuelle dans le glaucome chronique. *Ophthalmologica* 139 : *155–213* (1960).

ELSBERG, CH. & H. SPOTNITZ. The sense of vision: II. The reciprocal relation of area and light intensity and its significance for the localization of tumors of the brain by functional visual test. *Bull. Neur. Inst. N.Y.* 6 : *243–252* (1937).

ENGEL, F. L. Visual conspicuity, directed attention and retinal locus. *Vision Res.* 11 : *563–576* (1971).

ENGEL, S. Influence of a constricted pupil on the field in glaucoma. *Arch. Ophthal.* 27 : *1184–1187* (1942).

ENOCH, J. M. & R. N. SUNGA. Development of quantitative perimetric tests. *Doc. Ophthal.* 26 : *215–229* (1969).

—— —— & E. BACHMAN. Static perimetric technique believed to test receptive field properties. I. Extension of Westheimer's experiments in spatial interaction. *Amer. J. Ophthal.* 70 : *113–126* (1970).

—— & —— Neue Wege der quantitativen Perimetrie. *Graefes Arch. Ophthal.* 179 : *259–270* (1970).

ERCOLES, A. Contrast threshold for moving Landolt rings. *Atti. Fond. G. Ronchi.* 23 : 515 (1968).

—— Contrast threshold for perception of a moving target as a function of movement direction. *Atti. Fond. G. Ronchi.* 24 : *387–392* (1969).

ESTERMAN, B. Grid for scoring visual fields II. Perimeter. *Arch. Ophthal.* 79 : *400–406* (1968).

—— Grid for scoring visual fields I. Tangent Screen. *Arch. Ophthal.* 77 : *780–786* (1967).

EVANS, J. N. Angioscotometry. Modern Trends in Ophthalmology II. ed. A. Sorsby, Butterworth & Co., London, 141–149 (1948).

FANKHAUSER, F. Kinetische Perimetrie. *Ophthalmologica* 158 : *406–418* (1969).

—— & TH. SCHMIDT. Die Untersuchung des dunkeladaptierten Auges mit den Adaptometer Goldmann-Weekers. *Ophthalmologica* 133 : *264–275* (1957).

—— & —— Die Untersuchung der räumlichen Summation mit stehender und bewegter Reizmarke nach der Methode der quantitativen Lichtsinnperimetrie. *Ophthalmologica* 135 : *660–666* (1958).

—— & —— Die optimalen Bedingungen für die Untersuchung der räumlichen Summation mit stehender Reizmarke nach der Methode der quantitativen Lichtsinnperimetrie. *Ophthalmologica* 139 : *409–423* (1960).

—— & J. M. ENOCH. The effects of blur upon perimetric thresholds. *Arch. Ophthal.* 86 : *240–251* (1962).

—— & R. ROHLER. The physical stimulus, the quality of the retinal image and foveal brightness discrimination in one amblyopia and two normal eyes. *Doc. Ophthal.* 23 : *149–188* (1967).

—— & H. GIGER. Die perzeptorische Organisation von Punktfeldern. *Vision. Res.* 8 : *1349–1366* (1968).

FECHNER, P. U. & J. HAEFNER. Erfahrungen mit einem neuen Gerät zur Untersuchung des Gesichtsfeldes. *Klin. Mbl. Augenheilk.* 158 : *561–573* (1971).

—— Die Vermeidung des Akkomodationsspasmus bei der Behandlung jugendlichen Glaukompatienten. *Klin. Mbl. Augenheilk.* 158 : *112–116* (1971).

FERREE, C. E. An experimental examination of the phenomena usually attributed to fluxtuation of attention. *Amer. J. Psychol.* 17 : *81–120* (1906).

—— & G. RAND. An illuminated perimeter with campimeter features. *Amer. J. Ophthal.* 5 : *455–465* (1922).

—— & —— Effect of brightness of pre-exposure and surrounding field on breadth and shape of the colour fields for stimuli of different sizes. *Amer. J. Ophthal.* 7 : *843–850* (1924).

—— —— & N. M. MONROE. Studies in perimetry III. Errors of refraction, age and sex in relation to size of the form field. *Amer. J. Ophthal.* 12 : *659–664* (1929).

—— & —— The effect of relation to background on the size and shape of the form field for stimuli of different sizes. *Amer. J. Ophthal.* 14 : *1018–1029* (1931).

—— —— & C. HARDY. Refraction for the peripheral field of vision. *Arch. Ophthal.* 5 : *717–731* (1931).

—— —— & —— Refractive asymmetry in the temporal and nasal halves on the visual field. *Amer. J. Ophthal.* 15 : *513–522* (1932).

—— & —— The refractive conditions for the peripheral field of vision. The Physical and Optical Societies report of a joint discussion for vision. (1932).

—— & —— Interpretation of refractive conditions in the peripheral field of vision. A further study. *Arch. Ophthal.* 9 : *925–938* (1933).

—— —— & L. L. SLOAN. The effect of size of pupil on the form and colour fields. *J. gener. Psychol.* 10 : *83–99* (1934).

FIORENTINI, A. & T. RADICI. Binocular interaction. *Vision. Res.* 1 : *244–252* (1961).

FISHER, R. F. The variations of the peripheral field with age. *Doc. Ophthal.* 24 : *41–67* (1968).

332

FLAMANT, F. Étude de la repartition de lumière dans l'image rétinienne d'une fente. *Rev. Opt.* 34 : *433–459* (1955).

FORBES, M. Influence of miotics on visual fields in glaucoma. *Invest. Ophthal.* 5 : *139–145* (1966).

FRANCOIS, J. & G. VERRIEST. Contribution à l'étude des déficits périmétriques dans le glaucome. *Ann. Oculist* 187 : *985–1045* (1954).

—— & —— Conclusions des études sur le champ visuel central scotopique au moyen des tests de Livingston. *Ann. Oculist* 189 : *605–620* (1956).

—— —— & A. ISRAEL. Périmétrie statique coloré à l'aide de l'apparat de Goldmann. Résultats obtenus en pathologie oculaire. *Ann. Oculist* 199 : *113–142* (1966).

—— —— J. L. LAVALLEE & G. LEBRUN. Résultats en pathologie oculaire de la mesure de la durée d'adaptation locale dans les conditions d'une périmetrie statique avec fixation non stabilisée. *Bull. Soc. Belge Ophtal.* 153 : *713–723* (1969).

—— —— & A. ORTIZ-OLMEDO. Résultats en pathologie oculaire d'une périmétrie effectuée à l'aide d'objets plains et d'objets annulaires de mêmes surfaces. *Ann. Oculist* 203 : *109–130* (1970).

FRIEDMANN, A. I. Serial analysis of changes in visual field defects employing a new instrument to determine the activity of diseases involving the visual pathways. *Ophthalmologica* 152 : *1–12* (1966).

FRISEN, L. The cartographic deformations of the visual field. *Ophthalmologica* 161 : *38–54* (1970).

FRY, G. A. Retinal image formation: review, summary and discussion. *J. Opt. Soc. Amer.* 53 : *94–97* (1963).

—— Distribution of focused and stray light on the retina produced by a point source. *J. Opt. Soc. Amer.* 55 : *333–335* (1965).

—— & V. M. ROBERTSON. The physiological basis of the periodic merging of area into background. *Amer. J. Psychiol.* 47 : *644–655* (1935).

FUORTES, M. G. F., R. D. GUNKEL & W. A. M. RUSHTON. Increment thresholds in a subject deficient in cone vision. *J. Physiol.* 156 : *179–192* (1961).

GAFNER, F. & H. GOLDMANN. Experimentelle Untersuchungen über den Zusammenhang von Augendrucksteigerung und Gesichtsfeldschädigung. *Ophthalmologica* 130 : *357–377* (1955).

GALAN, F. Normal fields of vision with Goldmann perimetry. *Mod. Probl. Ophthal.* 6 : *52–61* (1968).

GERRITS, H. J. M. & G. J. M. E. N. TIMMERMAN. The filling in process of patients with retinal scotomata. *Vision Res.* 9 : *439–442* (1969).

GLANVILLE, A. D. & K. M. DALLENBACH. The range of attention. *Amer. J. Psychol.* 41 : *207* (1929).

GLEZER, V. D. The receptive fields of the retina. *Vision Res.* 5 : *497–525* (1965).

GLIEM, H. Das Verhalten der Fixationsbewegungen bei herabgesetzten Helligkeit des Fixationsobjektes. *Klin. Mbl. Augenheilk.* 150 : *334–341* (1967).

GLOSTER, J. Flash perimetry. *Brit. J. Ophthal.* 54 : *649–658* (1970).

GOLDMANN, H. Ein selbstregistrierendes Projektions Kugelperimeter. *Ophthalmologica* 109 : *71–79* (1945).

—— Grundlagen exakter Perimetrie. *Ophthalmologica* 109 : *57–70* (1945).

—— Demonstration unseres neuen Projektions Kugelperimeter samt theoretischen und klinischen Bemerkungen über Perimetrie. *Ophthalmologica* 111 : *187–192* (1946).

—— Beitrag zur Angioskotometrie. *Ophthalmologica* 114 : *147–157* (1947).

—— Discussion du rapport de Dubois-Poulsen. *Bull. Soc. Franç. Ophtal.* 65 : *38–42* (1952).

—— La périmétrie en Oto-Neuro-Ophthalmologie. *Confinia Neurol.* 14: *102–125* (1954).

—— Die Erzeugung von Röhrengesichtsfeldern bei Normalen. *Mon. Schr. Psychol. Neurol.* 108 : *233* (1943).

—— Lichtsinn mit besonderer Berücksichtigung der Perimetrie. *Ophthalmologica* 158 : *362–386* (1969).

GOUGNARD, L. Etude des sommations spatiales chez le sujet normal par la périmetrie statique. *Ophthalmologica* 142 : *469–486* (1961).

GOURAS, P. Primate retina: Duplex function of darkadapted ganglion cells. *Science* 147 : *1593–1594* (1958).

—— Rod and cone independence in the electroretinogram of the dark adapted monkeys parafovea. *J. Physiol.* 187 : *455–464* (1966).

—— The effects of light adaptation on rod and cone receptive field organization of monkey ganglion cells. *J. Physiol.* 192 : *747–760* (1967).

—— & K. KIRK. Rod and cone interaction in dark-adapted monkey ganglioncells. *J. Physiol.* 184 : *499–510* (1965).

GRAEFE, A. VON. Ueber die Untersuchung des Gesichtsfeldes bei amblyopische Affektionen. *Graefes Arch. Ophthal.* 2 : *258–298* (1856).

GRAHAM, C. H. Vision and visual perception, John Wiley and sons, New York (1966).

—— & R. MARGARIA. Area and intensity-time relation in the peripheral retina. *Amer. J. Physiol.* 113 : *299–305* (1935).

—— & E. H. KEMP. Brightness discrimination as a function of the duration of the increment in intensity. *J. Gen. Physiol.* 21 : *635–650* (1938).

GRAHAM, C., H. R. BROWN & F. MOTE. The relation of size of stimulus and intensity in the human eye. I. Intensity thresholds for white light. *J. Exp. Psychol.* 24 : *555–573* (1939).

GRAHAM, C. H. & N. R. BARTLETT. The relation of size of stimulus and intensity in the human eye: II. Intensity thresholds for red and violet light. *J. Exp. Psychol.* 24 : *574–587* (1939).

GRANIT, R. & W. A. DAVIES. Comparative studies on the peripheral and central retina IV. Temporal summation of subliminal visual stimuli and the time course of the excitatory effect. *Amer. J. Physiol.* 98 : *644–653* (1933).

GREVE, E. L. Een onderzoek naar de waarde van snelle methoden voor gezichtsveldonderzoek. *Belg. Tijdschr. Geneesk.* 11 : *567–581* (1970).

—— On static perimetry. Proc. of meeting of N.O.G. (1971), to be published in *Ophthalmologica.*

—— Perimetry in glaucoma. Communication presented at the joined meeting of the Irish and Dutch Ophthalmological Societies, Dublin (1972).

—— Multiple stimulus static perimetry. Proc. of Meeting of the Congres of Europ. Ophthal. Soc. Budapest (1972).

—— Single stimulus and multiple stimulus threshold. *Vision. Res.* 12 : *1533–1543* (1972).

—— & G. F. KINDS. Snelle methoden voor gezichtsveldonderzoek I en II. *Ned. Mil. Tijdschr. Geneesk.* 23; 1 *10–23*; II : *69–86* (1970).

—— & G. VERRIEST. Theorie en techniek van het gezichtsveldonderzoek. Uitgave Stichting Wetenschappelijk Gezichtsveldonderzoek, Amsterdam (1971).

—— & W. M. VERDUIN. Mass visual field investigation of 1834 subjects with supposedly normal eyes. *Graefes Arch. Ophthal.* 183 : *286–293* (1972).

—— P. J. M. BOS., R. MESKER & M. LEDEBOER. Static perimetry and fluorangiography in central serous choriopathy. Prof. of Meeting of N.O.G. (1972), to be published.

—— & M. WIJNANS. The statistical variation of results in static campimetry and its consequences for multiple stimulus campimetry. *Ophthal. Res.* 4 : *355–367* (1973).

—— W. M. VERDUIN & M. LEDEBOER. The two-colour threshold in static perimetry. Read at the sec. Int. Symp. on Recent advances in colour vision deficiencies.; Edinburgh (1973).

GRINDLEY, G. C. & V. TOWNSEND. Voluntary attention in peripheral vision and its effects on acuity and differential thresholds. *Quart. J. exp. Psychol.* 20 : *11–19* (1968).

—— & —— Visual search without eye movement. *Quart. J. exp. Psychol.* 22 : *62–67* (1970).

GROENOW, A. Über die beste Form der Gesichtsfeldschemata. *Arch. Augenheilk.* 31 : *75–84* (1895).

GRÜSSER, O. J., U. GRÜSSER-CORNEHLIS & M. D. LICKER. Further studies on velocity function of movement detecting class-2-neurons in the frog retina. *Vison. Res.* 8 : *1173–1185* (1968).

GUILFORD, J. P. Fluctuations of attention with weak stimuli. *Amer. J. Psychol.* 38 : *534–583* (1927).

GUNKEL, R. D. & P. GOURAS. Changes in scotopic visibility thresholds with age. *Arch. Ophthal.* 69 : *4–9* (1963).

HALLETT, P. E., F. H. C. MARIOTT & F. C. RODGER. The relationship of visual threshold to retinal position and area. *J. Physiol.* 160 : *364–373* (1962).

HAGEDOORN, A. & CH. VAN DEN BOSCH. A double-projection campimeter. *Amer. J. Ophthal.* 40 : *324–326* (1955).

HARGROVES, J. A. & R. A. HARGROVES. Bibliography of work on flashing lights (1911–(1969). *Vis. Res.* suppl. 2 (1971).

HARMS, H. Objektive Perimetrie. *Ber. Dtsche. Ophthal. Ges.* 53 : *63–70* (1940).

—— Die Adaptationsprüfung bei gleichbleibenden Lichtempfindlichkeit des Auges. *Ber. Dtsche. Ophthal. Ges.* 55 : *291–295* (1949).

—— Grundlagen Methoden und Bedeutung der Pupillenperimetrie. *Graefes Arch. Ophthal.* 149 : *1–68* (1949).

—— Entwicklungsmöglichkeiten der Perimetrie. *Graefes Arch. Ophthal.* 150 : *28–57* (1950).

—— Die praktische Bedeutung quantitativer Perimetrie. *Klin. Mbl. Augenhk.* 121 : *683–692* (1952).

—— Das menschliche Auge als photometer. Publicado en 'Coloquio sobre problemas opticos de la vision' Bermejo-Madrid. Tomo II 1–11 (1953).

—— Neue Methoden der Perimetrie. Zeitfragen der Augenheilk. Thieme Leipzig. (1954).

—— Quantitative Perimetrie bei Sella- nahen Tumoren. *Ophthalmologica* 127 : *255–261* (1954).

—— Die Bedeutung veränderlichen Gesichtsfeldstörungen. *Ber. Dtsche. Ophthal. Ges.* 59 : *308–315* (1955).

—— Möglichkeit und Grenzen der pupillomotorischen Perimetrie. *Klin. Mbl. Augenheilk.* 129 : *518–534* (1956).

335

—— Lichtsinnuntersuchung als grundlegender Funktionsprüfung des Auges. *Studium Generale* 6 : *347–354* (1957).

—— Vergleichende Untersuchungen über den Wert der statischen Lichtsinn-Perimetrie, Skiaskotometrie und Verschmelzungsfrequenz für die Erkennung beginnenden Gesichtsfeldstörungen beim Glaukom. Conciclium *Ophthalmologicum* 18 : *883–892* (1958).

—— Die Bedeutung einer einheitlichen Prüfweise aller Sehfunktion. *Ber. Dtsche. Ophthal. Ges.* 63 : *281–285* (1960).

—— Gesichtsfeldstörungen und ihre Bedeutung für die neurologische Diagnostik. *Dtsche. Zeitschr. Nervenheilk.* 187 : *423–445* (1956).

—— Die Technik der statische Perimetrie. *Ophthalmologica* 158 : *387–405* (1969).

—— & E. AULHORN. Vergleichende Untersuchungen über den Wert der quantitativen Perimetrie, Skiaskotometrie und Verschmelzungsfrequenz für die Erkennung beginnender Gesichtsfeldstörungen beim Glaukom. *Doc. Ophthal.* 13 : *303–332* (1959).

HARRINGTON, D. O. & M. FLOCKS. Visual field examination by a new tachystoscopic multiple pattern method. *Amer. J. Ophthal.* 37 : *719–723* (1954).

—— & —— The multiple pattern method of visual field examination (a five year evaluation). *Arch. Ophthal.* 61 : *755–765* (1959).

HARTLINE, H. K. Intensity and duration in the excitation of single photoreceptor units. *J. Cellular Comp. Physiol.* 5 : *229–247* (1934).

—— The response of single optic fibers of the vertebrate eye to illumination of the retina. *Amer. J. Physiol.* 121 : *400–415* (1938).

—— The effects of spatial summation in the retina on the excitation of the fibers of the optic nerve. *Amer. J. Physiol.* 130 : *700–711* (1940).

—— The receptive fields of optic nerve fibers. *Amer. J. Physiol.* 130 : *690–699* (1940).

—— Light quanta and the excitation of single receptors in the eye of limulus. Proc. Int. Conf. Photobiol. Torino, 193 (1957).

HEILMANN, K. Augendruck, Blutdruck und Glaukomschaden. Bücherei des Augenarztes 61 : (1972).

HENKE, G., R. RÖHLER., F. FANKHAUSER & G. WALLMANN. Untersuchungen der Sehschärfe und die Kontrastempfindlichkeit unter Berücksichtigung der Netzhaut Bildstruktur. *Optik* 23 : *56* (1965).

HILTON, G. The multiple pattern visual field screener: an evaluation. *Amer. J. Optom.* 35 : *314–320* (1958).

HUBEL, D. H. The visual cortex of the brain. *Scientific American* 168 : *1–11* (1963).

—— & TH. WIESEL. Receptive fields of single neurons in the cats striate cortex. *J. Physiol.* 148 : *574–592* (1959).

—— & —— Receptive field of optic nerve fibers in the spider monkey. *J. Physiol.* 154 : *572–580* (1960).

—— & —— Integrate activity in the cat's lateral geniculate body. *J. Physiol.* 155 : *385–398* (1961).

—— & —— Receptive fields, binocular interaction and functional architecture in the cat's visual cortex. *J. Physiol.* 160 : *106–154* (1962).

—— & —— Receptive fields and functional architecture of monkey striate cortex. *J. Physiol.* 195 : *215–243* (1958).

HUNTER, W. & M. SIEGLER. The span of visual discrimination as a function of time and intensity of stimulation. *J. Exp. Psychol.* 26 : *160–179* (1940).

IKEDA, M. Temporal summation of positive and negative flashes in the visual system. *J. Opt. Soc. Amer.* 55 : *1527–1534* (1965).

ISHII, cited in DUKE ELDER vol. II. The anatomy of the visual system. H. Kimpton, London (1961).

ISRAEL, A. Perimetric study of the blind spot, with static perimetry. *Mod. Probl. Ophthal.* 6 : *62–72* (1968).

JACOBS, G. H. Receptive fields in visual systems. *Brain. Res.* 14 : *553–573* (1969).

JACQUES, R. Ueber die Grösse des blinden Flecks bei aphakischen Augen. *Ophthalmologica* 113 : *365–374* (1947).

JAY, B. S. The effective pupillary area at varying perimetric angles. *Vision. Res.* 1 : *418–424* (1961).

JAYLE, G. E. Bases physiologiques et valeur clinique de la périmétrie qualitative et des isoptères équivalents d'adaptation. Le check-up périmétrique et l'Explorateur du sens lumineux. *Arch. Ophtal (Paris)* 20 : *685–705* (1960).

—— Le Check-up périmétrie. *Année Ther. Clin. Ophtal.* 11 : *67* (1960).

—— Note préliminaire sur la courbe de gradient relevée en luminance mésopique. *Bull. Soc. Ophtal. Fr.* 68 : *833–834* (1968).

—— La périmétrie mésopique exacte. *Ber. Dtsche. Ophthal. Ges.* 71 : *491–495* (1971).

—— & A. OURGAUD. Campimétrie du grand myope sans verre, avec correction habituelle et avec verres de contact. *Bull. Soc. Ophtal. Fr.* 53 : *513–515* (1953).

—— A. CROISY, .N. FRANCHINI., J. LEROUX & J. SAUVAN. La périmétrie en pratique ophthalmologique (A propos de 1680 champs visuels) *Arch. Ophtal.* 15 : *138–163* (1955).

—— G. BLET., L. AUBERT., R. BOYER & P. LOZIVIT. Note préliminaire sur l'intérêt de la campimétrie en pathologie oculaire. *Ann. Oculist* 189 : *108–166* (1957).

—— & L. AUBERT. Le Champ visuel mésopique en pathologie oculaire. Actualités Latines d'Ophtalmologie. Masson, Paris, 50–115 (1958).

—— —— R. BOYER & J. VOLA. Etude d'un isoptère photopique, mésopique et scotopique standard et de l'une de ses harmoniques photométriques avec ou sans flicker du fond relevé a l'explorateur de sens lumineux de Jayle et Blet. *Arch. Ophtal. (Paris)* 194 : *881–891* (1961).

—— J. VOLA., L. AUBERT & J. FANTIN. La périmétrie qualitative cinétique. Bases physiologiques et intérêt clinique. Le check-up périmétrique standard. *Cision. Res.* 3 : *253–267* (1963).

—— —— —— & G. BRACCINI. Etudes des seuils différentiels en périmétrie statique sur le méridien nasal inférieur. *Arch. Ophtal. (Paris)* 25 : *65–78* (1965).

—— & P. METGE. Champ visuel du glaucomateux. Notions récentes. *Année Ther. Clin. Ophtal.* 18 : *53–87* (1967).

—— & G. A. M. MARTIN. Caracteristique et intérêt de l'adaptocampimétrie. *Bull. Soc. Ophtal. Fr.* 68 : *170–173* (1968).

—— —— & B. MERMET. Note préliminaire sur la courbe de gradient relevée en luminance mésopique haute sur le méridian de 225°–450°. *Bull. Soc. Ophtal. Fr.* 68 : *833–834* (1968).

—— A. OURGAUD & P. METGE. La périmétrie statique circulaire dans le glaucome. *Arch. Ophtal. (Paris)* 29 : *513–520* (1969).

337

JONKERS, G. H. Quantitatieve en topografische perimetrie. *Ned. Tijdschr. v. Geneesk.* 94 : *2878–2883* (1950).

—— Perimetrie bij het aan de schemer en donker geadapteerde oog. *Ned. Tijdschr. v. Geneesk.* 95 : *1951–1954* (1951).

—— The isopters and the sensibility gradient of the dark adapted eye. Acta XVII Conc. Ophthal. III, 1786–1795 Toronto Press (1955).

KANEKO, A. Physiological and morphological identification of horizontal, bipolar and amacrine cells in goldfish retina. *J. Physiol.* 207 : *623–629* (1971).

KARN, H. W. Area and the intensity-time relation in the fovea. *J. Gen. Psychol.* 14 : *360–369* (1936).

KATZ, M. S. Brief flash brightness. *Vision. Res.* 4 : *361–373* (1964).

KAUFMAN, E. L., M. W. LORD., T. W. REESE & J. VOLKMAN. The discrimination of visual number. *Amer. J. Psychol.* 65 : *468–473* (1963).

MC KEE, S. & G. WESTHEIMER. Specificity of cone mechanisms in lateral interaction. *J. Physiol.* 256 : *117–128* (1970).

KELLER, M. The relation between the critical duration and intensity in brightness dicrimination. (Die Beziehung zwischen der kritischen Dauer und Intensität bei der Helligkeitsunderscheidung). *J. Exp. Psychol.* 28 : *407–418* (1941).

KISHTO, B. N. & R. SAUNDERS. Variation of visual threshold with retinal location. I. The central 20° of visual field. II. The fovea. *Vision. Res.* 10 : *745–767* (1970).

KLEMMER, E. T. The perception of linear dot patterns. *J. Exp. Psychol.* *468–473* (1963).

KOHLRAUSCH, A. Untersuchungen mit farbigen Schwellen Prüflichtern über den Dunkeladaptationsverlauf des normalen Auges. *Pflügers Arch. Ges. Physiol.* 196 : *113–117* (1922).

KOMMERELL, G. Binasale Refraktionsskotome. *Klin. Mbl. Augenheilk.* 154 : *85–88* (1969).

KRAUSKOPF, J. Light distribution in human retinal images. *J. Opt. Soc. Amer.* 52 : *1046–1050* (1962).

—— Further measurements of human retinal images. *J. Opt. Soc. Amer.* 54 : *715–716* (1964).

KUFFLER, S. W. Neurons in the retina: organization, inhibition and excitation problems. *Cold Spring Harbor Symposia on quantitative biology* 17 : *281–292* (1952).

KUHN, N. S. Glaucoma detection in industry. *Industr. Med.* 26 : *327–330* (1957).

LANDESBERG, D. Casuitische Mitteilungen II: Ausbruch von Glaucoom in Folge eines Streifschusses. Eigentümliche Gesichtsfeldbeschränkung. *Graefes Arch. Ophthal.* 15 : *204–210* (1869).

LANSFORD, T. G. & H. D. BAKER. Dark adaptation: an interocular lightadaptation effect. *Science* 164 : *1307–1309* (1969).

LAVERGNE, G. & M. T. DE CORTE. La détermination de l'exposant de sommation par la mésure de la fréquence critique de fusion. *Vision. Res.* 10 : *351–358* (1970).

LEGRAND, Y. Optique physiologique II. Lumière et couleurs. ed. de la 'Revue d'Optique' Paris, 296–297 (1948).

LEMMON, V. W. & S. M. GEISINGER. Reaction time under light and darkadaptation. *Amer. J. Psychol.* 48 : *140–144* (1936).

LEVELT, W. On binocular rivalry. Thesis. IZF-RVO-TNO Soesterberg (1965).

LEVICK, W. R., C. W. OYSTER & D. L. DAVIS. Evidence that Mc Illwain's periphery effect is not a stray light artifact. *J. Neurophysiol.* 28 : *555–559* (1965).

LICHTENSTEIN, M. & C. WHITE. Relative visual latency as a function of retinal locus. *J. Opt. Soc. Amer.* 51 : *1033–1034* (1961).

LIE, I. The momentary sensitivity contour of the retina, an approach to the study of attention. *Stud. Psychol.* 11 : *157–160* (1969).

LIEBMAN, P. A. & G. ENTINE. Visual pigments of frog and tadpole. *Vision Res.* 8 : *761–775* (1968).

LINFIELD, P. Industrial screening for the early detection of glaucoma. Read at the Int. Ophthal. Opt. Congress. April 1970.

LITH, G. H. M. VAN. Simultane Bestimmung der elektro-retinographischen und sensorischen Reizschwelle. *Vision. Res.* 6 : *185–197* (1966).

LONG, S. E. The effect of the duration of onset and cessation of light flash on the intensity time relation in the peripheral retina. *J. Opt. Soc. Amer.* 14 : *743–747* (1951).

LYNE, A. J. & C. I. PHILLIPS. Visual field defects due to opacities in the optical media. *Brit. J. Ophthal.* 53 : *119–122* (1969).

LUDWICH, E. & E. F. MC CARTHY. Absorption of visible light by the refractive media of the human eye. *Arch. Ophthal.* 20 : *37–51* (1938).

MAC FARLAND, R. A. Experimental evidence of the relationship between aging and oxygen want: In search of a theory of aging. *Ergonomics* 6 : *339* (1963).

MAC IIWAIN, J. T. Receptive fields of optic tract axons and lateral geniculate cells; peripheral extent and barbiturate sensitivity. *J. Neurophysiol.* 27 : *1154–1173* (1964).

MACKWORTH, J. F. The relation between the visual image and post-perceptual immediate memory. *J. Verb. Learn. Verb. Behav.* 2 : *75–85* (1963).

MAC MARTIN, L. S. & F. L. DIMMICK. Mapping the central scotoma of the dark adapted retina: comparison of a moving stimulus with a stationary presentation. MRL Report no. 150 8 : *94–112* (1949).

MAGIS, C. Du champ visuel. *Ann. Oculist* 190 : *322–358* (1957).

MALBRAN, J. Sobre la perimetria. *Ar. de. O.B.A.* 6 : *353–372* (1931).

—— Campo Visual, normal y patologico, ed. II El Alteneo, Buenos Aires (1936).

MANDELBAUM, J. & E. NELSON. Rod activity at photopic intensities. *Arch. Ophthal.* 63 : *402–408* (1960).

MANN, I. & F. W. SHARPLEY. The normal visual (rod) field of the dark adapted eye. *J. Physiol.* 106 : *301–304* (1947).

MARLOW, S. B. Visual field in chronic glaucoma: the effect of reduced illumination. *Arch. Ophthal.* 7 : *211–223* (1932).

MARKS, W. B. Visual pigments of single goldfish cones. *J. Physiol.* 178 : *14–32* (1965).

MASSIN, M. & J. PIOT. L'enregistrement du champ visuel des aphaques et des grands myopes au moyen des lentilles cornéennes. *Bull. Soc. Ophtal France* 63 : *161–173* (1963).

MARTIN, L. Binocular summation at the absolute threshold of peripheral vision. *J. Opt. Soc. Amer.* 52 : *1276–1286* (1962).

MAZZANTINI, L. Conclusione tra eta e estensione del campo visivo. *Boll. Oculist* 42 : (7) *407–422* (1963).

—— & A. WIRTH. Influenza del diametro pupillare sull' estenzione del campo visivo. *Boll. Oculist* 41 : *387–397* (1962).

—— & G. TOTA. L'acuità visiva e il campo visivo a bassa luminanza nelle alterationi maculair con appatente integrità funzionale. *Boll. Oculist* 44 : *909–923* (1965).

339

MELLERIO, J. Light absorption and scatter in the human lens. *Vision. Res.* 11 : *129–141* (1971).

MERTENS, J. J. Influence of knowledge of target location upon probability of observation of peripherally observable test flashes. *J. Opt. Soc. Amer.* 46 : *1069–1070* (1956).

MEUR, G. Contribution à l'étude des sommations spatiales retiniennes. *Ann. Oculist.* 198 : *436–447* (1965).

—— Etude des variations inter- et intra-individuelles des seuils absolus locale retiniens. *Vision. Res.* 5 : *435–442* (1965).

MEYTHALER, H. & W. RUPPERT. Vergleichenden Untersuchungen über den myopisierenden und miotischen Effekt von Pilocarpin und Aceclydine (Glaucostat). *Graefes Arch. Ophthal.* 181 : *234–245* (1971).

MICHAEL, C. R. Receptive fields of single optic nerve fibers in a mammal with an all-cone retina. *J. Neurophysiol.* 31 : *257–267* (1968).

—— Retinal processing of visual images. *Scientific American* 174 : *105–114* (1969).

MILLER, G. A. The magical number seven, plus or minus two. *Psychol. Rev.* 63 : *81–97* (1956).

MILLODOT, M. The effect of lenses on light transmission. *Amer. J. Optom.* 47 : *211–216* (1970).

MONJÉ, M. & R. OFFERMANN. Ueber die Empfindlichkeit der Netzhaut bei Refraktionsanomalien. *Graefes Arch. Ophthal.* 155 : *63–78* (1954).

MONTERO, V. M. & J. F. BRUGGE. Direction of movement as the significant stimulus parameter for some lateral geniculate cells of the rat. *Vision Res.* 9 : *71–87* (1969).

MOSES, R. A. Adler's physiology of the eye 5th edition C.V. Mosby. Saint Louis (1970).

MOTE, F. A. & A. J. RIOPELLE. The effect of varying the intensity and the duration of preexposure upon subsequent dark adaptation in the human eye. *J. Comp. Physiol. Psychol.* 46 : *49–55* (1953).

NIESEL, P. Die Streuung perimetrischen Untersuchungsergebnisse. *Ophthalmologica* 161 : *180–186* (1970).

NORTON, A. L., H. SPEKREIJSE, M. L. WOLBARSHT & H. G. WAGNER. Receptive field organisation of the S-potential. *Science* 160 : *1021–1022* (1968).

OBSTFELD, H. Spatial summation in static perimetry. *Ophthalmic Optician*, 11 : *214–229* (1971).

OGLE, K. N. Blurring of the retinal image and contrast threshold in the fovea. *J. Opt. Soc. Amer.* 50 : *307–315* (1960).

—— Foveal contrast thresholds with blurring of the retinal image and increasing size of test stimulus. *J. Opt. Soc. Amer.* 51 : *862–869* (1961).

—— Blurring of retinal image and foveal contrast thresholds of separated point light sources. *J. Opt. Soc. Amer.* 52 : *1035–1039* (1962).

OPPEL, O. Untersuchungen über die Verteilung und Zahl der retinalen Ganglionzellen beim Menschen. *Graefes Arch. Ophthal.* 172 : *1–22* (1967).

ØSTERBERG, G. A. Topography of the layer of rods and cones in the human retina. *Acta Ophthal (Kbh.)* Suppl. 6 (1935).

OURGAUD, A. G. & L. AUBERT. Adaptométrie topographique circulaire chez le sujet normal. *Bull. Soc. Ophtal. Fr.* 59 : *528–532* (1959).

OURGAUD, A. G., J. B. SARACCO., P. METGE & G. MARTIN. Confrontation entre la périmétrie statique méridienne et circulaire à 15° dans le glaucome primitif. *Bull. Soc. France Ophtal.* 81 : *480–492* (1968).

PANTLE, A. J. & W. SEKULER. Velocity-sensitive elements in human vision: psychophysical evidence. *Vision. Res.* 8 : *445–450* (1968).

PANTLE, A. & R. SEKULER. Contrast response of human visual mechanisms sensitive to orientation and direction of motion. *Vision. Res.* 9 : *397–406* (1969).

PATEL, A. S. & R. W. JONES. Increment and decrement visual thresholds. *J. Opt. Soc. Amer.* 58 : *696–699* (1968).

PAYNE, W. Visual reaction times on a circle about the fovea. *Science* 155 : *481–482* (1967).

PETER, L. The principles and practice of perimetry. ed. 3 Philadelphia, Lea & Febiger. (1931).

PFLÜGER, E. Wie verhalten sich einige Glaukom-Symptome zur Drucktheorie? *Ber. Dtsche. Ophthal. Ges.* 17 : *91–101* (1885).

PIERON, H. De la variation de l'énergie liminaire en fonction de la surface rétinienne excitée pour la vision foveale et de l'influence réciproque de la durée et de la surface d'excitation sur la sommation spatiale ou temporelle pour la vision foveale et périphérique. *C. R. Réanc. Soc. Biol.* 83 : *1072–1076* (1920).

PIPER, H. Ueber die Abhängigkeit des Reizwertes leuchtender Objekten von ihrer Flächen- bzw. Winkelgrösse. *Z. Psych. u. Physiol. Sinnesorg.* 32 : *98–112* (1903).

PIRENNE, M. Visual functions in man. In: The Eye II. The Visual Process. Parts I. ed. H. Davson, New York Academic Press, New York. (1962).

POLLOCK, W, T. The visibility of a target as a function of its speed of movement. *J. exp. Psychol.* 45 : *449–454* (1953).

POLYAK, S. L. The retina. Univ. of Chic. Press. (1941).

RATLIFF, F., H. K. HARTLINE & W. M. MILLER. Spatial and temporal aspects of retinal inhibitory interaction. *J. Opt. Soc. Amer.* 53 : *110–120* (1963).

REED, H. & S. M. DRANCE. The essentials of perimetry. Oxford University Press, London 2nd edition (1972).

REMPT, F., J. HOOGERHEIDE & W. HOOGEBOOM. Peripheral retinoscopy and the skiagram. *Ophthalmologica* 162 : *1–10* (1971).

RICCO, A. Relazione fra il minimo angola visuale e l'intensita luminosa. *Ann. Ottal.* 6 : *373–479* (1877).

—— Ueber die Beziehungen zwischen den kleinsten Sehwinkel und die Intensität. *Zentr. Blatt. Prakt. Augenheilk.* 1 : *122–126* (1877).

RIDDOCH, G. Dissociation of visual perceptions due to occipital injuries with a special reference to appreciation of movement. *Brain* 40 : *15–58* (1917).

RIGGS, L. A. Visual acuity. In Vision and Visual Perception .ed. C. H. Graham, John Wiley & Sons, New York, 321–349 (1966).

—— F. RATLIFF., J. C. CORNSWEET & T. D. CORNSWEET. The disappearance of steadily fixated visual test objects. *J. Opt. Soc. Amer.* 43 : *495–501* (1953).

—— J. C. ARMINGTON & F. RATLIFF. Motions of the retinal image during fixation. *J. Opt. Soc. Amer.* 44 : *315–321* (1954).

ROBERTS, W. Early diagnosis of primary glaucoma. *Amer. J. Ophthal.* 44 : *24–38* (1957).

ROBERTSON, L. T. Use of the Harrington-Pattern field screener in industry. *Trans. Amer. Acad. Ophthal.* 60 : *806–811* (1956).

ROCK, W. J., S. M. DRANCE & R. W. MORGAN. A modification of the Armaly visual field screening technique for glaucoma. *Canad. J. Ophthal.* 6 : *283–292* (1971).

RODIECK, R. W. & J. STONE. Analysis of receptive fields of cat retinal ganglion cells. *J. Neurophysiol.* 28 : *833–849* (1965).

RÖHLER, R. Die Abbildungseigenschaften der Augenmedian. *Vision. Res.* 2 : *391–429* (1962).

—— Bestimmung der Lichtverteilung auf die Netzhaut bei Abbildung einfacher Testobjekte. *Optik* 23 : *47–55* (1965).

RØNNE, H. Ueber das Gesichtsfeld beim Glaukom. *Klin. Mbl. Augenheilk.* 47 : *12–33* (1909).

RÖSSLER, F. 'Die Höhenstellung des blinden Fleckes in normalen Augen'. *Arch. f. Augenheilk.* 86 : *55–86* (1920).

ROUFS, J. Perception lag as a function of stimulus luminance. *Vision. Res.* 3 : *81–91* (1963).

—— On the relation between the threshold of short flashes, the flicker fusion frequency and the visual latency. *IPO Annual Progress Report* 1 : *69–77* (1966).

—— & H. J. MEULENBRUGGE. The quantitative relations between flash threshold and flicker-fusion boundary for centrally fixated fields. *IPO Annual Progress Report* 2 : *133–139* (1967).

RUSHTON, W. A. H. Les problèmes neurophysiologiques de la rétine des vertébrés. Symp. Int. Méc. Fond. Discr. Chrom. Paris (1958).

—— Increment threshold and dark adaptation. *J. Opt. Soc. Amer.* 53 : *104–109* (1963).

—— Visual adaptation. *Proc. Roy. Soc. (Lond.)* B 162 : *20–46* (1965).

RUDDOCK, K. H. The effect of age upon colour vision II. Changes with age in light transmission of the ocular media. *Vision. Res.* 47–58 (1965).

RUSHTON, W. A. H. & K. D. COHEN. Visual purple level and the course of dark adaptation. *Nature (Lond).* 173 : *301–302* (1954).

—— F. W. CAMPBELL., W. A. HAGINS & G. S. BRINDLEY. The bleaching and regeneration of rhodopsin in the living eye of the albino rabiit and of man. *Optica Acta* 1 : *183–190* (1955).

SAID, F. S. & R. A. WEALE. The variation with age of the spectral transmissivity of the living human crystalline lens. *Gerontologia* 3 : *213–231* (1959).

SALZER, F. Überblichsperimetrie. *Klin. Mbl. Augenheilk.* 78 : *6–15* (1927).

SCHMIDT, TH. Kurzes repetitorium der klinischen Perimetrie. *Ophthalmologica* 149 : *250–265* (1965).

—— Über die Verdopplung der Untersuchungsdistanz am Goldmann Perimeter. *Doc. Ophthal.* 26 : *286–294* (1969).

—— Perimetrie relativer Skotome. *Ophthalmologica* 129 : *303–315* (1955).

—— Über die Testmarkengeschwindigkeit und ein neues Registriergerät zum Goldmann Perimeter. *Ophthalmologica* 163 : *120–128* (1971).

—— & S. SCHMIDT-BERGHOFER. Über die Möglichkeiten einer genaueren Registrierung am Goldmann Perimeter. *Ophthalmologica* 151 : *435–439* (1961).

SCHMIDT, D., A. REUSCHER & G. KOMMERELL. Über das nasale Gesichtsfeld bei Strabismus fixus divergens. *Graefes Arch. Ophthal.* 183 : *97–105* (1971).

SCHOBER, H. Ein neues Weiss- und Farbenkampimeter mit einem auch zur Schielprüfung geeigneten Schirm. *Klin. Mbl. Augenheilk.* 115 : *149–157* (1949).

SCHUBERT, G. & H. BORNSCHEIN. Beitrag zur Analyse des menschlichen Elektroretinogramms. *Ophthalmologica* 123 : *396–413* (1952).

SEIDEL, E. Beiträge zur Frühdiagnose des Glaukoms. *Graefes Arch. Ophthal.* 88 : *102–157* (1914).

SEKULER, R. W. & L. GANZ. After effect of seen motion with a stabilized retinal image. *Science* 139 : *419–420* (1963).

—— E. L. RUBIN & W. H. CUSHMAN. Selectivities of human visual mechanisms for direction of movement and contour orientation. *J. Opt. Soc. Amer.* 58 : *1146–1150* (1968).

SHIGA, S. Visual field changes with loaded illumination. *Amer. J. Ophthal.* 66 : *245–263* (1968).

SLOAN, L. L. Instruments and technics for the clinical testing of light sense II. Control of fixation in the dark-adapted eye. *Arch. Ophthal.* 22 : *228–232* (1939).

—— Instruments and techniques for the clinical testing of light sense. III. An apparatus for studying regional differences in light sense. *Arch. Ophthal.* 22 : *233–251* (1939).

—— Rate of dark adaptation and regional threshold gradient of the dark adapted eye: physiologic and clinical studies. *Amer. J. Ophthal.* 30 : *705–720* (1947).

SLOAN, L. L. The threshold gradients of the rods and the cones: in the dark-adapted and in the partially light-adapted eye. *Amer. J. Ophthal.* 33 : *1077–1089* (1950).

SLOAN, L. L. An explanation for the poor performance of aphakic patients on the Harrington-Flocks screening test. *Amer. J. Ophthal.* 41 : *987–989* (1956).

—— Area and luminance of test object as variables in examination of the visual field by projection perimetry. *Vision. Res.* 1 : *121–138* (1961).

—— & D. J. BROWN. Area and luminance of test object as variables in projection perimetry. *Vision. Res.* 2 : *527–541* (1962).

—— The Tübinger perimeter of Harms and Aulhorn. *Arch. Ophthal.* 86 : *612–623* (1971).

SPEKREYSE, H., L. H. VAN DER TWEEL & D. REGAN. Interocular sustained suppression: correlations with evoked potential amplitude and distribution. *Vision Res.* 12 : *521–526* (1972).

—— See NORTON et al.

SPERLING, G. The information available in brief visual presentations. Psychol. Monographs 74 : no. 11 (1960).

SPERLING, H. G. & C. L. JOLLIFFE. Intensity-time relationship at threshold for spectral stimuli in human vision. *J. Opt. Soc. Amer.* 55 : *191–199* (1965).

SPILLMAN, L. & G. V. GAMBONE. A test of the Mac Illwain effect in man. *Vision. Res.* 11 : *751–755* (1971).

SPRING, K. M. & W. G. STILES. Variation of pupil size with change in the angle at which the light stimulus strikes the retina. *Brit. J. Ophthal.* 32 : *340–346* (1948).

SPRING, K. H. & W. G. STILES. Apparent shape and size of the pupil viewed obliquely. *Brit. J. Ophthal.* 32 : *347–354* (1948).

STILES, W. G. Colourvision: the approach through increment threshold sensitivity. *Proc. Nat. Ac. Sciences* 45 : *100–114* (1959).

—— & B. H. CRAWFORD. The luminous efficiency of rays entering the eye pupil at different points. *Proc. Roy. Soc. (Lond.)* 112B : *428–450* (1933).

STONE, J. & M. FABIAN. Specialized receptive fields of the cat's retina. *Science* 152 : *1277–1279* (1966).

STURR, J. F. Neural limitations of visual excitability VIII Binocular convergence in cat geniculate and cortex. *Vision. Res.* 6 : *401–418* (1966).

SUNGA, R. N. & J. M. ENOCH. A static perimetric technique believed to test receptive field properties. III. Clinical trials. *Amer. J. Ophthal.* 70 : *244–274* (1970).

343

—— & —— Further perimetric analysis of patients with lesions of the visual pathways. *Amer. J. Ophthal.* 70 : *403–422* (1970).

SUTCLIFFE, R. L. The Fincham-Sutcliffe screening scotometer. *Optician* 145 : *261–287* (1963).

—— & H. C. BINSTEAD. The development of improved methods of examining visual fields with special reference to routine visual field screening. Trans. Int. Ophthal. Optic. Congress. Hofner, New York. 379–401 (1961).

SWAN, W. On the gradual production of luminous impressions on the eye and other phenomenons of vision. *Trans. Roy. Soc. Edin.* 16 : *581–602* (1849).

THIEBAULT, F., L. GUILLAUMAT & P. BREGEAT. L'hémianopsie relative. *Rev. Neur.* 77 : *129* (1945).

THOMAS, J. P. Relation of brightness contrast to inducing stimulus outputs. *J. Opt. Soc. Amer.* 53 : *1033–1037* (1963).

—— Brightness-contrast effects among several points of light. *J. Optom. Soc. Amer.* 55 : *323–327* (1965).

—— & C. W. KOVAR. The effect of contour sharpness on perceived brightness. *Vision. Res.* 5 : *559–564* (1965).

TRAQUAIR, H. M. Clinical detection of early changes in the visual field. *Arch. Ophthal.* 22 : *947–967* (1939).

—— The nerve fiber bundle defect. *Trans. Ophthal. Soc. U.K.* 64 : *3–23* (1944).

—— Clinical perimetry. Henry Kimpton London. 7th edition. (1957).

TROXLER, D. Uber das Verschwinden gegebener Gegenstände innerhalb unseres Gesichtskreisses. *Ophthal. Bibliothek* 2 : *51–53* (1804).

VERPLANCK, W. S. Previous training as a determinant of response dependency at the threshold. *J. Exp. Psychol.* 46 : *10–14* (1953).

—— & J. COTTON. The dependence of frequencies of seeing on procedural variables: I. Direction and length of series of intensity-ordered stimuli. *J. Gen. Psychol.* 53 : *37–47* (1955).

—— & S. BLOUGH. Randomized stimuli and the non-independence of successive responses at the visual thresholds. *J. Gen. Psychol.* 59 : *263–272* (1958).

VERRIEST, G. Studie over de achromatische gezichtsfuncties in de congenitale sensoriele anomalieën van het menselijk oog bij en sommige amphibia en reptilia. Dr. W. Junk B.V. Den Haag (1960).

—— L'influence de l'âge sur les fonctions visuelles de l'homme. *Bul. de l'académie royale de medicine de Belgique* VIIe série; tome XI; no. 8. p. *527–577* (1971).

—— & A. ISRAELS. Application du périmètre statique de Goldmann au relève topografique des seuils différentiels de luminances pour de petits objets colorés projetés sur un fond blanc. *Vision. Res.* 5 : *151–174* (1965).

—— & J. L. LAVALLÉE. Les variations de la durée d'adaptation locale chez les sujets normaux et dans les conditions d'une périmétrie statique avec fixation non stabilisée. *Revue d'Optique* 12 : *533–552* (1966).

—— & A. ORTIZ-OLMEDO. Etude comparative du seuil différentiel de luminance et de l'exposant de sommation spatiale pour des objets pleins et pour des objets annulaires de mêmes surfaces. *Vision. Res.* 9 : *267–292* (1969).

—— P. PADMOS & E. L. GREVE. Calibration of the Tübingen perimeter for colour perimetry. Proc. Sec. Int. Symp. on Recent advances in colour vision deficiencies. Edinburgh (1973).

344

WALD, G. Participation of rods and cones in visual responses. *J. Opt. Soc. Amer.* 51 : *241–243* (1961).

WARRINGTON, E. Disorders of visual perception in patients with cerebral lesion. *Neuropsychologica* 5 : *253–266* (1967).

WEALE, R. A. The aging eye. H. K. Lewis & Co Ltd. London (1903).

—— Visual function of the retinal periphery. Proc. XIII CIE congres Zurich (1955).

—— Problems of peripheral vision. *Brit. J. Ophthal.* 40 : *392–415* (1956).

—— Retinal summation and human visual thresholds. *Nature (Lond.)* 181 : *154–156* (1958).

WEEKERS, J. Contribution à l'étude de la périmétrie statique. *Arch. Ophthal. (Paris)* 29 : 47–56 (1969).

WEEKERS, R. & M. HUMBLET. L'angioscotome physiologique. *Ophthalmologica* 110 : *43–59* (1945).

—— & F. ROUSSEL. Utilisation de la campimétrie en lumiere attennée pour la mésure de l'adaptation retinienne à l'obscurité. *Ophthalmologica* 110 : *242–258* (1945).

—— & —— Introduction à l'étude de la fréquence de fusion en clinique. *Ophthalmologica* 112 : *305–319* (1946).

—— & G. LAVERGNE. Applications cliniques de la périmétrie statique *Bull. Soc. Belge Ophtal.* 119 : *418–430* (1958).

WEINSTEIN, C. & A. ARNULF. Contribution à l'étude des seuils de perception de l'oeil. *Commun. Inst. Opt.* 2 : *1–43* (1946).

WELT, M. Etude sur les rapports entre les dimensions de la tache aveugle de Mariotte et des angioscotomes et la tension artérielle rétinienne. *Ophthalmologica.* 190 : *137–158* (1945).

WENCKER, B. L'analyseur périmétrique quantitatif de Friedmann ses applications en pratique ophthalmologique. Thèse Paris. (1970).

WERBLIN, F. & J. DOWLING. Organization of the retina of the mudpuppy, Necturus maculosus II intracellular recording. *J. Neurophysiol.* 32 : *339–355* (1969).

WESSING, A. Fluoreszenzangiographie den retina, Thimee Verlag Stuttgart (1968).

WESTHEIMER, G. Spatial interaction in the human retina during scotopic vision. *J. Physiol.* 181 : *881–894* (1965).

—— Lateral inhibition in the human rod retina. Performance of the eye 1966. Low luminances. Ex. Med. Int. Congr. no. 125 53–56.

—— Spatial interaction in human cone vision. *J. Physiol.* 190 : *139–154* (1967).

—— Bleached rhodopsin and retinal interaction. *J. Physiol.* 195 : *97–105* (1968).

—— Visual acuity and spatial modulation thresholds. In: Handbook of Sensory Physiology VII/4: Visual Psychophysics. ed. D. JAMESON, L. M. HURVICH, Springer, Berlin, 170–187 (1972).

—— & F. W. CAMPBELL. Light distribution in the image formed by the living human eye. *J. Opt. Soc. Amer.* 52 : *1040–1046* (1962).

WEYMOUTH, F. Visual sensory units and the minimal angle of resolution. *Amer. J. Ophthal.* 46 : *102–113* (1958).

WHITTLE, P. & P. D. C. CHALLANDS. The effect of background luminance on the brightness of flashes. *Vision. Res.* 9 : *1095–1110* (1969).

WILSON, M. E. Spatial and temporal summation in impaired regions of the visual field. *J. Physiol.* 189 : *189–208* (1967).

WOLFF, E. The anatomy of the eye and orbit. Oxford Med. Publ. (1948).

—— Glare and age. *Arch. Ophthal.* 64 : *502–514* (1960).

—— Studies of the shrinkage of the visual field with age. Annual Meeting of Highway Research Board. 17–19 (1966).

—— & J. GARDINER. Sensitivity of the retinal area in one eye corresponding to the blind spot in the other eye. *J. Opt. Soc. Amer.* 53 : *1437–1440* (1963).

YARBUS, A. L. The perception of a stabilized retinal image. *Biofizika* 1 : *435–437* (1956).

ZAPPIA, R. J., J. M. ENOCH., R. STAMPER,. J. Z. WINKELMAN & A. I. GAY. The Riddoch-phenomenon revealed in non-occipital lobe lesions. *Brit. J. Ophthal.* 55 : *416–420* (1971).

ZEHNDER-ALBRECHT, S. Zur standardizierung der Perimetrie. *Ophthalmologica* 120 : *253–270* (1950).

ZUEGE, P. & S. M. DRANCE. Studies of dark adaptation of discrete paracentral retinal areas in glaucomatous subjects. *Amer. J. Ophthal.* 64 : *56–63* (1967).

INDEX

Kinetic perimetry and Visual Field Analyser, 196
Kinetic perimetry in visual field defects, 107

L

Law of Bloch, 37
Laws of spatial summation, 31
Lens, 206, 208
Light sensitivity, 5, 49
Local adaptation, 41
Local adaptation and temporal summation, 38
Localized reduction of sensitivity, 223
Luminance, critical, 110
Luminance, distribution of, 12
Luminance before examination, 10
Luminance, logarithmic steps of, 11
Luminance maximum, 110
Luminance range in multiple stimulus presentation, 200
Luminance of stimulus, 11
Luminance of stimuli of Visual Field Analyser, 182

M

Marginal contrast gradient, 210
Maximum luminance, intensity for, 220
Mesopization, 206, 208
Mesopic adaptation levels, 64, 208
Mesopic adaptation and preretinal factors, 71
Mesopic adaptation and pupil, 206
Mesopic campimetry, 66
Mesopic examination and ametropia, 65
Mesopic kinetic examination, 66
Mesopic level of adaptation, 28
Mesopic perimetry and glaucoma, 68
Mesopic sensitivity curve, definition, 28
Method of Armaly, 200
Method of constant stimuli, 5, 6
Method of Gloster, 202
Method of Harrington-Flocks, 171
Method of limits, 5, 6
Method of measurement, 5
Miosis, senile, 145
Miotics, 214
Miotics and myopia, 214
Movement and kinetic perimetry, 49
Movement, standardization of, 14
Movement of stimulus, 13, 42
Movement, successive lateral spatial summation, 52, 79

Multiple stimuli and angioscotomata, 169
Multiple stimuli and cerebral lesions, 169
Multiple stimuli and configurations of stimuli, 199
Multiple stimuli in detection phase, 291
Multiple stimuli and differential light sensitivity, 199
Multiple stimuli and 'Gestalt' psychological phenomena, 163
Multiple stimuli and higher perceptual functions, 169
Multiple stimuli and individual sensitivity, 161
Multiple stimuli and infraliminal stimuli, 162
Multiple stimuli and intensity of a defect, 162
Multiple stimuli and intra-individual variations, 161
Multiple stimuli, maximum number of stimuli, 165
Multiple stimuli and neural interaction, 163
Multiple stimuli, number of stimuli, 199, 305
Multiple stimuli, position, 305
Multiple stimuli, optimum procedure, 199
Multiple stimuli, pseudo-variation, 168
Multiple stimuli, range of luminance, 200
Multiple stimuli and reliability of the visual field examination, 168
Multiple stimuli and screening, 198
Multiple stimuli and simultaneous perception, 160
Multiple stimuli and simultaneous threshold approach, 160
Multiple stimuli and supraliminal stimuli, 162
Multiple stimuli, luminance, 200
Multiple stimuli and threshold, 160, 168, 305, 307
Multiple stimuli and defects, 169
Mydriatics and visual field examination, 215
Myopia and miotics, 214

N

Nasal constriction, 276
Nasal defects, 260, 268, 284

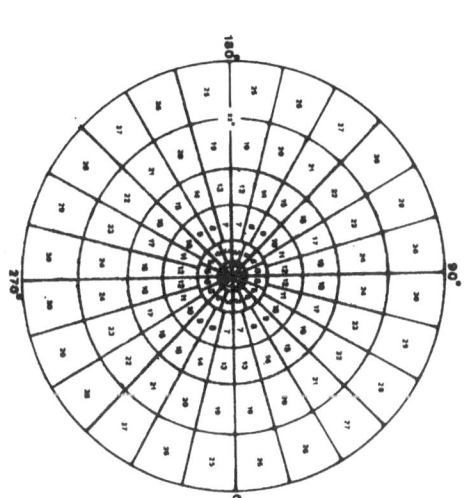

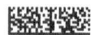